MAD SCIENCE

MAD SCIENCE

Psychiatric Coercion, Diagnosis, and Drugs

Stuart A. Kirk, Tomi Gomory, & David Cohen

Transaction Publishers
New Brunswick (U.S.A.) and London (U.K.)

Library of Congress Catalog Number: 2012035176
ISBN: 978-1-4128-4976-0
Printed in the United States of America

Library of Congress Cataloging-in-Publication Data

Kirk, Stuart A., 1945-
Mad science : psychiatric coercion, diagnosis, and drugs / Stuart A. Kirk, Tomi Gomory, and David Cohen.
    p. ; cm.
    Includes bibliographical references and index.
    ISBN 978-1-4128-4976-0 (alk. paper)
        I. Gomory, Tomi. II. Cohen, David, 1954- III. Title.
        [DNLM: 1. Diagnostic and statistical manual of mental disorders.
2. Mental Disorders--history--United States.   3. Mental Disorders--drug therapy--United States.   4. Psychiatry--history--United States. WM 11 AA1]
616.89'075--dc23
                                                                        2012035176

Contents

Preface

Over the last fifty years in the United States, there has been a massive expansion of the psychiatric enterprise. According to one source (Frank & Glied, 2006), the principal group of mental health professionals in 1950 used to be made up of about seven thousand psychiatrists. Today, using US Department of Labor (2012) figures and selecting professions with the terms *psychiatric, mental health, substance abuse,* as well as *clinical psychologists* and *mental health* and *substance abuse social workers,* we have an army of at least six hundred thousand mental health professionals. By adding psychiatric nurses and a number of other counseling and therapeutic occupations and their supporting staff, such as medical records keepers and various mental health technicians, the number would easily top one million. Not surprisingly, the amount spent on what are called mental health services has also exploded, from about $1 billion in 1956 (Frank & Glied, 2006) to $113 billion today (Garfield, 2011).

The people who are the target of these services—those from infancy to senescence who are considered mentally ill, who consider themselves mentally ill, and who are encouraged to seek mental health services—is at an all-time high. According to the latest American Psychiatric Association methods of diagnosing mental illness, nearly one hundred million people, 25 to 30 percent of the US population, have a mental illness during any one year (Frank & Glied, 2006, pp. 10–11), and half of the population will have a mental illness during their lifetime. This massive expansion of recognized illness, professional manpower, and services was accompanied by the rise of state and federally funded programs that provide most funding for mental health services. A growing number of private health insurance policies also provide psychiatric coverage. Surrounding this expansion is the pharmaceutical industry, which has immersed the entire mental health service system in a tidal wave of prescription psychoactive drugs, oxygenated by multibillion-dollar lucre, most of it also paid for by public funds.

Many psychiatric authorities claim that these developments are signs of major medical progress: the growing humanitarianism of an enlightened society caring for those in need; the advances in methods of accurately identifying and diagnosing all those suffering from psychiatric illness; and the scientific breakthroughs in understanding and treating mental illness biochemically.

If this grand explanation of progress was accurate, then the following should also be true. There would be less mental illness in America now than in 1950. Those with mental illness would be much more likely to recover with treatment than before. Those who are now called the severely mentally ill, who formerly would have been involuntarily committed to state asylums, would now be more effectively and humanely treated. The use of coercion as a psychiatric intervention would be a method of the distant past. The techniques of diagnosing mental illness would be more accurate, and *valid*, than methods used previously. Diagnosis would rest on biological markers rather than conversation as the "biological basis" of the currently more than three hundred types of mental illnesses would have been substantiated or disconfirmed. As a result, the remaining actual bodily illnesses formerly called mental illnesses or mental disorders would be the concern of medical specialties such as neurology or endocrinology. We would have confirmed methods of preventing and curing these illness that could be employed by any mental health practitioner. With at least one in four American women and one in seven American men today receiving psychoactive drugs by prescription, there would be solid evidence that these drugs effectively treat the problems for which the Food and Drug Administration approves them.

If you believe that even one of the above signs of progress has occurred, the review and analysis presented in *Mad Science* will be eye-opening, if not disturbing. None of these confirming developments has occurred. Of course, many in the public and in the mental health professions think that major "advances" in diagnosis and treatments of mental disorders have occurred and are continually occurring. Agencies such as the National Institute of Mental Health and organizations such as the American Psychiatric Association regularly tout such advances, which are then widely echoed by the media. Many, perhaps a majority of adults today, believe that the problem of mental illness is fundamentally a medical problem whose solution lies, through conventional medical research, in identifying its causes and devising effective treatments (e.g., targeting brains and genes). Most people view modern drug treatments as an undisputed improvement (more effective and safer) over any previous interventions designed for those considered mentally ill. Moreover, many people believe (or perhaps merely hope) that those labeled severely mentally ill—and those who treat them—now operate in an atmosphere of cooperation without the use coercion.

In this book we offer a radically different interpretation of the character of the massive American psychiatric and mental health expansion and how it came to be. The discrepancy between the views held by the public and many professionals on the one hand and the actual evidence on the other hand brought the authors of this book together. Our goal was to understand and describe how psychiatric research and science of the past half century have shaped the public understanding of expressions such as "mental illness" or "mental disorder" and of the effectiveness of psychiatric treatment. Much of the psychiatric research that has fueled the expansion of the mental health enterprise has not contributed to a science of madness. Instead, it has fueled mad science, which rests on unverified concepts, the invention of new forms of coercion, unremitting disease mongering, the widespread use of treatments with poorly tested and misleading claims of effectiveness, and rampant conflicts of interest that have completely blurred science and marketing. This is the "madness" of American psychiatry, and of psychiatry in much of the world.

We begin by examining the prevailing language of disease and medicine and its effect on views about the nature of madness and how it ought to be controlled or managed. By critically assessing whether the claims of scientific advances are supported, we track the fate of those labeled the severely or seriously mentally ill as they are ushered into purportedly more humane "community treatment" in which coercion has become redefined as scientifically-elucidated therapy. We examine the nature of the "epidemic of mental disorders" that was manufactured by the ever-expanding boundaries of mental illness contained in the *Diagnostic and Statistical Manual of Mental Disorders*, the well-promoted and profitable guidebook to madness that has allowed those with institutional and financial interests to claim that existential, interpersonal, and troublesome problems in living are actually diagnosable brain diseases. We then connect these developments to the explosive growth in the use of prescribed psychoactive substances, developed and relentlessly promoted by the pharmaceutical industry and delivered to willing and unwilling persons by licensed physicians and their collaborators in the other mental health professions.

Although the order of the chapters reflects in part the chronological development of coercion, diagnosis, and drug myths in psychiatry, readers should feel free to read chapters 2 to 7 in any order they wish. Each chapter, as it turns out, contains a mix of historical observations, conceptual and critical analysis, and discussions that, we hope, dovetail nicely and occasionally overlap with the other chapters and should augment readers' appreciation of the interrelatedness of the various topics. We recommend, however, that chapter 8 be read last, as it draws upon all that preceded.

Our Collaboration

Before we began working on this book, we had barely met or worked together. We are from diverse origins: one—a Hungarian child refugee fleeing the failure of that small country's 1956 fight for freedom from the tentacles of the Soviet Union—grew up in New York City's Greenwich Village. The second—a French-speaking Sephardi emigrant from Morocco and then Canada—lives and works in Florida. The third—with German and Lebanese ancestors—was raised in California. Our moral and religious upbringings and our political views are dissimilar, and we are in different stages of our personal lives and careers. We have lived in different states for most of our professional careers. We all happened to be married fathers and professors of social welfare with interests in human distress, misbehavior, and madness; and we each pursued doctoral studies at Berkeley, although in different decades. We have each practiced as mental health clinicians, taught at universities, conducted research, and published on mental health topics.

What really brought us together, however, was that we were each writing critically about psychiatric claims that were at odds with the best empirical evidence, especially the evidence cited by the claims-makers themselves. Each of us struggled to understand how gross misinterpretations of research evidence were allowed to promote vast policies and practices under the rubric of mental health progress. Was good science being misused? Was bad science being propagated? Were equivocal findings being exaggerated for some institutional advantage? Were fake findings being manufactured? Was there merely widespread lack of knowledge and/or gullibility by the public and mental health professionals, hoping to solve an age-old problem? Or was there some even larger, more nebulous enterprise, a sort of mass delusion or self-deception? What was going on? Although working individually, none of us had kept his individual doubts a secret. Quite the contrary, we had each been actively engaged for many years in writing, speaking, and debating with our opposition in professional journals and media outlets. We began meeting together in 2004 in New York City and conversing about madness and the madness institutions. In that process, we saw that a broader context was needed to fully understand the relationship of psychiatric science to psychiatric practice and policy.

This book arose from our conversations, of our effort to tell a broader, more compelling story than we had told individually. The book is truly a collaborative effort. We took seriously Alexandre Dumas' motto for *his* three musketeers, "One for all and all for one"—the order of authorship representing only an administrative convenience. We spent obsessive months imagining the structure of the book and ceaselessly reworked that preliminary structure until publication. Although one person had to author a first draft of each chapter using a collectively developed outline, the chapters were read, revised, edited, and re-read by each of us. Sections of content were swapped among chapters. Ideas advanced by one of us were sometimes deleted by others or borrowed and expanded. In the end, we all have our fingerprints on practically every paragraph.

While we developed the book, we presented some of its ideas in academic and professional gatherings, most recently at University of California at Los Angeles and at Berkeley; the University of Brussels; Florida International University; University of Tartu, Estonia; University of Pecs, Hungary;

University College Cork, Ireland; and in France, Universities of Poitiers, Bordeaux, Paris-Descartes, and Paris-Diderot. Most surprising was not that our views were challenged, but that so many participants shared our concerns about the direction of modern American psychiatry.

Our Benefactors and Helpers

For reasons that will become abundantly clear, our work on this book did not enjoy any direct financial support from the psychiatric-pharmaceutical complex. Instead, we relied on the support of our universities to pursue our inquiry and on the tolerance of our colleagues for our perspective, which at times runs counter to their views. In addition, the Marjorie Crump Endowed Chair at UCLA covered a few of the expenses of finishing our project. Finally, a sabbatical stipend from Florida International University and the Fulbright-Tocqueville Chair Award to David Cohen in 2011–2012 allowed him to devote time to this project.

In addition to our supportive academic institutions, many small enterprises from coast to coast unknowingly supported our efforts. Several times a year we met for days of intensive discussion and to examine our evolving work. We gathered in coffeehouses and restaurants as we argued, bantered, and brainstormed our way through umpteen drafts of chapters. These small, local establishments provided the ambience, sustenance, service, and espresso for our work, some of them on more than one occasion. For their tolerance of our antics and appropriation of their tables, it is only fitting that, in gratitude, we thank a few of them by name. In Greenwich Village (NYC): Café Dante on Macdougal Street with its legendary Latte Macchiato *Strong*. In Santa Fe (NM): Café Pasquals, Coyote Café, Downtown Subscription, Mucho Gusto, Plaza Café, and Rio Chama. In South Beach (FL): Big Pink and News Café. In Big Sur (CA): Deetjens Big Sur Inn and the Ripplewood Café. In Tallahassee (FL): Z. Bardhi's Italian Cuisine and Samrat Indian Restaurant. In Ojai (CA): Ojai Emporium Café, and the Ojai Roasting Company. In New Orleans (LA): Lafitte's Blacksmith Bar.

We are hardly the first to raise critical questions about the mental health enterprise. For intellectual inspiration we drew on dozens of authors whose work we cite repeatedly in the text. In addition, we also asked other scholars to review and comment on draft chapters and discussed our work with others. Their advice and suggestions were wise, constructive, and unfailingly helpful, although we have undoubtedly disappointed some of them by not fully adopting their suggestions or addressing their concerns. Our gratitude to Lauren Dockett, Eric Engstrom, François Gonon, Nikki Hozack, David Jacobs, Herb Kutchins, Jeffrey Lacasse, Bruce Levine, Joanna Moncrieff, David Oaks, Pascal-Henri Keller, the late Thomas Szasz, Robert Whitaker, and several anonymous reviewers. A special thanks to Professor Eileen Gambrill of the University of California, Berkeley, who shaped our early academic careers by stimulating a critical attitude toward all conventional assumptions that apply to the study of and responses to human travail. Finally, we were encouraged early in our project by the late Professor Irving Louis Horowitz, the founder of Transaction Publishers, who reviewed our book prospectus in 2010. Unfortunately, he passed away the week before our full manuscript was submitted. We are indebted to him, Mary E. Curtis, the president, and the other editors at Transaction for providing a welcoming home for our book.

Finally, we have deep personal gratitude for those close to us who encouraged our work and provided the emotional support that sustained us. While they bear no responsibility for our book, their lives were certainly affected by our entanglement with *Mad Science*. Stuart acknowledges and deeply appreciates the tolerance, support, and humor of Carol Ann Koz, who was not blind to what life with him would be like when he began another book. Tomi could not be the engaged academic critic that he is without the uncritical, loving support of his life partner Fran and the very best and sweetest two daughters any father could be privileged to love, Aniko and Rozsa. He owes to those three much more than he could ever express. Throughout his career, David's most dedicated support and encouragement has come from his wife Carole and their children, Saskia and Bernard.

Inevitably, coauthoring a book involves time, complexities, and frustrations. Yet, the three of us agree that the deep, meaningful relationships that we formed among us constitute the major benefit of our effort.

Stuart Kirk, Ojai, CA
Tomi Gomory, Tallahassee, FL
David Cohen, Miami Beach, FL

References

Frank, R. G., & Glied, S. A. (2006). *Better but not well: Mental health policy in the United States since 1950.* Baltimore: Johns Hopkins University Press.

Garfield, R. L. (2011). *Mental health financing in the United States: A primer.* Washington, DC: Kaiser Commission on Medicaid and the Uninsured.

US Department of Labor. (2012). Occupational employment and wages—May 2011. Bureau of Labor Statistics. Retrieved from: http://www.bls.gov/news.release/archives/ocwage_03272012.pdf

1

Illusions of Psychiatric Progress

Introduction

Madness poses fundamental problems for every society, past and present. The terms used to describe it—*lunacy, insanity, mental disease, mental illness, nervous breakdown, emotional* or *psychological distress, mental disorder*—carry a cargo of cultural meanings and spawn countless social reactions. Although each of these terms invokes a different understanding, the concept and the category of madness serve an essential purpose: they help those not so categorized to feel better about themselves and their presumed normalcy, while at the same time they earmark others as violating society's expectations and deserving to be targeted by professional and state intervention.

Madness also safely subsumes and "explains" behavioral strangeness and violence that threaten social order, such as, for example, apparently unprovoked mass shootings by solitary individuals harboring deep grudges. The word *madness* represents some reality that triggers images for everyone, but hardly any two individuals would agree about its essence. Perhaps madness has no essence; perhaps it is only a linguistic black hole. Psychiatric historians and others, however, relying on their own personal histories and presumptions (often unacknowledged), have usually attempted to tell coherent and optimistic tales affirming the belief that medicine has virtually solved the mystery of madness and has validated it as yet another affliction of nature—a disease.

The current psychiatric establishment, exemplified by the US National Institute of Mental Health (NIMH) and the American Psychiatric Association (APA), wants the public to believe that disturbing behaviors result from brain diseases, that scientific research moves ever closer to finding causes and cures for these diseases, and that patients should be treated by approved, expertly-trained therapists applying certified, evidence-based treatments. This medical language and medicalized apparatus is a bid for authority over a long-disputed territory of distresses and misbehaviors. The language implies that errors of the past have given way to steady progress in understanding madness

1

and treating it effectively. The claim for authority covers an immense range of human emotion, suffering, and behavior, including experiences that can severely frighten a person or those around them, such as panic, immobilizing despondency, having unusual perceptions, or acting violently in response to (possibly imagined) threats. But the bulk of the behavioral territory claimed by the modern professions addressing madness—including psychiatry, psychology, and social work—covers more common experiences, such as feeling irritable, sad, or very sensitive; having difficulty concentrating; feeling inept; working too much or too little; sleeping too much or too little; eating too much or too little; or feeling discomfort in ordinary social situations. Contemporary psychiatry claims that these diverse feelings and behaviors—from the rare and extreme to the common and mild—are symptoms of mental disorder, signs of underlying physiological dysfunction, requiring medical treatment.

In contrast, we will argue that the fundamental claims of modern American psychiatry[1] are not based on well-tested research but on science that is itself a bit mad: misconceived, flawed, erroneous, misinterpreted, and often misreported. Using the cover of scientific medicine, psychiatry has managed to become the leading legally chartered profession for the management of misery and misbehavior reframed as an illness (i.e., mental illness). We will demonstrate that the touted achievements of psychiatry in the past half century—keeping disturbed people out of psychiatric hospitals for extended periods, developing a novel and easily applied diagnostic approach embodied in the modern *Diagnostic and Statistical Manual of Mental Disorders (DSM)*, and using "safe and effective" drugs as the first-line intervention for every ill and misfortune—are little more than a recycled mishmash of coercion of the mad and misbehaving, mystification of the process of labeling people, and medical-sounding justifications for people's desires to use, and professionals' desires to give, psychoactive chemicals. Obviously, then, this book questions the notion that these psychiatric achievements constitute *progress*. We argue that until society come to grips with the unscientific nature of the management of madness, it will perpetuate a "mental health" system that serves the interests of professional and corporate elites while it exacerbates the very problems it claims to tackle.

Mental health professionals and the public have been well apprised of the notable achievements of psychiatry this past half century: the near-closing of state asylums in order to provide "evidence-based" care in the community, the expansion of the category mental illness via the renovation of the *Diagnostic Manual of Mental Disorders* (especially since *DSM-III*), and the invention and marketing of new psychoactive drugs. These achievements have often been described as paradigm shifts that have shaped the current mental health system. Undoubtedly, their role in shaping this system cannot be taken lightly. However, we argue that these achievements constitute a trio of illusions, spawned more by the misuse than the progress of science.

And, as illusions often do, they have unleashed a torrent of unanticipated adverse consequences, even as they have benefited organized psychiatry, pharmaceutical companies, and the proponents of the "mental health movement."

As with the "unexpected" collapse of Wall Street in 2008, Americans may yet again, much to their consternation, come to realize that a huge social institution is not as sound as its best and brightest continually claim. The mental health enterprise, like some banks, is continually propped up by government, the profession, and the media because it has become too big to fail. Yet there is no question to us that it has failed and continues to fail daily. Our hope in this book is that society may yet learn to minimize psychiatric coercion and excuses, to offer help to those who need it, and to minimize the manipulation and distortion of science.

On the Language of Madness

> Social scientists have to decide, every time they do research, what to call the things they study. If they choose the terms decided on by the interested and powerful parties already involved in the situations they are studying, they accept all the presuppositions built into that language.

> (Becker, 2007)

As the sociologist Howard Becker reminds us in the quotation above, we should be skeptical about the rhetoric used by powerful parties and the assumptions that they may bootleg into public discourse. It is advice that we intend to follow throughout this book. Let's begin by examining how the National Institute of Mental Health (NIMH), the federal government's leading mental health agency, speaks of madness. Here is a typical excerpt from its website in 2008:

> The mission of NIMH is to reduce the burden of mental and behavioral disorders through research on mind, brain, and behavior. Mental disorders are brain disorders and that means that achieving progress requires a deeper understanding of the brain and behavior.

> Since our inception in 1946, NIMH has been the lead agency for research on mental disorders. Through our research, enormous gains have been made over the decades, including: establishing that mental disorders are complex brain diseases and demonstrating that medications and behavioral therapies can relieve suffering and improve daily functioning for many people. Recent groundbreaking discoveries from mapping of the human genome, sophisticated studies of the brain, and investigations of cognition and behavior have provided powerful new insights and approaches.

3

Science now provides opportunities that promise to deliver for each of these needs. Success will require an understanding of the underlying processes in brain and behavior—from neurons to neighborhoods—to make the discoveries that point the way to new diagnostics and interventions and, eventually to recovery, prevention, and cure. (From Strategic Planning Reports, NIMH website, 2/15/08)[2]

NIMH is explicit about madness: the behaviors are "brain diseases" managed by "therapies" while science moves closer to finding a "cure." The language of biomedicine pervades today's official views: *disease, genetics, medications, behavioral therapies, rehabilitation, cure, recovery*. It is as if none of these terms are contested or misleading. And yet great confusion exists at NIMH and throughout the scientific establishment about what behaviors express brain disorders, how they come about, how they should be managed, and by whom. As we will see, many experts believe that no scientific evidence exists to describe the vast array of behaviors corralled in the rubric of mental disorders as "brain diseases." What NIMH presents as a simple equation is a political, not a scientific, pronouncement. For fifty years, the bureaucratic language about madness has contained many convoluted, vague, or tautological attempts at definition, as exemplified by the definition of "serious emotional disturbances" in children taken from the President's New Freedom Commission on Mental Health (2002):

> *A serious emotional disturbance* is defined as a mental, behavioral, or emotional disorder of sufficient duration to meet diagnostic criteria specified in the DSM-III-R that results in functional impairment that substantially interferes with or limits one or more major life activities in an individual up to 18 years of age. Examples of functional impairment that adversely affect educational performance include an inability to learn that cannot be explained by intellectual, sensory, or health factors; an inability to build or maintain satisfactory interpersonal relationships with peers and teachers; inappropriate types of behavior or feelings under normal circumstances; a general pervasive mood of unhappiness or depression; or a tendency to develop physical symptoms or fears associated with personal or school problems. (Retrieved 10-17-12 from: http://govinfo.library.unt.edu/mentalhealthcommission/reports/FinalReport/FullReport.htm)

The President's Commission appears to eschew the terms *brain disorder* or *brain disease* in describing children's behaviors. It opts to use "serious emotional disturbance" instead, admittedly a more neutral term, but its meaning is itself obscure. For example, the passage leads to confusion by defining serious emotional disturbance "as a mental, behavioral, or emotional disorder," suggesting that three distinct types of "disorders" constitute emotional disturbance, without a wisp of explanation about the nature of the distinctions. To shore up the ambiguities, the passage borrows language from the *DSM* and elsewhere regarding "duration" and "functional impairment" that lead to various inabilities and inappropriate behaviors, feelings, fears, or unhappiness—plunging the reader into the depths of current psychiatric diagnostic murkiness. This type of descriptive obscurity would be unacceptable, for example, to cancer researchers trying to distinguish pathological from normal cells, suggesting that despite the official modern vocabulary of madness, we are leagues away from the logic of medicine. In fact, the more ambiguous the terms used to demarcate mental disorder from no mental disorder, or emotional disturbance from emotional stability, the more behavioral territory can be annexed under the jurisdiction of the mental health professions.

In 1980 the APA published its first serious official attempt to grapple with a definition of *mental disorder*, the current popular term. This occurred in the third edition and all subsequent editions of what is regularly referred to as the psychiatric Bible, the *Diagnostic and Statistical Manual of Mental Disorders (DSM)*, readying itself for its seventh face-lift, *DSM-5*, scheduled for release in 2013. Admitting that "there is no satisfactory definition that specifies precise boundaries" (p. 5) for mental disorder, the *DSM* (APA, 1980) offered the following guidance:

> In DSM each of the mental disorders is conceptualized as a clinically significant behavioral or psychological syndrome or pattern that occurs in an individual and that is typically associated with either a painful symptom (distress) or impairment in one or more important areas of functioning (disability). In addition, there is an inference that there is a behavioral, psychological, or biological dysfunction, and that the disturbance is not only in the relationship between the individual and society. (When the disturbance is *limited* to a conflict between an individual and society, this may represent social deviance, which may or may not be commendable, but is not by itself a mental disorder.) (p. 6)

Almost every phrase in this cumbersome definition has been criticized (Kutchins & Kirk, 1997). One critic (Wakefield, 1992) noted in a widely cited article that the *DSM* defined *disorder* as a dysfunction, but without any attempt to suggest what a dysfunction is. Wakefield's subsequent attempts to define *dysfunction* have, in turn, also been questioned as constituting speculative hypotheses about the functions of human evolution (Bolton, 2008; Boyle, 2002; Lilienfeld & Marino, 1995; McNally, 2011). More recently, a group of psychiatric researchers (Rounsaville et al., 2002), working under the auspices of the APA in preparation for *DSM-5*, concluded that *mental disorder* as defined in *DSM* is not an exact term and "is not cast in a way that allows it to be used as a criterion for deciding what is and is not a mental disorder" (p. 3), and that there is a "contentious" debate about "whether *disease, illness, and disorder* are scientific biomedical terms or are socio-political terms that necessarily involve a value judgment" (p. 3, emphasis in original). And finally, they report that the current *DSM* "...is based on a falsely optimistic assumption: that psychiatric disorders are discrete bio-medical entities with clear . . . boundaries" (p. 8). In other words, even these prominent psychiatric researchers, trying to improve or fine-tune diagnosis of the presumed entities that make up the very subject matter of psychiatry, disagree not only with *DSM* but with the professed certainties of NIMH's "brain diseases."

The definition of madness remains in disarray. This dilemma has become abundantly clear as the American Psychiatric Association struggles to produce *DSM-5*, which will be discussed in greater detail in chapter 5. Particularly revealing is an article titled "What Is a Mental/Psychiatric Disorder: From *DSM-IV* to *DSM-V*," written to guide *DSM-5* (Stein et al., 2010). The authors concede the following: there are disagreements about the term *mental disorder*; the "clinically significant" *DSM* criterion for mental disorders is tautological and difficult to operationalize; the boundaries between normal and pathological are complex and contentious; and the concept of dysfunc-tion is controversial and involves speculative theoretical assumptions about human evolution. Undeterred, the authors suggest adding additional criteria that are themselves problematic. First, "any disorder in DSM should have diagnostic validity" on the basis of a number of key validators, which they admit are variable and may not be readily available, but "in their absence . . . other evidence of diagnostic validity is helpful." Second, any disorder in *DSM* "should have clinical utility," another potentially tautological or meaningless criterion that would exclude almost no human distress, because someone somewhere can always claim that an effective treatment for it exists. Allen Frances, the chairperson of the *DSM-IV* Task Force (who presided over an enormous expansion of the mental disorder vocabulary and population), surprisingly summarized the definitional difficulties in the plainest terms: "There is no definition of a mental disorder. It's bullshit. I mean, you just can't define it" (Greenberg, 2011).

In 2007, in one of his many statements about the nature of "mental ill-nesses as brain disorders," Thomas Insel, the director of NIMH, expressed less-than-usual certainty. He speculated that mental disorders *may* result from brain lesions (i.e., some damaged areas of tissue), *may* eliminate the distinction between neurology's focus on the brain and nervous system and psychiatry's traditional focus on thoughts and behaviors, and *may* arise from abnormal activity in "brain circuits," even without detectable lesions (Insel, 2007). Naturally, these conjectures *may* turn out to be wrong. Nevertheless, they form part of Insel's active campaign to push the NIMH even more deeply into framing and pursuing madness as a biomedical entity and to convert psy-chiatry into a neuroscience discipline (Insel et al., 2010; Insel & Quirion, 2005), or at least the trappings of one. There is nothing new in Insel's claims about madness as brain disease: they have been made for over two hundred years (Bynum, 1974). That such claims are still being put forth, rather than their precise empirical basis described succinctly for public verification, illustrates how little progress the biopsychiatric approach has made in understanding or elucidating madness.

Three powerful organizations—the NIMH, the President's Commission, and the APA—offer us three official languages to define and describe *mental illness*. The major institutional players in the field, including the pharmaceutical industry, have so expanded the kinds of behaviors and emotions now considered symptoms of mental disorder that the term has lost coherence, if it ever possessed any. For example, common behaviors among schoolchildren, such as fidgeting with hands and feet, difficulty awaiting turn, running about, and blurting out answers before questions are completed, now make up actual diagnostic criteria of the mental disorder named Attention-Deficit/Hyperactivity Disorder if they occur "often" (but that last qualifier is completely undefined) (APA, 1994, pp. 83–85). Yet this incoherence has not led to a loss of legitimacy or power for these major players. To the contrary, the varieties of meaning and confusion have only helped to expand the psychiatric enterprise.

If we undertook a broader survey of psychologists, social workers, philosophers, historians, and social scientists who study mental illness about what madness might be and how it should be handled by society, the level of disagreement would rise dramatically. NIMH and others try to smooth over these disparities, to view the whole issue as a matter of brain disorders requiring medical interventions. We will show in later chapters that the science for such a sweeping conclusion remains feeble, although the political effort is exceedingly powerful.

The way in which language has been used to designate madness and its management distorts as much as it illuminates the nature of the subject. We face the same continuing dilemma: how to illuminate without foreclosing questions that haven't been sufficiently answered or pretending that consensus and clarity exist when they do not. No supportable or practical resolutions to this dilemma exist. Words are human artifacts; their meanings change over time to adjust to changing cultural norms, everyday practices, or new knowledge. We have chosen to adopt the custom of many historians and sociologists who use various rubrics to discuss phenomena that range from minor social deviance (e.g., smoking marijuana or conning others) to serious personal distress and suffering (such as feelings of worthlessness, overwhelming fear, or grossly disturbing behavior). Although all are viewed as symptoms of mental disorders in the *DSM*, as a matter of convenience we will very reluctantly use conventional terms for madness interchangeably—*mental disease, mental illness,* and *mental disorder*—without making presumptions about their underlying nature or particular causes and despite the fact that

7

these terms often seem incoherent to us. We do, however, admit a preference for two general groupings of human difficulties that we believe encompass as well as any other the psychological disarray and the disruption of relationships that most people often attribute to madness or refer to when they speak of *madness* or *mental disorder*.

What Is Meant by *Madness*?

The process of transmogrifying the notion of madness into a medical disease has been essentially linguistic: it has involved verbally funneling an exceedingly heterogeneous group of individuals needing complex, individualized management or assistance into one category describing people burdened with a medical illness and requiring technical attention from mental health professionals. The pedagogic effort has been hugely successful (everyone seems to know what mental illness looks like and that it requires treatment), whereas the scientific effort to validate madness as a medical entity far less so (no one knows what a mental illness is). For example, a leading contemporary biological researcher of schizophrenia, psychiatrist Nancy Andreasen (1999), thus commented:

> At present the most important problem in schizophrenia research is not finding the gene or localizing it in the brain and understanding its neural circuits. Our most important problem is identifying the correct target at which to aim our powerful new scientific weapons. Our most pressing problem is at the clinical level: defining what schizophrenia is. (p. 781)

Given this obvious definitional uncertainty, here is our own view of what is subsumed by the term *mental illness*. It is a label used to characterize and organize the many different behaviors that have become the targets of a "biomedical industrial complex" (Gomory et al., 2011). They include at least two broad types of problems that should be distinguished, although people may experience or manifest both. On the one hand, there is personally perceived *distress*: usually situational, life stage-related difficulties in coping with life's and society's demands that often appear as inability or unwillingness to pursue personal goals or to interact smoothly with other people. When people experience personal distress, they typically seek or accept help voluntarily from whatever sources they believe will best address these difficulties. Personal distress usually directly burdens no one outside of friends, peers, immediate family, and co-workers and causes little public notice, nor does it trigger formal public intervention, although when people fail to meet various personal and social obligations while they are distressed, there are indirect social and economic consequences.[3]

On the other hand, there is *misbehavior*: visibly deviant, uncooperative, morally offensive or socially disruptive behaviors. These behaviors threaten and therefore mobilize the immediate interpersonal network or the larger society to forcefully restrain and then exclude (and perhaps re-educate) the offending individual (who may be acting from a variety of possible motives, or from no discernable motive). Although many people who so misbehave may cross over into frankly criminal activities, and may therefore also experience simultaneous or successive management by the criminal justice system, many do not.

Both these categories of behavior fall into what sociologist Andrew Abbott (1988) described as the *personal problems jurisdiction*, an arena vigorously competed for by several helping professions in the late nineteenth and early twentieth centuries. These professions included psychiatry, social work, neurology, the clergy, and a nascent clinical psychology. The struggle for professional supremacy over this jurisdiction was won by psychiatry. Abbott pointedly thinks that psychiatry's success rested particularly on its ability to construct a persuasive medicalized rhetoric that combined both social control and therapeutic care, even though "[o]f its treatments, only incarceration had any effect, and that made the psychiatrists little different from the jailers they had replaced, despite their reference to the medical model of science, treatment and cure" (p. 295).

In its effort to gain leadership, the failure of psychiatry (and society) to carefully distinguish between *personal distress* and *public misbehavior* and between the responses necessary for properly addressing each, conflated caring and coercing under the single rubric of "mental health practice." Efforts to care and efforts to control became hopelessly mixed, and as a small late eighteenth-century system focused on a small number of misbehaving individuals evolved into a gigantic twentieth-century biomedical industrial complex, the consequences for those distressed, those misbehaving, and for our society expanded correspondingly.

People Seeking Help

Scholars can afford to be skeptical about the pronouncements of experts and authorities on mental illness, but the general public often becomes engaged with the psychiatric establishment when struggling to contend with personal and family distress. When individuals and families are in crisis, they must make a series of judgments: How unpleasant is the difficulty to me or others I care about? If I ignore it or wait, will it resolve itself over time or get worse? Is the difficulty due to my own mistakes or inadequacies or to challenges thrust on me by circumstances or the actions of others? Can I rectify the difficulty through diligence, self-control, and perseverance? Would I benefit from asking friends or family for advice, or should I seek professional advice? If I seek professional advice, whom should I turn to first—a member of the clergy, attorney, nurse, social worker, psychologist, family counselor, or medical doctor? Should I first speak to someone who experienced a similar difficulty and found a way to resolve it?

These questions raise complicated issues that involve assessments of self, guesses about what is likely to happen if no action is taken, and estimates of the future consequences of taking different courses of action. These issues, in turn, are heavily constrained by the options available in one's community, society, and culture. People with similar troubles may handle them in very different ways. Although scientific knowledge cannot indicate the best way for people to proceed when troubled, those who enter the current mental health system seeking help are likely to face a bewildering array of professional beliefs, theories, treatments, and controversies—and may also find themselves completely removed from decision making about their lives or the lives of their relatives.

Let us explore three examples of how people who seek help for themselves or for their children become involved with the mental health system and the consequences their actions bring.

Case 1: Treating "Brain Disease"

The first time the parents noticed anything wrong with their son, Mi, was in the summer of 2004 when, following a fever, the twenty-one-year-old had trouble sleeping and often felt sick. He was depressed and moody, according to his mother. Mi stopped going to work at the glass factory where he was an intern. His parents then sought advice from several medical doctors. Some suggested that Mi had "mental problems"; some reviewed brain scans and told his father that there was little to worry about. Nevertheless, when Mi's parents, worried that their son's condition might worsen, saw a newspaper article about the purported success of a new brain surgery, they withdrew their life savings, borrowed additional money, and traveled to the hospital mentioned in the article to seek treatment.

Upon seeing Mi for the first time, the doctor demanded the full payment, asked them to sign a page-long diagnostic report (that the parents later claimed they had never read and described as bogus). Mi was placed on a gurney, strapped down, and taken away, presumably for more diagnostic tests. The report by the hospital, however, makes no mention of further tests but instead describes how frames were fixed onto Mi's head, holes drilled into his skull, and a seven-inch needle heated to 180 degrees Fahrenheit and inserted by the physician into the young man's brain for about one minute to destroy selected areas of brain tissue. At three o'clock that afternoon, nurses wheeled the son out of the elevator. The doctors told the parents the surgery had gone as planned. Mi vomited during that night, blood ran from both ears, and, for five subsequent days, he slipped in and out of consciousness. His right arm was limp and his speech was slurred.

Mi's treatment inflicted irreversible brain damage. He is still depressed and withdrawn. His parents regret their decision to take him to the hospital. The surgeon who performed the operation on the day he met Mi claims that the surgery went well and that Mi was fine when he left the hospital. The surgeon said he has performed nearly one thousand such procedures for patients with schizophrenia, depression, and epilepsy.

Case 2: The Full Treatment

David was a handsome, smart, and happy youngster who grew up in a middle-class neighborhood, the son of an executive for an international transportation company. His troubles apparently surfaced when he was twenty-two, after he had enrolled and withdrawn from three different universities. His father first suspected a drug problem. David wouldn't talk, claimed to see things, believed people were out to get him. He could not hold a job for more than a day. On the advice of a personal physician, his father took David to a psychiatrist, who diagnosed him with acute paranoid schizophrenia. On the advice of this professional, his parents obtained a court order and had David committed to a psychiatric hospital, where he was kept for forty days, until the family's insurance coverage ended.

David's psychiatric treatment continued. Over the ensuing years, he was repeatedly evaluated by psychiatrists and was forcibly hospitalized approximately twenty times in different psychiatric hospitals, among the best available in the region. His family also obtained a court order to treat David involuntarily as an outpatient, but he regularly managed to elude those who were supposed to monitor his medication usage. He received many drugs commonly used to treat psychiatric patients: lithium, Depakote (valproate), Haldol (haloperidol), Seroquel (quetiapine), and Zyprexa (olanzapine). He also received electroshock treatment. Often against his parents' wishes, David was released from these hospitals after being evaluated as not posing a danger to himself or others.

When his mother was placed in a nursing home, David visited her frequently but caused such commotions that the nursing home staff became uncomfortable. His father moved his mother to three different care facilities because of David's disruptive and threatening behavior. The police took him by force to a hospital after he threatened to kill people at one of these nursing homes. He left that hospital but, because he was still acting threateningly, his father called the police and David was committed to another university-affiliated hospital, where he stayed for a while. Several months later, he got in a fight with a hospital guard where his mother had been transferred, and he was arrested again. He was examined by a doctor who said he did not need to be kept at the hospital. His father's ardent efforts with the police and hospital personnel to keep David incarcerated in a psychiatric hospital failed, and David was released the next day. Several weeks later, David was charged with murdering a female psychotherapist and attempting to murder a psychiatrist who was her colleague.

Case 3: "Bipolar Is a Lifetime Diagnosis"

Diana was anguished in trying to understand what was happening to her sixteen-year-old son Benjamin, who was sad, afraid, not sleeping, and doing poorly in school. Where could she turn for help? She contacted Benjamin's teachers for their observations of his class performance; then she turned to his pediatrician and to mental health professionals for advice. A psychologist recommended by the school's principal concluded that the boy was "deeply depressed" and referred them to a psychiatrist for a medication evaluation. "The psychiatrist was another nice man, young, in an attractive office," she reported. The psychiatrist asked them to fill out questionnaires. When she mentioned to the doctor that her own mother had been hospitalized once with a "nervous breakdown," had seen a therapist and seemed to recover, the psychiatrist showed great interest in this family history. After forty-five minutes, the psychiatrist looked at Benjamin and said: "You're bipolar. It will only get worse over time unless we begin to medicate you now. I'm prescribing Abilify." When asked, the doctor said that Benjamin would have to take the medication for "the rest of his life. Bipolar is a lifetime diagnosis."

Madness and Institutional Dynamics

Each of these help-seeking efforts occurred in a broad social and institutional context. While each individual and family has a unique personal history and particular circumstances and resources, all encountered the sometimes dehumanizing reality of the bureaucracies that govern psychiatric care. Throughout psychiatric history, institutions and procedures that appear reasonable responses to madness by most members of society in one era are often viewed as brutal and ineffective in the next because of the evolving mores and the democratization of the human experience over time (e.g., women becoming recognized as entitled to equal human rights as men). Our current arrangements are also likely to suffer in hindsight. Contemporary jurisdiction over those presumed or pronounced mentally ill is assigned to hospitals, courts, police, insurance companies, the prescribers and the manufacturers of psychiatric drugs, the psychiatric professional organizations that regulate practitioners, and the government agencies that fund and shape mental health care, as well as to individual therapists governed by professional ethical codes and state licensure requirements. The bureaucracies, their requirements, regulations, and funding needs—often more than the so-called illnesses—are crucial to understanding how each of these cases unfolded. Let's examine some additional details about how the institutional dynamics shaped the interventions in these three cases, which have all been described extensively and published in leading American newspapers, sometimes by several reporters working together.

Case 1: Treating Brain Disease

The patient was Mi Zhantao. His surgery, reported in the *Wall Street Journal* (Zamiska, 2007), was performed by Dr. Yifang Wang at No. 454 Hospital of the People's Liberation Army in Nanjing, China. The *Journal* explained that a financial incentive exists to perform these surgeries. When Beijing began privatizing health care in the 1980s and dismantling the social welfare safety net that characterized that nation, both patients and hospitals had to "fend for themselves." Almost 10 percent of Hospital No. 454 revenues come from these surgeries, which the hospital promoted aggressively in pamphlets and feature stories, presumably like the one that came to the attention of Mi's parents. Other Chinese hospitals have developed similar surgical profit centers. The assertions that troublesome behaviors are due to brain disease provide a medical rationale for brain surgery. China's health-care financing system provided an external financial inducement to Chinese hospitals and physicians to perform surgery, even when its efficacy is highly questionable and the consequences on patients are devastating.

A smug Westerner may dismiss this harmful intervention as an example of paternalistic medicine in a rapidly mutating country with a tradition of deferring to authorities. Yet, according to the *New York Times*, in the last decade in the United States, more than five hundred people have undergone experimental procedures involving burning holes into their brains and other forms of brain surgery for mental illnesses including obsessive-compulsive disorder, depression, and anxiety. The treatments are often ineffective or harmful (Carey, 2009, 2011).

Case 2: The Full Treatment

For nearly two decades, David Tarloff's disturbing behaviors were well-known to his family, to medical and psychiatric professionals, and to the police. During these years—before his arrest a few days after the murder in New York City of therapist Kathryn Faughey and the wounding of psychiatrist Kent Shinback—Mr. Tarloff received the full gamut of modern psychiatric evaluations and treatments. His psychiatric records run over ten thousand pages (Jacobs, 2010). By no means is Mr. Tarloff someone who has been *neglected* by the psychiatric service system. Rather, he has been both a willing and unwilling recipient of standard psychiatric interventions for many years. That system was so interested in and concerned about Mr. Tarloff and so convinced that he needed what the system had to offer that it repeatedly restrained him, secluded him, and forced drugs and shock treatments on him, with the approval of his family, though as far as we can tell Mr. Tarloff was never accused, tried, or found guilty of any offense. Although his motivations for the killing and assault remain uncertain, Dr. Shinback was possibly the intended target, as he was among the first mental health professionals, seventeen years earlier, to have diagnosed Mr. Tarloff as schizophrenic and have him committed to a psychiatric facility.

Shortly after Mr. Tarloff's arrest in February 2008, the court at first declared him mentally competent to stand trial. Then, it forced him to take medications (Eligon, 2008a), and after several months declared him incompetent to be tried (Eligon, 2008b). After two years of attempts to begin the trial, psychiatrists and his own lawyer convinced court judges that David was still not mentally fit enough to assist in his own defense (Eligon, 2010a, 2010b). As one newspaper headline summarized it: "In Tarloff Trial, Both Sides Agree: Lock Him Up" (Eligon, 2010b). In late 2012, state psychiatrists found Tarloff fit to stand trial. His lawyers did not contest the claim. One of them stated: "The case is not so much about whether he remains in custody—it's about where he remains in custody" (Peltz, 2012).

Case 3: Bipolar Is a Lifetime Diagnosis

Benjamin's story, as told by his mother, a writer (Wagman, 2006), appeared in the *Los Angeles Times*. Initially in the help-seeking process, both mother and son were relieved and optimistic because a diagnosis had been made and a drug treatment prescribed. When they filled the prescription, however, they were startled and confused by the list of adverse effects on the product label. They googled the drug and became "terrified." The prescribed drug, branded as Abilify, had not been tested in children or teenagers. A forty-five-minute appointment with a psychiatrist had pushed Benjamin toward an expected lifetime of drug consumption with likely harmful short-term effects and unknown long-term effects.

The mother called a cousin—also a psychiatrist—for a second opinion. Her cousin was astounded. "It was a ridiculous diagnosis, he ranted, impossible after one office visit, especially for a teenager with no prior history." He directed her to seek out other mental health professionals. Eventually, after hundreds of phone calls, she found another mental health professional to see Benjamin at a university clinic. Benjamin began seeing this therapist for weekly psychotherapy sessions, as that therapist did not think medications were necessary. Benjamin slowly began to feel better, the mother reports, and the following year he went off to college. "As parents," Diana acknowledges, "we will do anything to help our children, to keep them from pain, to make them feel better. But we also are at the mercy of professionals." In this case, a well-educated, resourceful working mother was confused by conflicting diagnoses and treatment advice from mental health professionals and startled that one of them could so cavalierly prescribe to her son a drug that no validated body of evidence had suggested was indicated for his troubles and that could seriously harm him to boot. She and other family members in these cases feel that they are victims of a psychiatric system that doesn't always protect or help them.

These cases identify problems that point to fundamental confusions about how our society has defined troublesome behaviors, shaped diagnoses, and formulated policies to "treat" these behaviors. In Nanjing, New York, and Los Angeles, distraught parents sought mental health professionals for help with their children. The patients received diagnoses and the parents received treatment recommendations that they presumed utilized solid scientific evidence and sound clinical judgment. But the parents quickly learned that psychiatric judgments are not always sound or scientific, nor do they necessarily aim to protect the best interests of the patient.

The parents of Mi, David, and Benjamin feel rightfully aggrieved by the diagnosis or the treatment advice they received for their sons. Their complaints, however, should have extended far beyond the clinicians they encountered to the web of government officials, mental health advocates, health care and insurance policy-makers, scientists, pharmaceutical company executives and their marketing personnel and lobbyists—all of whom share responsibility for these families' devastating experiences in seeking help. These families have, indeed, been at the mercy of professionals, even very distant professionals from Madison Avenue.

Yet we would be off the mark if we portrayed families as uniformly helpless. There is no simple way to characterize the stances, resources, and desires of families and individuals vis-à-vis the psychiatric system. Families and individuals understand and try to deal with crises and distress in a variety of ways. Obviously, some individuals who are treated as mental patients have problems in living. Others are victimized by their families or by society. Still others want to be seen as medically ill patients, including those who wish to avoid responsibility for their misbehavior or for a burdensome situation or duty. Exploring all of the ways that people encounter the psychiatric system would take us far afield. As our examples above have suggested, some people seek mental health services and others have services imposed on them. Some are able participants. They possess well-honed critical skills, prepare themselves adequately before meeting with any professional, have the means to ask for second and third opinions, or have definite ideas about helping themselves or their members that keep them out of the orbit of institutional psychiatry. Yet it is fair to say that most do not. They lack the resources, abilities, and critical thinking skills that might constitute some form of advance protection from exploitation, or they have learned to trust socially- or government-accredited experts. Many other factors come into play when people consider seeking help, including their fear of being stigmatized, blamed, or shamed for how one's children have turned out. Parents are particularly vulnerable to psychiatric authority when they are coping with a troubled child.

Seen from a distance, however, it is probably fair to characterize the relations between accredited mental health experts and families as a dance in which each dancer alternately takes the lead. Families respond and listen to experts, but experts certainly respond and listen to families. The formation and development of the politically powerful National Alliance on Mental Illness (NAMI), formerly the National Alliance for the Mentally Ill, is a case in point, at least at the policy level. From an initial grouping of 184 relatives of diagnosed people in 1979, energized by the wish to overcome the stigma they felt at the hands of family-blaming mental health professionals, its membership purportedly had grown to eighty thousand by 1989, when it constituted one of the most powerful lobbies in Washington. When Congress allocated an additional $40 million to NIMH for conducting schizophrenia studies in 1988, the then-NIMH director publicly credited NAMI's "tremendous lobbying effort" for this decision (McLean, 1990, 2010). NAMI has remained an extremely powerful association of family members and a key promoter of biological discourse on distress and misbehavior in the United States.

NAMI's prominence, however, may not result directly from its "grassroots" support among the mentally ill and their families, as its promotional literature claims. For example, in its 2010 annual report, NAMI states that it provides "support, education and empowerment for more than 500,000 members and supporters" (p. 16). This is certainly a most impressive figure for any grassroots organization, but when one of us (TG) contacted NAMI for an exact membership figure in early 2012, the organization's membership services replied the following in an email: "The 250,000 members and supporters number is the publishable number that we can provide but we do not have exact numbers that we can provide at this time" (Elizabeth Monrad, Information Coordinator, NAMI, personal email communication April 12, 2012).When we reviewed NAMI's consolidated financial statements for 2006 through 2010 (publicly available on its website) for total annual membership dues collected, we calculated an annual average of approximately 10,500 dues-paying members ($35 per membership) over that period. We conclude that NAMI's statements conflating members and supporters exaggerate by twenty-five- to fifty-fold its actual membership. So if NAMI is not quite the "grassroots" organization representative of the mentally ill citizens of the United States and their families, who does it represent? According to the *New York Times* (Harris, 2009), "drug makers from 2006 to 2008 contributed nearly $23 million to [NAMI], about three-quarter of its donations." In that news report, NAMI's executive director Michael Fitzpatrick expressed contriteness and "promised that industry's share of the organization's fund-raising would drop 'significantly' next year." The latest figure available (2010) on NAMI's website shows that pharmaceutical companies provided over $4.1 million out of total contributions of $6.7 million (62 percent of the total donations to NAMI), about 10 percent less than the figure cited in the *New York Times* a year earlier.

In this book we have chosen to focus our critique on psychiatric professionals rather than on the dynamics of help seeking by individuals and families. We think that the evolution of the mental health system over the last fifty years is important to understand, and we want to particularly highlight the role of what we label "mad science." Our examination is made possible because the rules and standards to which scientists, scholars, researchers, and practitioners are held are more public—matters of public discussion and accountability—than are rules for personal life.

Let us provide an illustration of our approach to examining the mental health system and how institutional actors, such as professional groups, federal research institutes, the pharmaceutical industry, and established family lobbies operate together to shape individuals' experiences when they seek psychiatric help. Let us explore the expanded institutional context of Wagman's saga about Benjamin.

Prescription for Insanity

The day after Wagman's distressing story appeared in the *Los Angeles Times*, a full-page, multicolored advertisement was displayed in the Health section of the same paper (November 6, 2006, section F10). The two-inch banner headline read: "Treating Bipolar Disorder Takes Understanding." The top half of the ad, in large print, offered a purported diagnosis: "You've been up and down with mood swings. You want to move forward." The ad continued: "Maybe ABILIFY can help: control your symptoms of bipolar mania; stabilize your mood; reduce your risk of manic relapse." The ad implied that if you experience distinct mood changes and want to move forward—and who doesn't?—you are likely to suffer from *something* called bipolar mania.

The ad then claims that some scientific consensus exists about how ABILIFY "works" in the body: "ABILIFY may work by adjusting dopamine activity, instead of completely blocking it and by adjusting serotonin activity. However, the exact way any medicine for bipolar disorder works is unknown." Why dopamine or serotonin might need adjusting because one's mood changes, however, can be left unsaid. What specific sort of adjusting would actually be done by the chemical also need not be stated. The ad does not indicate that this drug is not approved by the Federal government's drug-approval agency for children or adolescents. Then, before presenting a half page of small-print warnings about possible adverse effects, including death, it makes the perfunctory pitch: "Ask your healthcare professional if once-a-week ABILIFY is right for you." In the smallest of print, one learns that the ad was placed by two multinational pharmaceutical companies: Bristol-Myers Squibb and Otsuka Pharmaceutical. Of course, seeking advice from health-care professionals was exactly what Diana Wagman tried exhaustively to do, but the experienced professionals sharply disagreed on how to help.

Why would a drug company make a pitch to the lay public about a presumable psychiatric disease, one that even baffles the experts? And why would a company advertise to the public a drug that no layperson could legally obtain without the permission and prescription of a physician? As the ad admits, no one has any evidence regarding how or why Abilify "works"—even here it is implied that it *does* work, though what this means is left to the copywriters. Moreover, as two of our cases illustrated, professionals do not agree on how to define mental illnesses, on exactly what kind of phenomena they are, on what causes them, or on how they should be treated—or even if they exist as entities at all. And certainly, professionals, including the makers of Abilify, don't understand the pharmacology of these drugs. (To be more precise, the makers of Abilify have an exquisitely honed understanding of the pharmacology of their drug, but no understanding of how that pharmacology influences the hypothesized entity *bipolar mania*.) Lay and professional ignorance about these matters is the norm, not the exception. But it is precisely this level of ignorance that the pharmaceutical industry exploits to make billions of dollars. The federal regulatory agency, the Food and Drug Administration (FDA), rather than protect the public from the marketing campaigns of pharmaceutical firms, is seen by many critics (Angell, 2004; D. Healy, 2012) as ineffectual, for example, approving Abilify for use with children in February 2008. In addition, in 2007 Bristol-Myers paid $515 million to settle a lawsuit filed by the federal government over accusations of fraud in which the drug company employed a kickback scheme to defraud Medicare and Medicaid. Several years later California regulators filed suit, accusing Bristol-Myers of bribing doctors and pharmacists to use its products, including Abilify (Helfand & Lifsher, 2011).

One week after Wagman told her story, the *New York Times'* mental health reporter, Benedict Carey, wrote a long article, "What's Wrong with a Child? Psychiatrists Often Disagree" (2006). He reported that many other families echo Wagman's laments. Parents seeking help for their children receive shifting and confusing diagnoses accompanied by different regimens of drug treatment; mental health professionals acknowledge that there is confusion in the field; and advice given to parents is subject to diagnostic and treatment fads. Bipolar disorder, in particular, was described as being "wildly overdiagnosed." Carey reports that Jane Costello, a psychiatry professor at Duke University, stated that "the system of diagnosis in psychiatry was 200 to 300 years behind other branches of medicine" and that "on an individual level, for many parents and families, the experience can be a disaster."

One year later, the American Medical Association's leading psychiatric journal, the *Archives of General Psychiatry*, published a report that confirmed what many clinicians and journalists had already discovered: namely, that there has been an explosion of diagnoses of bipolar disorder for youth and adults. The report, however, offered no conclusive judgments from acknowledged experts as to why this had occurred (Moreno et al., 2007). In fact, the increase in the use of the bipolar diagnosis was so astounding that the national press immediately reported it (Carey, 2007; Gellene, 2007).

In a survey of outpatient office visits to physicians, a team of researchers at Columbia University found that youth received bipolar disorder diagnoses *forty times more frequently* in 2002–2003 than ten years prior, 1994–1995. The number of adults receiving bipolar diagnoses doubled during the same period. Nine out of ten children and adults diagnosed received psychotropic medications. This was a staggering increase in bipolar disorder diagnoses, and yet the researchers stumbled in offering possible explanations: the disorder had been seriously under-diagnosed before; the disorder is over-diagnosed currently; bipolar overlaps symptomatically with other common disorders such as ADHD; clinicians and researchers do not agree on how to recognize bipolar disorder in children, or recognize it better and earlier in a child's life; and so on. The most plausible explanation for the explosion of the use of bipolar diagnoses was not mentioned by the research team: the generously funded and well-crafted marketing campaigns by drug companies providing financial incentives to psychiatrists and the public to make bipolar diagnoses among children and to prescribe psychotropic medications such as Abilify (D. Healy & Le Noury, 2007).

Only two days after media reports of the epidemic of bipolar disorder among children, the Business section of the *Los Angeles Times* ("Sales of Antipsychotic Drugs for Kids Surge," September 6, 2007, section C6) reported that sales of antipsychotic drugs for children had exploded. Johnson & Johnson, AstraZeneca, and Pfizer were the beneficiaries of the doubling of prescriptions for children from 2003 to 2006, making children the fastest-growing segment of the $11.5 billion US market for antipsychotic drugs, which were not then even approved by the FDA for children. Joseph Woolston, chief of child psychiatry at Yale University Hospital, was quoted by the *Los Angeles Times* calling the trend "the juvenile bipolar juggernaut" and a "big problem."

Remarkably, twenty years ago children were never diagnosed with bipolar disorder (or its prior *DSM-II* moniker: manic depressive illness/psychosis). Bipolar disorder was only reserved for adults and, even then, to very few. Manic depression/bipolar was viewed as an exceedingly rare affliction. By 2006, however, the experiences of young Benjamin Wagman were common. What we suggest actually occurred is not an illness epidemic, but rather what the British describe as disease mongering—the manufacturing of diseases and disease explanations by those with a financial interest in opening new markets for their medical products (Moynihan, Heath, & Henry, 2002). The explosion in the psychiatric labeling of children, many younger than five years, has been so dramatic that it is now routinely the subject of media comment (Groopman, 2007; M. Healy, 2007). These exposés typically review the rapid spread of labeling children and youth as mentally ill, the confusion among psychiatrists about what these labels represent, and the trial and error prescription of powerful drugs pushed by Big Pharma without anyone knowing whether they truly help children or what the lifetime negative consequences may be. John March, a child psychiatrist at Duke University, offers a partial defense of the increase: "I think the increase shows that the field is maturing when it comes to recognizing pediatric bipolar disorder," but acknowledges that the controversies reflect "that we haven't matured enough" and that bipolar diagnosis for young children "may or may not reflect reality" (Carey, 2007). Is such ambiguity from a professional leader truly an informed opinion? Does Dr. March display any more insight into the prescribing situation than anyone else?

Gabrielle Carlson, a professor of psychiatry at Stony Brook University School of Medicine, describes plainly how the drug companies pressure psychiatrists: "We are just inundated with stuff from drug companies, publications, throwaways, that tell us six ways from Sunday that . . . we're missing bipolar" and encouraging parents with difficult children to seek relief in that diagnosis (Carey, 2007). She estimated that only one out of five children referred to her with bipolar diagnoses actually had it (a seemingly finer-grained critical judgment, but one which ignores that the bipolar disorder diagnosis cannot be validated), and in some cases the diagnosis was given in order to obtain insurance reimbursement (Gellene, 2007).

In an extensive analysis of how drug companies can "create a culture that legitimizes practices that would otherwise appear extra-ordinary," David Healy and Gabrielle Le Noury (2007) suggest, using the medical language of psychiatry, that we may have witnessed "a variation on Munchausen's syndrome, where some significant other wants the individual to be ill and these significant others derive some gain from these proxy illnesses" (p. 219). We will have much to say about these issues in chapters 6 and 7.

Defenders of this psychiatric expansionism argue that there is now more accurate recognition of mental disorder in children and adults and a need for a majority of the US population to seek psychiatric help, particularly by consuming daily doses of expensive psychoactive drugs. For example, Mani Pavuluri, director of the Pediatric Mood Disorders Program at University of Illinois at Chicago, said the label "bipolar disorder" was often better than any of the other diagnoses typically given to difficult children: "These kids that have rage, anger, bubbling emotions that are just intolerable for them" and that it is "good that this is finally being recognized as part of a single disorder" (Carey, 2007).

Within the psychiatric establishment, which has enormously benefited from these erroneous claims, signs of skepticism are emerging nonetheless. Perhaps members of that establishment recognize that public gullibility, although easily manipulated, is not limitless. Perhaps that is why even Thomas Insel, the director of NIMH, called the increase in bipolar diagnoses "worrisome" (Gellene, 2007). Yet the authors of the article in the *Archives of General Psychiatry* that uncovered the exploding use of bipolar diagnoses avoided mentioning the most likely explanation: that the rise of bipolar diagnoses may be attributed to how psychiatric researchers, in conjunction with the drug companies, turned clinicians into pawns of the drug salespeople and tarnished clinicians' reputations, credibility, and independence (Angell, 2004; Barber, 2008; Petersen, 2008). Insight and recognition of these matters has come quite late in psychiatry.

By 2008 a congressional investigation (spearheaded by Senator Charles Grassley of Iowa) had uncovered that prominent university psychiatrists, who had salient roles in promoting psychoactive drugs, had been secretly accepting hundreds of thousands of dollars from drug companies, in violation of federal and university regulations (Harris & Carey, 2008). The most prominent American child psychiatrist, Joseph Biederman of Harvard Medical School and Massachusetts General Hospital, considered the undisputed "inventor" of childhood bipolar disorder—which arguably triggered both the bipolar epidemic in children and their treatment with antipsychotics—had received over a million dollars in payments from drug companies (as had two of his close Harvard colleagues and former mentees, Thomas Spencer and Timothy Wilens). This occurred while receiving funds simultaneously from the NIMH to scientifically evaluate the products of these same drug companies, a fact Biederman failed to disclose to his Harvard employers as required by that university. This revelation spawned another cascading mini-scandal within American psychiatry and child psychiatry. A full three years later, the famed doctors' Harvard employers reported taking "appropriate actions" to discipline them: they were barred from receiving money for any outside activity for one year, required to obtain their employers' approval before receiving any outside money for two years, and to undergo additional ethics training, and would not be promptly considered for further advancement (all three are already full professors, the most senior of academic designations) (Silverman, 2011).

It's a Mad, Mad, Madness Establishment

Today millions of people like the parents of David, Benjamin, and Mi turn to medical professionals for help with personal troubles. They expect experts to possess scientifically informed opinions, to make skilled judgments, and to apply evidence-supported treatments that will not harm. Moreover, people believe the experts will assist in a personally disinterested way, in which the client's best interests are paramount and safeguarded. The psychiatric establishment, in its flood of press releases and presidential commissions, constantly warn of the dire consequences if people do not recognize their own mental diseases early and seek approved medical diagnoses and treatments. The families of David, Benjamin, and Mi were the victims of these messages.

The stories of people encountering the mental illness establishment that we have reported in this chapter might be dismissed by some as rare instances of medical malpractice. Unfortunately, misdiagnosis (or plain diagnosis), misinformation, disinformation, coercion, and harmful treatments are troublingly common occurrences within standard practice. They are the accumulated outcome of a series of psychiatric failures: the unquestioned belief that all the problems identified are medical problems; misuses of medical authority in implementing harmful treatments (e.g., with Benjamin and Mi); inadequately informing patients and family about options or the limits of psychiatric knowledge and authority (e.g., with David, Benjamin, and Mi); the long tradition of using involuntary treatment in psychiatry as well as questionable assumptions about its efficacy (e.g., David); misconduct and conflict of interests among many of the actors in the mental health system; the misuse of psychiatric diagnoses, which appear ill-informed, unreliable, and useless as guides to effective care; and, finally, the incredibly intricate ways in which the pharmaceutical industries have confounded thinking about human troubles and individualized psychiatric treatment and what professionals believe they ought to do as their first response to narratives or observations of distress and misbehavior.

These problems and their assumptions are often intertwined, and claims of major psychiatric breakthroughs remain profound illusions, built on flawed and misinterpreted research, and worse. Naturally, we suggest that continuing to believe in these illusions actually retards progress in understanding troubled people and in developing less harmful and coercive ways of helping them. We expect our claims that the mental health field has been shaped by psychiatric illusions of progress to be skeptically considered by many mental health professionals. Skepticism in psychiatric matters is appropriate, for there is much to be skeptical about. But the skepticism, which usually has come from outside critics, is now almost openly expressed by those at the pinnacles of the psychiatric establishment.

Earlier in this chapter we introduced Thomas Insel, the current director of the NIMH and his attempts to focus his institute on the operation of brain circuits, from which he thinks future breakthroughs will come. In justifying the new neuroscience direction for NIMH, Insel was recently impelled to make some profoundly important admissions about the state of psychiatric knowledge and practice. In a 2009 article in the *Archives of General Psychiatry*, he admits that the gap between biological knowledge and mental health care—a gap he would like to close—may be getting wider, not narrower (Insel, 2009). To close the gap, he believes, requires that the current state of psychiatry be accurately appraised. He offers the following assessment.

First, he argues, "There is no evidence for reduced morbidity or mortality from any mental illness" from new psychiatric medications developed over the last twenty years, in striking contrast to the "steadily decreasing mortality rates of cardiovascular disease, stroke, and cancer" (p. 129).

Second, despite increases of 20 to 33 percent in the rate of people in psychiatric treatment, there has been "no change in the prevalence of mental illness between 1992 and 2002" and "no evidence for decreased disability." In fact, Insel asserts that "while more people are receiving treatment, fewer than half of those who are treated receive treatments for which there is any evidence base" (p. 129).

Third, even when what he considers appropriate and evidence-based treatment is offered (e.g., the latest medications), they often fail to help. As documented in a series of NIMH-sponsored studies of thousands of patients in dozens of clinical sites, improvements are more the exception than the rule, and many patients simply discontinue taking their medications (see chapter 6). Insel states that, "While psychosocial interventions have received far less marketing attention than pharmacological treatments, the results are arguably more encouraging" (p. 129).

Fourth, he admits that "despite 5 decades of antipsychotic medication and deinstitutionalization, there is little evidence that the prospects for recovery have changed substantially in the past century." The data, he concludes, "on prevalence, treatment, and mortality indicate that mental illness remains an urgent, unmet public health concern" (p. 130).

Insel's summary of the limited progress made in the prevention or treatment of mental illness over the last fifty years can be interpreted in several ways. For example, Insel might be correctly recognizing that no outstanding neuroscience discoveries have improved the treatment of mental disorders, but he also might be hinting that the biomedical approach is still in its infancy and eventually the understanding and treatment of madness as a disease will be scientifically transformed and many disorders will be effectively treated medically. Insel's statements would thus constitute an admission of the difficulties faced, leading up to a plea for more time and money to confirm the grand biomedical hypothesis of psychiatry and develop medical cures.

An alternative reading is that, while Insel correctly admits the lack of progress in understanding and treating madness and even in alleviating any of its burdens on patients and their families, he fails to consider that the failure may result from madness not being, for the most part, a biomedical problem. This simple hypothesis may explain why, after a hundred years of pursuing the neuroscience hypothesis, so little (actually, nothing) has been discovered of any direct relevance to clinical psychiatric practice. That Insel does not even entertain this hypothesis in print—even if only to dismiss it—suggests that the NIMH is not a scientific institute. (See our discussion of "science" ahead.) His criticisms of the state of current knowledge, instead of prompting a reanalysis of the nature of distress and misbehavior, reconfirms to him, at least in written statements intended for public consumption, that psychiatry is on the right biomedical track. In the chapters that follow, we attempt to discuss an alternative hypothesis: that much of psychiatric research actually *undermines the biomedical hypothesis* of brain disease as an explanation of madness.

Understandably, as the director of NIMH, Insel must be concerned about the future of his agency. Given NIMH's commitment to the "mental illnesses are brain diseases" conjecture, it is unsurprising for him to move more vigorously into studying even more subtle and hard-to-measure areas of brain circuitry and to mount large studies to gauge infinitesimal statistical variations in genetic profiles, while continuing to promise that the age-old puzzles of madness will be solved. So, despite acknowledging that fifty years of biomedical research on madness has uncovered no causes of mental illnesses and a dismal record of effective treatments, Insel rallies the biomedical faithful by urging *more of the same.*

Perhaps we ought to examine the past more critically before moving forward with more of the same. How did fifty years of psychiatric failure get accepted as success and progress by major psychiatric institutions? Until we can better understand how the mental health professions arrived at their present medicalized views regarding madness and its management, we are unlikely to find meaningful alternatives. Our aim in this book is to examine how the science of madness—the research, publications, and professional organizations—became mad science: research that was viewed uncritically, distorted, and misinterpreted to serve institutional purposes. We will examine three fundamental changes in mental health care as exemplars of mad science: the nature of deinstitutionalization and community treatment, changes in the methods of diagnosis, and the nature and uses of psychoactive drugs.

These changes have been described as reforms, revolutions, progress, innovations, and paradigm shifts. Many ardent proponents of these reforms were motivated by the desire to create better and more humane care for troubled people, which they fervently believed could be done, but always by building upon or extending the view of madness as disease. Between the early 1960s and 1980 the scope, shape, and understanding of mental illness and its treatment were significantly altered in ways familiar not only to mental health professionals but to the lay public as well. What is less well recognized is that the three "reforms" were mutually reinforcing and were initially justified on the basis of scientific studies that were seriously flawed and misused, but these flaws were not easily spotted. As with many other complex issues in which scientists weigh in heavily (climate change, effects of pesticides, genetic determinism, energy policy, national security) the public relies, understandably since most of its members lack the training or time to investigate such issues in detail, on the media and the experts to interpret the studies. Even well-trained experts often rely on the judgments of scientific authors or scan only the summaries (abstracts) of articles. In short, the current landscape of the mental health industry—its conceptions and services—are built on a trio of scientific claims that appeared at first to mark significant progress. Decades later, these claims of progress appear illusory. We intend to trace this evolution.

It is noteworthy that during the decades in which these three momentous changes were implemented, psychiatry did not lack critics from within and from without. Indeed, the major challenge to the validity of the central psychiatric notion, mental illness—against which psychiatry was forced to respond over the next decades by "remedicalizing" itself—was published in 1961: *The Myth of Mental Illness* (Szasz, 1961). It was followed by numerous critiques of psychiatric philosophies and practices and their harmful effects on people and social institutions (Armstrong, 1993; Breggin, 1991; Cohen, 1990; Conrad & Schneider, 1980; Fisher & Greenberg, 1997; Goffman, 1961; Kirk & Kutchins, 1992; Kittrie, 1973; Modrow, 1992; Robitscher, 1980; Ross & Pam, 1995; Scheff, 1966; Torrey, 1974; Wilson, 1997)[4]. How psychiatry actually dealt with (or ignored) the issues raised by these and many other scholars and practitioners is described in the rest of this book.

What Is Science?

Since much of our book is devoted to discussions involving science as if it were the best approach to devise better understandings and explanations of the workings of our physical and human world, it is fitting to offer briefly our own view of what proper science is. To begin with, science is a human enterprise and therefore highly fallible. Scientists are not a special class of individuals free from error, able to set biases aside, able to be completely objective, or concerned mostly with searching for the truth. As the sociologist of science Thomas Kuhn suggested, most scientists are "normal scientists," a phrase by which he meant scientists who do not question the current assumptions of the reigning theoretical paradigm and are mostly not interested in getting at fundamental truths, but rather who less ambitiously try to solve smaller-scale everyday problems (which he called puzzles) within the current paradigm. Normal scientists leave the bigger questions to an elite group of scientific authorities recognized by their peers. One of these bigger questions is the question of when a shift in the scientific paradigm should occur. Usually the shift happens, according to Kuhn, when members of the old elite die out or retire and are replaced by young Turks; when a consensus is reached among them that a shift is called for; or when observations from the everyday puzzles that are directly at odds with expected findings accumulate to such an extent that these contradictory observations can no longer be ignored. But any of these factors succeed only if an alternative paradigm is readily available to take its place.

One of Kuhn's main contributions to the history and sociology of science has been to draw attention and scholarship to the personal nature of activities of scientists: that is, the extent to which the work of scientists is like the work of all humans: shaped by personal beliefs, commitments, capabilities, skills, and social and cultural expectations. But as the authors of this book we are not Kuhnians in any strict sense. We are more in line with those who might call themselves falsificationists (exemplified by the work of Karl Popper). That is, we see all theories (explanations, which include proposed solutions, interventions, programs, and policies) regarding the world and human behavior as tentative efforts to explain or predict that world, that must be rigorously criticized (through vigorous debate) and evaluated (by means of logical and transparent experimental tests) before being offered more generally. And even after being implemented, stringent evaluations should be regularly conducted on these theories and interventions, keeping in mind that future application of apparently successful theories or treatments and solutions may turn out ultimately to be more harmful than helpful.

The social science methodologist Donald Campbell suggested that:

> [s]cience requires a disputatious community of "truth seekers." The ideology of the scientific revolution agrees with Popper's . . . epistemological sociology of science. . . . Truth is yet to be discovered. Old beliefs are to be systematically doubted . . . The community of scientists is to stay together in focused disputation, attending to each others' arguments . . . mutually monitoring and "keeping each other honest." (Campbell, 1988, p. 290)

Open and frank attempts to falsify the hypothesized explanations lead, through trial and error, to better and more comprehensive explanations, allowing us tentatively to claim progress. We will demonstrate in the subsequent chapters the failure of mad science to meet any of these standards.

Psychiatric Coercion, Diagnosis, and Drugs

We will begin with a brief history of attempts to understand and treat mental disease and the claims about the effectiveness of community treatment. We then turn to an analysis of the revolution in defining mental disorders that began with the publication of the third edition of the *Diagnostic and Statistical Manual of Mental Disorders (DSM)* in 1980. Finally, we review the puzzling scientific terrain of psychoactive drugs.

Coercion and Deinstitutionalization

The movement of people out of state psychiatric hospitals and into various forms of care and control in the community or into other institutions, called deinstitutionalization, was the most important policy and institutional change in psychiatry in the twentieth century. Community care consisted of a potpourri of services (e.g., coordination of health and welfare benefits by a case manager), treatments (crisis intervention, medication monitoring, brief hospitalizations, counseling), and facilities (group homes, board and care residences, nursing homes, jails and prisons). During the 1960s and 1970s there was a sizeable emptying of state asylums for the mad, which had many determinants—exposés in the media about inhumane confinement in massive facilities, skepticism about the effectiveness of custodial treatment, misgivings about involuntary commitment, growing cost of hospital care, and the shift to federal funding for community treatments, as well as new hopes spurred by the introduction of newer psychoactive drugs. Whereas coercion had been a major component of psychiatric practice in state asylums, there was hope that community treatment, by using the new psychoactive drugs to control the mad and misbehaving, could operate without obvious coercion. Proponents of deinstitutionalization justified it as a method of providing more efficient, effective, and humane treatment for the "chronically mentally ill" than warehousing them in large, oppressive facilities. The stated goals of deinstitutionalization were to reintegrate the mad into their communities, normalize their circumstances, and improve their quality of life.

In chapter 2 we provide a succinct history of the rise of community treatment and public psychiatry in America and how private troubles for individuals and families have become concerns, first of communities, then states, and, finally, the federal government. But throughout that evolution in responsibility, the language of madness has also changed decisively into a language of medical disease. In reviewing the history of madness in America, it is notable that the major historians have trapped themselves in a medical vocabulary that, while it arguably shapes or reflects professional and public views, impairs their ability to provide an objective account of this history.

We extend this story in chapter 3, where we will examine what we believe is the mainstay of psychiatry—coercion—and its community-based use that often goes by the persuasive-sounding moniker of evidence-based practice (EBP). EBP is derived from a currently popular but seemingly already fading movement in medicine called evidence-based medicine (EBM). EBM claims to identify the most effective medical treatments through a series of workgroups that evaluate the research literature on treatments and rank them based on their effectiveness through a methodological protocol that includes the use of statistical methods. In selecting effective medical treatments, EBM is argued to be superior to the traditional reliance on the expertise of individual doctors and the wishes of their patients. We examine the evidence regarding both EBM's and EBP's claimed superiority and find it wanting. To demonstrate EBP's failure, we include a close review of the evidence on assertive community treatment (ACT), touted and promoted enthusiastically by a coterie of academic experts as one of only six evidence-based, gold-standard psychosocial interventions in mental health. Our analysis shows how the claim for the benefits of community treatment over state mental institutions rests on the use of administrative tactics and medically and socially sanctioned coercion (currently renamed "leverage"). Exaggerating the presumed effectiveness of a heavily marketed ACT helped to divert attention from the sorry plight of those supposedly reintegrated into the community. Jails, inhumane group facilities, and the streets have been the major community environments for the chronically mad for the past few decades. Community treatment's failure to deliver on its promises can be seen by the increasing efforts of psychiatric experts to justify and legitimize coercion as treatment.

Diagnosis

The second major psychiatric development, discussed in chapters 4 and 5, was a response to criticisms that psychiatric diagnoses lacked validity and were unreliably used by clinicians: in layman's language, they were inaccurate. These flaws were potentially ominous for psychiatry as a respected medical profession but were for years rarely discussed because providing scientific evidence was not necessary for psychiatry to carry out its functions. Nevertheless, in the interest of improving the scientific and political standing of their profession and to counteract psychiatric critics, a handful of psychiatrists in the mid-1970s strategically used the vulnerability of the diagnostic system to revolutionize psychiatric diagnosing, culminating in the 1980 publication of the third revision of the *DSM*, which provided what appeared to be more *scientific* detail and guidance for clinicians in making diagnoses.

Unlike the shift to community care, no one had clamored for change in the *DSM*, and few laypeople even knew it existed. The new *DSM* promised a descriptive diagnosis—using symptoms alone, without the need to understand any presumed underlying causes or dynamics—to defining mental illness. Although fully aware of the limitations of descriptive diagnosis, its proponents continually affirmed its advantages and their belief that its adoption was a necessary step in investigating and then discovering the biological bases of madness and misbehavior and in "remedicalizing" psychiatry. The heralded *DSM-III* hugely enhanced psychiatric authority, as it formalized a vast expansion of the behaviors, states, circumstances, and emotions indicating mental disorder. This expansion, in turn, was used to create a manufactured epidemic of mental illness in the United States.

All interested parties relentlessly exploited the new *DSM*—the pharmaceutical industry for economic gain; related professional and consumer groups (e.g., National Alliance for the Mentally Ill, Children and Adults with Attention Deficit Hyperactivity Disorder) vying to share in the reborn power and prestige of psychiatry; and the public, seduced by the ease and appeal of wielding diagnoses on themselves, just like the experts. The territory of madness thus was greatly enlarged, and many mental disorders became banal, even normal. When psychiatric experts (Kessler et al., 1994; US Dept. of Health and Human Services, 2011) declared that half the US population would qualify for a psychiatric diagnosis in their lifetime, validly distinguishing disorder from normality became largely irrelevant, since practically everyone could be viewed as potentially "in need of treatment."

The popular fascination with the *DSM-III* hid the fact that any evidence for its superiority over any previous diagnostic approaches was seriously flawed, as *DSM-III* barely made a dent in the acknowledged reliability and validity problems of diagnoses. Today, as the fifth edition of *DSM* is being prepared for publication in 2013, a firestorm of criticism has erupted (from, among others, the former chief architects of *DSM-III* and *DSM-IV*) about the continuing expansion of the concept of mental disorder, its extremely flimsy scientific and medical basis, and the disastrous consequences that widespread use of this medical concept has had on understanding the troubles of real people seeking help from mental health experts.

Drugs

The third fateful illusion regarding modern madness concerns psychoactive drugs, which we discuss in chapters 6 and 7. While deinstitutionalization and the *DSM* brought images of mental disorder into every neighborhood, the promotion of modern psychoactive drugs capitalized on the public's desire for medicalized yet familiar solutions to life's difficulties. Psychoactive drug cultures are nothing new, given that vast numbers of people have always used drugs to relieve their personal distress, to work more efficiently, to enhance pleasure, and to find meaning in life. The novelty lies in the successful campaign by the mental health establishment to convince people that their appreciation of psychoactive drugs *proved* that their unwanted emotions and behaviors were symptoms of mental disorders and, moreover, that whatever psychoactive drugs their physicians prescribed were *specific* treatments for these disorders.

The campaigns began with the industry promotion of amphetamines (such as Benzedrine) to physicians as antidepressants in the 1940s, closely followed by the marketing success of the benzodiazepines in the 1960s (such as Librium and Valium). In parallel, the arrival of the stupor-producing antipsychotics in the 1950s (led by Thorazine) radically changed the insane asylums and wedded psychiatry (then still largely operating and viewed as a custodial enterprise) to a future with drugs. Waves of new-and-improved "selective serotonin reuptake inhibitors" (led by Prozac and Paxil), "atypical antipsychotics" (led by Risperdal and Zyprexa), "mood stabilizers" (led by Depakote and Neurontin), and the resurgence of stimulants (led by Ritalin and Adderall) expanded and strengthened convictions that solving the problem of mental illness (now seen as affecting large segments of the populations of post-industrialized nations) meant making the drug *du jour* as widely available as possible. It did not seem to matter that the promoted drugs differed little—as substances affecting feeling, thinking, and behaving and regularly inflicting physical harm—from the banished and forbidden drugs on which authorities simultaneously waged a century-long war.

The misuse of science and research in the pursuit of profits from drug sales has been phenomenal, with no stakeholder guiltless. While the new drugs changed expectations and perceptions, the documented helpfulness of psychiatric treatment has remained unchanged, despite fifty years of widespread psychiatric drug prescriptions. In comparison with the pre-modern drug era, no significant improvements on any indicator of any major mental disorder, including depression, schizophrenia, and bipolar disorder have been demonstrated in studies that have been conducted relatively free of industry design or funding, as we will document in later chapters (and as the director of the NIMH states explicitly). Still, the marketing of medications has resulted in the daily drugging of an unprecedented number of children, youths, and adults, converting every mental health practitioner into a potential or actual drug dispenser. At the same time, the power of placebo, which could account for most of what passes as treatment "effectiveness," and the stupendous failings of clinical drug trials to inform about the actual, genuine effects of psychoactive drugs remain barely acknowledged. Moreover, producing and recycling drugs created new opportunities to invent *DSM*-style diseases and to market more drugs, making diagnoses more important to Big Pharma than they had ever been to clinicians or patients.

In chapter 8, we recapitulate our arguments and attempt to discern a way ahead. First, we reflect on our potential biases and how we attempted to counter them. Next, we identify what we think are the crucial characteristics of mad science. We then call for a de-emphasis of the current biomedical control over the understanding and management of the mentally ill in favor of a broad nonmedical system of personal assistance and supports to those seeking help, along with an essential decoupling of coercion from services. The helping enterprise does not need to pretend that coercion is treatment or that people must be treated against their wishes, and society must cease expecting those it considers healers to police and sequester the distressed and misbehaving. We also call for a decoupling of diagnosis from the eligibility and provision for services. There is no inherent need for diagnosing people as medically defective or pathological with hollow diagnoses in order to offer and to fund information, help, advice, counseling, support, and other personal, vocational, or housing services (that is, the bulk of what are called mental health services). There is also no meaningful empirical or rational distinction between (currently) legal and (currently) illicit psychoactive drugs, and no self-evident justification for allowing any group that claims unique expertise or responsibility to control how people use drugs to relieve their distress or reduce their misbehavior. We think that psychiatric practitioners have demonstrated—especially over the past half-century—that they regularly fail to exercise independent, informed judgment about the worth and usefulness of the various psychoactive medications under their purview.

Although rampant conflicts of interest among psychiatric leaders and institutions make it extremely difficult to disentangle knowledge from propaganda, this has always been so in the history of psychiatry and of the helping professions. We will suggest that the monopolistic reign of psychiatric experts over therapeutic resources for troubled and misbehaving people should be abolished. This will require clear-headedness about the illusions that have encouraged us to believe that the sometimes tragic challenges and troubles of human life—of living with our self and with other people—are symptoms of eradicable brain diseases falling under the jurisdiction of medicine. This does not mean that human existence cannot be improved or made more palatable. Moreover, medicine certainly has a place in a more truly humane system of services for people in need. But we question whether the current system, dominated by state-sanctioned psychiatric definitions, coercion, and prescription psychoactive drugs and distorted by financial conflicts of interest, is serving the public very well. This book is a hard-headed examination of the mad science that has created these psychiatric illusions and failures of the past and present, so that we might begin to move in new directions in the future.

Notes

1.   It's far beyond the scope of this book to examine psychiatry from an international comparative perspective. Nonetheless, the peculiar form of American psychiatric thinking that we describe in the book—which views distress and misbehavior as symptoms of conventional medical diseases, the discovery of their (unknown) etiologies requiring first and foremost the categorization of their presenting problems, and their treatment requiring the medical prescription of centrally active chemicals—has had a major influence on psychiatric thinking and practice throughout the world. The publication of *DSM-III* in 1980 (the third edition of the *Diagnostic and Statistical Manual of Mental Disorders* of the American Psychiatric Association), and its widespread dissemination and translations, fostered and in turn was fostered by globalization, including the expansion of markets for psychiatric drugs by multinational pharmaceutical companies. As it continues to become exported far and wide, this style of American psychiatry undoubtedly contributes to reducing the number of different existing vocabularies and models of madness, much like opening roads and transforming forests into farms in the Amazon Basin undoubtedly reduces biodiversity. A similar thesis is made by Watters, 2010.

2.   A similar but more elaborate recent statement from NIMH (April 24, 2012) may be found at: http://wwwapps.nimh.nih.gov/about/strategic-planning-reports/index.shtml.

3.   Personal distress becomes of public concern when people seek "health" insurance to cover the costs of treatment for personal difficulty (which currently requires them to receive a clinical diagnosis of a psychiatric disorder), or when chronic or unacknowledged personal distress leads to misbehaviors that physically or emotionally damage other people.

4.   Writings critical of psychiatric thinking and practice run in the hundreds if not thousands. Two bibliographies displaying the breadth and varieties of critiques are available at the following websites: Philosophy of Psychiatry Bibliography (http://www.uky.edu/~cperring/PPB2.HTM) and Critical Psychiatry Website (http://www.mentalhealth.freeuk.com/article.htm). But we caution that the mainstream psychiatric literature is considerably larger.

References

Abbott, A. (1988). *The system of professions: An essay on the division of expert labor*. Chicago: University of Chicago Press.

American Psychiatric Association. (1994). *Diagnostic and statistical manual of mental disorders, Fourth edition (DSM-IV)*. Washington, DC: American Psychiatric Association.

American Psychiatric Association. (1980). *Diagnostic and statistical manual of mental disorders, Third edition (DSM-III)*. Washington, DC: American Psychiatric Association.

Andreasen, N. (1999). A unitary model of schizophrenia: Bleuler's "fragmented phrene" as schizencephaly. *Archives of General Psychiatry, 56*(9), 781–787.

Angell, M. (2004). *The truth about the drug companies: How they deceive us and what to do about it*. New York: Random House.

Armstrong, L. (1993). *And they call it help: The psychiatric policing of America's children*. Reading, MA: Addison-Wesley.

Barber, C. (2008). *Comfortably numb: How psychiatry is medicating a nation*. New York: Pantheon Books.

Becker, H. S. (2007). *Telling about society*. Chicago: University of Chicago Press.

Bolton, D. (2008). *What is mental disorder? An essay in philosophy, science, and values*. New York: Oxford University Press.

Boyle, M. (2002). *Schizophrenia: A scientific delusion?* (2nd ed.). East Sussex, UK: Routledge.

Breggin, P. R. (1991). *Toxic psychiatry: Why therapy, empathy, and love must replace the drugs, electroshock, and biochemical theories of the "new psychiatry."* New York: St. Martin's Press.

Bynum, W. F. (1974). Rationales for therapy in British psychiatry: 1785–1830. *Medical History, 18*, 317–334.

Campbell, D. T. (1988). The experimenting society. In E. S. Overman (Ed.), *Methodology and epistemology for social science: Selected papers—Donald T. Campbell* (pp. 290–314). Chicago: University of Chicago Press.

Carey, B. (2006, November 11). What's wrong with a child? Psychiatrists often disagree. *New York Times*, http://www.nytimes.com/2006/11/11/health/psychology/11kids.html?ref=benedictcarey

Carey, B. (2007, September 4). Bipolar illness soars as a diagnosis for the young. *New York Times*, http://www.nytimes.com/2007/09/04/health/04psych.html?ref=benedictcarey

Carey, B. (2009, November 27). Surgery for mental ills offers both hope and risk. *New York Times*, http://www.nytimes.com/2009/11/27/health/research/27brain.html?ref=benedictcarey

Carey, B. (2011, February 14). Wariness on surgery of the mind. *New York Times*, http://www.nytimes.com/2011/02/15/health/15brain.html?ref=benedictcarey

Cohen, D. (1990). *Challenging the therapeutic state: Critical perspectives on psychiatry and the mental health system. Journal of Mind and Behavior* (Special double issue), *11*(3 & 4).

Conrad, P., & Schneider, J. W. (1980). *Deviance and medicalization: From badness to sickness.* St. Louis: C.V. Mosby.

Eligon, J. (2008a, June 11). Bellevue is allowed to medicate suspect. *New York Times*, http://www.nytimes.com/2008/06/11/nyregion/11tarloff.html?ref=davidtarloff

Eligon, J. (2008b, November 9). Suspect in psychiatrist's killing ruled unfit for trial. *New York Times*, http://www.nytimes.com/2010/11/10/nyregion/10tarloff.html?ref=davidtarloff

Eligon, J. (2010a, October 18). Mistrial for schizophrenic in killing of psychologist. *New York Times*, http://cityroom.blogs.nytimes.com/2010/10/18/mistrial-declared-in-tarloff-murder-case/?ref=davidtarloff

Eligon, J. (2010b, October 17). In a schizophrenic's trial, both sides agree. *New York Times*, http://www.nytimes.com/2010/10/18/nyregion/18tarloff.html?ref=davidtarloff

Fisher, S., & Greenberg, R. P. (1997). *From placebo to panacea: Putting psychiatric drugs to the test.* New York: John Wiley & Sons.

Gellene, D. (2007, September 4). Youths may be over-diagnosed as bipolar. *Los Angeles Times*, A13.

Goffman, E. (1961). *Asylums: Essays on the social situation of mental patients and other inmates.* Garden City, NY: Anchor Books.

Gomory, T., Wong, S. E., Cohen, D., & Lacasse, J. R. (2011). Clinical social work and the biomedical industrial complex. *Journal of Sociology & Social Welfare, 38*, 135–166.

Greenberg, G. (2011, January). Inside the battle to define mental illness. *Wired*, http://www.wired.com/magazine/2010/12/ff_dsmv/

Groopman, J. (2007, April 9). What's normal? The difficulty of diagnosing bipolar disorder in children. *New Yorker*, 28–33.

Harris, G. (2009, October, 22). Drug makers are advocacy group's biggest donors. *New York Times*, A23.

Harris, G., & Carey, B. (2008, June 8). Researchers fail to reveal full drug pay. *New York Times*, http://www.nytimes.com/2008/06/08/us/08conflict.html?pagewanted=all

Healy, D. (2012). *Pharmageddon.* Berkeley: University of California Press.

Healy, D., & Le Noury, J. (2007). Pediatric bipolar disorder: An object of study in the creation of an illness. *International Journal of Risk & Safety in Medicine, 19*, 209–221.

Healy, M. (2007, November 5). The push to label. *Los Angeles Times*, F1, F6–8.

Helfand, D., & Lifsher, M. (2011, March 19). Drug giant accused of fraud, bribes. *Los Angeles Times*, B1, B4.

Insel, T. R. (2007). Neuroscience: Shining light on depression. *Science, 317*, 757–758.

Insel, T. R. (2009). Translating scientific opportunity into public health impact. *Archives of General Psychiatry, 66*(2), 128–133.

Insel, T. R., Cuthbert, B., Garvey, M., Heinssen, R., Pine, D. S., Quinn, K., et al. (2010). Research domain criteria (RDoC): Toward a new classification framework for research on mental disorders. *American Journal of Psychiatry, 167*(7), 748–751.

Insel, T. R., & Quirion, R. (2005). Psychiatry as a clinical neuroscience discipline. *JAMA, 294*(17), 2221–2224.

Jacobs, S. (2010, October 12). Jury selection begins in trial of man who admitted to killing psychiatrist. *DNAinfo.com. Manhattan Local News.* Retrieved from http://www.dnainfo.com/20101012/upper-east-side/jury-selection-begins-trial-of-man-who-admitted-killing-psychiatrist

Kessler, R., McGonagle, K., Zhao, S., Nelson, C., Hughes, M., Eshleman, S., et al. (1994). Lifetime and 12-month prevalence of *DSM-III-R* psychiatric disorders in the United States: Results from the National Comorbidity Survey. *Archives of General Psychiatry, 51*, 153–164.

Kirk, S. A., & Kutchins, H. (1992). *The selling of DSM: The rhetoric of science in psychiatry.* Hawthorne, NY: Aldine de Gruyter.

Kittrie, N. N. (1973). *The right to be different: Deviance and enforced therapy.* New York: Penguin.

Kutchins, H., & Kirk, S. A. (1997). *Making us crazy: DSM: The psychiatric bible and the creation of mental disorders.* New York: Free Press.

Lilienfeld, S. O., & Marino, L. (1995). Mental disorder as a Roschian concept: A critique of Wakefield's "harmful dysfunction" analysis. *Journal of Abnormal Psychology, 104*, 411–420.

McLean, A. (1990). Contradictions in the social production of clinical knowledge: The case of schizophrenia. *Social Science and Medicine, 30*, 969–985.

McLean, A. (2010). The mental health consumers/survivors movement in the United States. In T. L. Scheid & T. N. Brown (Eds.), *A handbook for the study of mental health* (2nd ed., pp. 461–477). Cambridge: Cambridge University Press.

McNally, R. J. (2011). *What is mental illness?* Cambridge: Harvard University Press.

Modrow, J. (1992). *How to become a schizophrenic: The case against biological psychiatry.* Lincoln, NE: Writer's Club Press (2003 edition).

Moreno, C., Laje, G., Blanco, C., Jiang, H., Schmidt, A. B., & Olfson, M. (2007). National trends in the outpatient diagnosis and treatment of bipolar disorder in youth. *Archives of General Psychiatry, 64*(9), 1032–1039.

Moynihan, R., Heath, I., & Henry, D. (2002). Selling sickness: The pharmaceutical industry and disease mongering. *British Medical Journal, 324*, 886.

National Alliance on Mental Illness. (2010). *2010 NAMI annual report.* Arlington, VA: National Alliance on Mental Illness.

Peltz, J. (2012, August 15). David Tarloff, man charged in meat-cleaver murder of Kathryn Faughey, found fit for trial. *Huff Post New York.* Retrieved from http://www.huffingtonpost.com/2012/08/15/david-tarloff-man-charged-meat-cleaving-murder-fit-for-trial_n_1785780.html

Petersen, M. (2008). *Our daily meds: How the pharmaceutical companies transformed themselves into slick marketing machines and hooked the nation on prescription drugs.* New York: Farrar, Straus and Giroux.

Robitscher, J. (1980). *The powers of psychiatry.* Boston: Houghton-Mifflin.

Ross, C. A., & Pam, A. (1995). *Pseudoscience in biological psychiatry.* New York: John Wiley & Sons.

Rounsaville, B., Alcarcon, R., Andrews, G., Jackson, J. S., Kendell, R. E., & Kendler, K. (2002). Basic nomenclature issues for *DSM-V.* In D. J. Kupfer, M. B. First, &

D. A. Regier (Eds.), *A research agenda for* DSM-V (pp. 1–29). Washington, DC: American Psychiatric Association.

Scheff, T. J. (1966). *Being mentally ill: A sociological theory.* Chicago: Aldine.

Silverman, E. (2011, July 2). Harvard docs disciplined for conflicts of interest. *Pharmalot.* Retrieved from http://www.pharmalot.com/index-ad-new .html?gotourl=http://www.pharmalot.com/2011/07/harvard-docs-disciplined-for-conflicts-of-interest/

Stein, D. J., Phillips, K. A., Bolton, D., Fulford, K. W. M., Sadler, J. Z., & Kendler, K. S. (2010). What is a mental/psychiatric disorder? From *DSM-IV* to *DSM-V. Psychological Medicine, 40*(11), 1759–1765.

Szasz, T. (1961). *The myth of mental illness: Foundations of a theory of personal conduct.* New York: Hoeber-Harper.

Torrey, E. F. (1974). *The death of psychiatry.* New York: Penguin.

US Department of Health and Human Services, C. f. D. C. a. P. (2011). *Mental illness surveillance among adults in the United States.* Retrieved. from www.cdc.gov/mmwr/pdf/other/su6003.pdf

Wagman, D. (2006, November 5). One diagnosis away from despair. *Los Angeles Times.* http://articles.latimes.com/2006/nov/05/opinion/op-wagman5

Wakefield, J. C. (1992). Disorder as harmful dysfunction: A conceptual critique of *DSM-III-R*'s definition of mental disorder. *Psychological Review, 99*, 232–247.

Watters, E. (2010). *Crazy like us: The globalization of the American psyche.* New York: Free Press.

Wilson, J. Q. (1997). *Moral judgment: Does the abuse excuse threaten our moral system?* New York: Basic Books.

Zamiska, N. (2007, November 2). In China, brain surgery is pushed on the mentally ill. *Wall Street Journal,* pp. 1, 10.

2

The History and Historians of Madness

And in my solitude in England, doubting my vocation and myself,
I drifted into something like a mental illness. This lasted for much of
my time in Oxford. . . . I was in a state of psychological destitution
when—having no money besides—I went to London after leaving
Oxford in 1954, to make my way as a writer. Thirty years later, I can
easily make present to myself again the anxiety of that time: to have
found no talent, to have written no book, to be null and unprotected
in the busy world.

V.S. Naipaul, Nobel laureate

Introduction

Thousands of volumes have been written over the centuries about the true nature and definition of *madness*. Yet, as the medical historian Roy Porter notes, our current definitions depend on the same tautology used in the sixteenth century, when Shakespeare wrote famously in Hamlet, "What is't but to be nothing else but mad?" (2002, p. 1). Porter's own definition, the "generic name for the whole range of people thought to be in some way, more or less, abnormal in ideas or behaviour" (1987a, p. 6) adds nothing of consequence but suggests that the word *madness* does have a useful purpose: namely, to capture within a reassuringly resonating and apparently comprehensive category all those "abnormal" people who significantly disturb society and sometimes themselves. Porter importantly notes that "even today we possess no . . . consensus upon the nature of mental illness—what it is, what causes it, what will cure it. That is true even amongst psychiatrists. . . . Short of the discovery tomorrow of the schizophrenia gene, these controversial issues will not be quickly settled" (1987a, pp. 8–9, see also Andreasen, 1997; Grob, 1983, p. 36; Scull, 1993, pp. 391–394). Despite heroic or, depending on who is doing the judging, desperate and enormously expensive research efforts over many decades, no genes or reliable pathophysiology that maps schizophrenia or any other "mental disease" has been found

37

(Andreasen, 1997; Bentall, 1990; Boyle, 2002; Kupfer, First, & Regier, 2002). But even if such pathophysiology were found and some current "mental disorders" relegated to true physiological pathologies (neurological diseases) and disappear from psychiatric concern (as occurred, say, with epilepsy, general paralysis of the insane, and pellagra), at best only some people currently diagnosed as afflicted with a mental disorder would be identifiable by relevant biomarkers. The rest would remain mystifyingly *mad*.

A multiplicity of theories about madness has been proposed. Is it medical disease; a person's unfortunate, incompetent handling of greater and lesser problems in living; social labeling of disapproved behavior; social construction tout court; or, more provocatively, merely a word for a semantic category referring to all manner of behavior peculiar enough to be publically disturbing at any given time? The hypothesized causes, determinants, or contributing factors are as perplexingly varied. Are the mad mad because of unbearable social pressures; because of mental, physical, hereditary, genetic, or environmental vulnerabilities; or because of some as yet unfathomable combination of all of these (Read, Mosher, & Bentall, 2004)?

Neither the many theories nor the implied causes of madness have been scientifically validated, perhaps because mad science rests on hundreds of constantly shifting diagnostic categories of "mental illness," which have little in common (addressed in chapters 4 and 5). Fifty years of scientific efforts revising these categories, quantifying them, and statistically calculating perceived differences among them may not be the best analytic approach for understanding what is subsumed under the word *madness* and its many linguistic analogs. As the developmental economist Sir Peter Bauer (1981, pp. 262–266) argues, overreliance on numbers and mathematics devalues a fundamental component of scientific development, namely, conceptual analysis. Those elements of the social world that can be quantified have taken precedence over those less amenable to quantification.

Despite the failure of scientific attempts to validate the nature or causes of madness, groups with enormous political, ideological, and economic clout have taken up one theory about madness in particular: that it is medical/bodily disease. This disease theory is supported by the government mental health bureaucracy under the leadership of the National Institute of Mental Health, the pharmaceutical companies, mental health lobby groups, the organized profession of psychiatry, and hundreds of thousands of providers of mental health services from all professional stripes. Their successful effort to reify this medical theory, which we argue is at best only a useful analogy or explanatory metaphor whose depths already have been plumbed to no scientific avail, endangers further efforts to understand whatever contents the category of madness may hold.[1]

But as we dive into the murky historical waters in search of the hypothesized essence or even the specific content of madness, we emphasize that before anything else, madness is a word. Like all words, it is a human artifact stitched together to represent or echo something (abstract or concrete) related to human behavior or one's perception of this behavior. As a linguistic sign, *madness* becomes available for our critical manipulation, but like all linguistic signs it need not be anchored to particular aspects of the material world. The word *trees*, for example, does not directly locate any specific tree in the observable world, nor does it specify what the particular limiting attributes of the categorical term trees are. It serves as a label for collecting many disparate types of plants judged to belong under the category "trees," though these plants may share few common elements other than their category name (for example banana trees and oak trees). Such a category might best be called "disjunctive." According to Bruner, Goodnow and Austin (1986), "[w]hat is peculiarly difficult about . . . a disjunctive category is that [any] two of its members, each uniform in terms of an ultimate criterion [for example being living organisms], may have no defining attributes in common" (p. 156).

Words and categories matter. The philosopher Immanuel Kant proposed that categorizing is a fundamental and necessary act of human survival: it helps us to make sense and perhaps to respond and control the mysterious nonhuman noumena (*das Ding an sich*, the thing in itself) that makes up the "out there" that another philosopher, William James (1890), described as "one great blooming, buzzing confusion" (p. 462).

To recapitulate, words are semiotic tools, but they do not have any fixed meaning or direct connection to material reality or enjoy any consensus about their usefulness. They are open to variable definitions and interpretations often dependent on the learning history and cultural background of the definer. So it is with the word *madness*, because it is a word first and foremost and because as such it has no immanence, its meaning being primarily determined by those responding to it. Indeed, the history of social responses to madness suggests an abundance of possible meanings, some contradicting others (e.g., devil possession versus pathological personality organization versus brain disease versus inept training for social life versus a metaphoric haven for escaping from wrenching difficulties). Trying to define what madness *really* is—or what its verbal siblings such as mental disease, mental illness, or mental disorder *really* are—has been and may continue to be a failure. Based on the poor track record of progress in objectively validating madness or its contemporary semantic substitutes, we might consider admitting that ideas and behaviors, even the strange, troubling, and frightening ones we call mad, are *just that*: *ideas and behaviors*.

Unusual and scary behaviors of our own or those of others that attract our attention and elicit powerful emotions typically challenge us to provide an explanation for their existence. If no obvious explanation is found, often the best that we can do in response to our need for knowing why is to manufacture a word or phrase as an explanation that can safely contain all that puzzling and frightening content to provide ontological comfort in order to regain the existential stability we lost as a result of our encounter. In short, madness is a disjunctive category label. The term *mad* has been that universal remedy for disturbing behaviors for hundreds of years. It is a linguistic black hole that (metaphorically) sucks in all peculiar human behavior that society cannot digest or normalize but still feels compelled to explain in order to control. The word serves, on the one hand, to instruct reassuringly the normal that genuine boundaries distinguish the mad from the rest of us. On the other hand, the word strikes a cautionary note about what might happen if the normal are not vigilant and transgress.

The word also serves to limit inquiry. Its invocation appears to explain by mere assertion, though of course it cannot. "Why is John's behavior bizarre?" Answer: "He is mad (mentally ill)." "How can we be sure that John is mad (mentally ill)?" Answer: "He exhibits bizarre behavior." This circular process can be recognized by the logical thinker as tautological. However, the strength of the various institutions aligned to support and validate that logically erroneous judgment—such as government (National Institute of Mental Health), business (pharmaceutical industry), the professions (psychiatry, psychology, social work, nursing), and the academy (distinguished professors from the helping professions conducting research)—effectively discourages exploring alternative explanations for John's bizarre behavior.

In what follows, we present an overview of how the age-old social problem of madness was transformed into the contemporary medical problem of mental illness. We also discuss the attendant attempts to ameliorate this problem in America, as reported by prominent historians of madness. We then conclude with a discussion of the possible impact of the personal beliefs regarding madness of these very historians on the shaping of their historical accounts.

In the Beginning

The ancient Greeks were perhaps the first to discuss the problem of madness. For them it probably meant the loss of reason. The early Greek myths and legends focused on external rather than internal events to explain human action. They told of how heroes were subjected to the will of the gods who punished from on high, cursed, and sometimes drove them into madness (Porter, 1987a, p. 10). The Greek philosophers considered reason to be the noblest faculty of man. Socrates' "know thyself" represented the highest expression of this ideal through the use of self-critical reason (Popper, 1998). For the Greeks, this faith in reason to successfully negotiate the human predicament was counterbalanced by its opposite, *unreason*, seen as a major threat to human survival. Conceived as made up mostly of powerful primitive forces often dark and destructive—but sometimes constructive (*divine* madness to explain genius for example)—madness challenged the understanding of human behavior as being reasonable behavior. Such early Greek notions have significantly shaped our contemporary Western thought. Western civilization embraces the centrality of reason for ethical and scientific development while simultaneously battling to minimize the impact of irrationality because of its assumed causal role in the "senseless" tragedies that constantly confront humankind (Porter, 1987a).

The Greeks, Porter (1987a) argues, citing another psychiatric historian, Bennett Simon, originated the West's two principal ways of viewing and treating irrationality. The first sees the human condition as a struggle over "great unbearable elemental conflicts of life" (p. 12), such as love, hate, jealousy, and greed, and as efforts to cope with their powerful emotions of *unreason*, relying principally on spoken language to heal the soul or psyche. Theater in ancient Greece illustrates how treatment under this conception of irrationality could have proceeded. Greek dramatists such as Euripides, in plays like *Medea* and *Hippolytus*, through dramatic renderings of the individual's personal struggles against himself and others, brought the demons within to the public-at-large. Not only could the complex circumstances, conflicts, and emotions required for possible self-discovery be personified on the stage, but an opportunity was presented for ritual healing of *unreason* through communal *catharsis* of the audience. The professional rhetoric (its form and content calculated to persuade and gain agreement) later used by priests in the confessional and the "talking cure" practiced by psychotherapists in modern times are direct descendents of this tradition (see Vatz & Weinberg, 1994).

The Greek physicians associated with the Hippocratic school developed the other major way of responding to madness. They relied on their earlier contention that epilepsy, rather than being a sacred and supernatural disease delivered by the gods, had more mundane physical causes. They claimed that madness too was just another medical condition caused by humoral imbalances affecting various organs including the heart and brain (Porter, 1987a, p. 12). These two approaches to madness, rendered by Porter as "madness as badness and madness as sickness" (1987a, p. 13), are diametrically at odds with one another and to this day not reconciled, but they remain the models used to conceptualize irrational and frightening behavior and its treatment.

The other constant in "mad treatment," at least from the late seventeenth century when nation-states began to assume some formal social welfare responsibilities vis-à-vis their citizens, has been the formal, state-supported, bureaucratic coercion of public dependents. This emerged as marginal groups, consisting of criminals, the angry jobless, the unemployable, and the religious extreme, all exhibiting "dangerous and delinquent traits," were increasingly seen as needing separation from the rest of society to prevent social unrest. They were first cast as "disturbing" the social order due to their unconventional thinking and behavior, but because this kind of behavior might be seen as appropriate criticism of the state by the discontented and powerless, it was soon followed by their being recast as personally disturbed. The calculated separation of these fringe groups from society by authorities recast them as alien in thinking and feeling as well, justifying their forced confinement (Porter, 1987a, pp. 14–16).

The deviant behaviors subsumed under the "madness as badness" model potentially justify coercive responses because the deviant's negative behavior may be seen as intentional and harmful to the polity's welfare, requiring forceful control by society since the perpetrator has no intention of controlling himself. The criminal justice system is society's apparatus to confront this form of aberrant behavior. However, the second model, "madness as illness," does not necessarily suggest the same straightforward imposition of state-sanctioned force. Illnesses (at least in more modern scientific views) are usually seen as involuntary events that happen to people and over which no self-control is posited. It is ordinarily assumed that ill individuals desire to be rid of illnesses and to seek treatments or cures proactively. The selection and acceptance of medical treatment in medical practice therefore is viewed as the prerogative of the person seeking help. The apparent disregard of this general rule by the imposition of *involuntary treatment* when the medical model is used to address madness presents a dilemma. The dilemma relates to how "science" is employed in the explanation and treatment of madness.

Does science and its rigorous empirical approach for fact-finding support the psychiatric claim that the troubling behaviors subsumed under various mental illnesses are real medical entities, but which, unlike other real medical entities, can nevertheless be subjected to the routine use of coercion as treatment? Or does the language and imagery of scientific medicine serve to justify the use of force by the professions vying for control over the highly politicized and contested turf of what sociologist Andrew Abbott calls "the personal problems jurisdiction" (Abbott, 1982)? Part of the answer may be informed by how mad treatment evolved in the United States.

From Social Concern to Medical Treatment

Colonial Americans' views of madness were shaped by those of their European predecessors relying on the two models developed by the Greeks. Theirs was a metaphysical mélange combining "religious, astrological, scientific and medical elements" (Grob, 1994b). For over two hundred years, from colonial times till the mid-eighteenth century, America's mad folk were just one of many dependent groups designated as the "poor." The mad were viewed simply as one segment of the population appropriate for community concern and care; others were orphans, widows, the aged, the sick, and the physically disabled. What mattered in obligating the local community to provide public assistance was each subgroup's state of poverty leading to their dependency, not the particular causes or manifestation of their dependency (Grob, 1973; 1994b; Scull, 1985).

The community response to inexplicable, troubling behavior threatening the public safety on occasion prompted legally sanctioned coercion. Gerald Grob describes the case of a colonial soldier who murdered his mother but was found not guilty because he was adjudicated insane. The court required that he be confined for the rest of his life in a small room built for that purpose by his father, with the public bearing the cost (Grob, 1994b, p. 16).

Very few people were considered to be mad during the early colonial period, although almost no hard data are available and most of our information is anecdotal (Grob, 1973, chapter 1; also Viets, 1935, p. 395). Communities where the mad resided at first had no special facilities for their care, with families and occasionally other community members taking responsibility for their welfare. Later, as the general population and dependent populations grew, the insane were offered the same services provided all worthy dependents (almshouses and outdoor relief). The first almshouse in America was built in Boston in 1662 (Grob, 1973). Some of these mad folk worked productively, and the community generally accepted their accompanying bizarre behavior as one of the vagaries of life. Until the middle of the eighteenth century, medical considerations "played virtually no role" in how the "distracted" were handled (Grob, 1994b, p. 17).

The mad started to be formally institutionalized during the early part of the eighteenth century. Boston, one of the larger colonial communities, as early as 1729 sought to develop a separate structure for housing the mad, partly to reduce the physical conflicts arising when the sane and controllable and the mad and uncontrollable poor were housed haphazardly together (Grob, 1994b, p. 17, also Scull, 1985, p. 27). Several other communities shortly thereafter began to erect "hospitals." These facilities were specifically designed for the care of the destitute ill, including the insane, and were meant to reflect the community's continuing commitment to a special personal relationship with this group. But due to gradual demographic shifts and population increases, families and friends who originally bore the brunt of the care for mad community members were less able to take care of their own, and these hospitals served as professionally run "surrogate households" that "would help to train medical personnel" who would try, but rarely succeed, in curing "the sick stranger, the ill-kept resident, and wandering insane" (Rothman, 1990, p. 45). The first such official hospital was established in Philadelphia in 1752. It should be emphasized that these hospitals were more a segregating managerial response to the perceived problems of poverty and its impact on the health and welfare of the community "rather than to changes in medical theory and practice" (Grob, 1973, p. 16). The very first hospital exclusively for mad people was started in Williamsburg, Virginia, in 1773 (Grob, 1973).

The urban population of America steadily grew from just 5.1 percent of the total population in 1790 to 19.8 percent by 1860 (Rothman, 1990, p. 327, note 1). The increased societal and individual stress and displacement that resulted required the bureaucratic reorganization of the existing social welfare structure, including the approach to the care of the mad.

The Community—Cause or Cure of "Mental Illness?"

The specific type of organized care developed for the mad in the early 1800s and modeled on the approach taken earlier in England was the community-based decision to confine them to suburban or rural asylums (later government-funded state mental hospitals) to avoid the toxic stress of urban living (Grob, 1994a, 1990). The Asylum for the Relief of Persons Deprived of the Use of their Reason, opened by the Quakers in 1817 in the City of Brotherly Love, Philadelphia (Whitaker, 2002, p. 25) is often identified as our first nineteenth-century asylum; however, New York Hospital (opened in 1792) in 1808 constructed a building that was known as the New York Lunatic Asylum (Ozarin, 2006). The approach at these asylums was to remove the person, usually *forcibly*, from the hubbub and corruption of urban life, which was deemed to be primarily responsible for their *insanity* and, through the well-organized *rustic* asylum experience, allow for respite and healing before returning if possible to one's community (Rothman, 1990).

The three principles of asylum treatment that famously became *moral treatment* were, first, the rapid removal of the insane from the community; second, assuring that the confining institutions were at a sufficient physical distance from the inmate's community; and, third and most important, fulfilling, "[t]he charge of the asylum . . . to bring discipline to the victims of a disorganized society" (Rothman, 1990, p. 138). To impart order without brutality was the stated aim of moral treatment. The Quakers' original or ideal version of this approach in America around 1817 required that the asylum would be situated in a rural setting, housing no more than about 250 people (Whitaker, 2002, p. 25) under the governance of a paternal superintendant who might be a lay or medically trained individual. This individual would have a close personal relationship with each inmate and would help guide them together with supportive staff back to *reason* through simple, regimented, socially useful yet healthy physical work maintained by a ward system based on rewards and punishments (Whitaker, 2002).

Over time, the reality of nineteenth-century asylums turned out to be very different than originally conceived. Their populations routinely exceeded their optimal capacities, often by many hundreds of residents. The superintendents managing these asylums were primarily trained in designing, organizing, and administering them, not in the art and science of coping with behavioral disturbance. As Rothman notes, "[The superintendent's] skills were to be those of the architect and the administrator, not the laboratory technician"

(1990, p. 134). The title of a leading textbook on insanity published in 1854 by one of the more influential superintendents, Thomas Kirkbride, of the Pennsylvania Hospital for the Insane (*On the Construction, Organization, and General Arrangements of Hospitals for the Insane, with Some Remarks on Insanity and Its Treatment)*, reveals what professional areas were thought to be important and in what order.

Even the oft-stated goal of moral treatment, to eliminate harsh physical punishment or restraint, must be viewed skeptically. The renowned nineteenth-century French alienist, Philippe Pinel, one of the inventors of the *traitement moral* and considered to be a visionary who "unchained"[2] the incarcerated mad, also believed that successful treatment depended on the employment of psychological terror and fear to gain the compliance of the insane (see his description in Pinel, 1962, pp. 63–91). Moral treatment at its core was coercive because it was practiced on *involuntary* inmates, not willing, help-seeking participants free to come and go at their leisure, and used "the pervasive authority of the alienist, and his ability to link classification with a system of rewards and punishments, constitut[ing] an extraordinarily powerful new form of 'moral machinery,' a superior mode of *managing patients*" (Scull, 1993, p. 379).

The reality was that these patients were confined against their will in (eventually) large physical plants architecturally designed to separate the inmates into a series of wards that demanded various levels of psychological and physical conformity. Making progress in this system required obedience and proper behavior by the patients. Failure to follow the rules dramatically undermined the patient's social status, institutional privileges, and personal wellbeing by the forced transfer to more remote and less respectable and comfortable wards. Total control by the alienists/moral managers over the physical and social environment of the inmates was the mechanism that imposed discipline. Moral treatment originally was marketed by its proponents as a more humane approach for working with the mad, theoretically relying on minimal physical restraint (if one overlooks their forced sequestering in the asylums) while emphasizing other methods of behavioral control. By the end of the nineteenth century, it had transformed into a bloated, highly dysfunctional system utilizing physical punishment and that had almost no resemblance to its original psychological reeducation approach. Moral treatment became the rallying point for progressive political activists promoting the growth of government intervention in the care of the insane under the cover of medical science.

The Growth of the Bureaucratic Medical Management of Mental Health

Scientific medicine became a reality only in the mid-nineteenth century. German physician Rudolf Virchow's research, demonstrating the central role of cell pathology in human disease processes, offered for the first time medical treatment that reliably ameliorated certain physical diseases (Porter, 1997, pp. 304–347). The new scientific medical model of disease that developed as a result consists of reported (subjective) symptoms, measurable or palpable physiological signs, and demonstrable physical lesions. It replaced the ancient Greek humoural theory of health and illness prevalent until that time. Humoural theory speculates that the human organism contains four body humours, blood, phlegm, black bile, and yellow bile (choler), the balancing of which is necessary for good health (Porter, 1997, p. 9). (The intellectual debris of the humoural theory can be found in current speculations that "chemical imbalances" in the human brain cause assorted mental disorders.) The new medical disease model emboldened alienists to claim that "mental illness" was just like other medical disease entities even though "no evidence could in fact be produced to show that insanity had a somatic origin" (Scull, 1993, p. 241).

Benjamin Rush, a signer of the Declaration of Independence whose portrait appears on the emblem of the American Psychiatric Association and is considered to be the father of American psychiatry, in 1812 published the first American psychiatric textbook, *Medical Inquiries and Observations upon the Diseases of the Mind.* In it he declares "that the cause of madness is seated primarily in the blood-vessels of the brain" (pp. 11–17). Rush's statement might be the first published American psychiatric assertion that "mental illnesses" are brain diseases. This position was also held by most of Rush's contemporaries in Europe and America, even though little pathological work was undertaken to identify brain differences between normal and insane people (Rothman, 1990, p. 110). Such claims gradually shifted the thinking about the nature of treatment itself.

The early-nineteenth-century reports claimed impressive successes for moral treatment. "At McLean Hospital, 59 percent of the 732 patients admitted between 1818 and 1830 were discharged as 'recovered,' 'much improved,' or 'improved.' Similarly 60 percent of 1841 patients admitted at Bloomingdale Asylum (the successor to the New York Lunatic Asylum) in New York between 1821 and 1844 were discharged as either 'cured' or 'improved'" (Whitaker, 2002, p. 27). This success raised expectations about the possibility of effective nonmedical treatment for insanity. As popular support grew for lay asylum treatment, physicians, feeling threatened by the potentiality of professional marginalization, intensified their efforts to acquire medical jurisdiction over these asylums. In 1824 the Connecticut State Medical Society successfully lobbied for government and private funding and built the Hartford Retreat with Dr. Eli Todd as the medical superintendent in charge. Todd argued that earlier asylum treatment had "placed too little reliance upon the efficacy of medicine . . . and hence their success is not equal to that of other asylums in which medicines are more freely employed [and as a result his institution will be adhering] . . . to the lofty conceptions of truly combined medical and moral management" (Whitaker, 2002, p. 28). As states funded public asylums, they generally supported this integrated medical/moral approach, which also led to the increased use of physical interventions. Bloodletting, physical restraint, and psychological terror, originally promoted by Rush, became key treatment components (Porter, 1997, p. 500). By 1844, thirteen physicians in charge of asylums had organized into the Association of Medical Superintendents of American Institutions for the Insane, becoming in 1921 the American Psychiatric Association. One of their declared goals was to make sure that asylums would always have doctors as their executive officers and superintendents.

The traditional roles of hospitals as poor relief institutions for the transient or homeless sick, safe havens for the indigent dying, and places for custodial care of almshouse inmates sane and mad, also began to change to better fit the emerging, nineteenth-century scientific worldview. Hospitals became experimental way stations for the new notions of scientific medicine, curative interventions, and scientific research (Leiby, 1978, p. 61). These progressive ideas provided the empirical justification for recasting some hospitals into state asylums or hospitals for the insane. The earlier general social control mechanisms of poor relief could now be merged with the more recent "scientific" claims of psychiatry about the mad, boosting both its police powers and professional stature.

This shift in the United States from the early colonial voluntary concern about social dependents to the "scientific" approach for managing human problems in the late nineteenth century turned out in practice to consist largely of acts of bureaucratic categorizing and management. The collection and analysis of quantifiable data about various dependent groups served to confirm the rationality of administrative and bureaucratic activity. The individuals who helped develop public policy regarding these groups were confident that their centralized decisions would "promote . . . rationalization and systemization . . . to enhance the presumed effectiveness of public and private institutions" (Grob, 1983, pp. 81).

The scientific management of madness under this approach, in the United States and elsewhere, required renaming and categorizing disturbing behaviors as diseases and symptoms of diseases. This led to the development in several countries of various diagnostic systems for asylum practice and record-keeping. In Germany, the psychiatrist Emil Kraepelin published his first textbook of psychiatry in 1883, containing his descriptive nosological work, which remained one of the most influential. "Indeed, his textbook can be seen as the forerunner of today's *Diagnostic and Statistical Manuals*" (Porter, 1997, p. 512). Kraepelin's influence is discussed in more detail in chapter 4.

The successful nineteenth-century transition from lay to medical control of madness in America energized the mental health reform movement as it sought to convince the population and state governments to establish more mental hospitals. One of the leading progressive proponents of hospital treatment was Dorothea Dix. She herself experienced an emotional collapse at the age of thirty-four that was in her era diagnosable as moral insanity (Gollaher, 1995, p. 105). As part of her recovery, she spent about fifteen months in England, staying at the home of William Rathbone, III, a close friend of Samuel Tuke, the grandson of the great English Quaker William Tuke, who developed the by-then famous York Retreat, providing moral treatment for the English mad. Samuel Tuke's youngest son, Daniel Hack Tuke, was in charge of Dix's recovery (spent in part at the Retreat), and he tutored Dix on the Retreat's principles (Gollaher, 1995, p. 357). As a result she "adopted them as the basis for most of her later ideas about asylums and psychiatric treatment" (p. 112).

Dix's intentions were admirable. She wanted to help a group of deeply troubled individuals who were often treated miserably by the prevailing penal authorities. Her solution was to go from state to state in an attempt to convince the legislators to fund public insane asylums. She claimed, relying on apparently irrefutable data, that insanity was curable, that effective treatment was at hand, and that only the funding of enough public institutions to take care of the indigent lunatics would eliminate this grave social problem. So effective was she that thirty-two state mental hospitals were either founded or enlarged as a direct result of her lobbying (Leiby, 1978, p. 67).

Well intentioned as her approach was, it left something to be desired. To argue her cause Dix relied on false statistics and dubious claims about the curative powers of treatment. She apparently made no effort to examine or question the scientific data because it supported her assumptions about "mental illness" (Scull, 1981, p. 112). Rothman (1990) reports, "these statistics were inaccurate and unreliable. Not only was there no attempt to devise criteria for measuring recovery other than release from an institution [which was, as we will discuss in chapter 3, an administrative decision] but in some instances a single patient, several times admitted, discharged and readmitted entered the list as five times cured" (p. 131).

This focused lobbying effort by Dix and fellow progressives to organize and institutionalize publicly funded hospital care for the insane was a resounding success, serving as an early example of how good intentions and enthusiasm for change in psychiatric treatment overrides evidence. By 1880, about 140 public and private mental hospitals were managing about 41,000 individuals (about 90 percent were in public care). Notably, even at the end of the nineteenth century the mad still represented a very small portion of social dependents, making up less than 0.2 percent of the general population. The census of 1880 listed 91,997 insane people in the United States out of a total population of fifty million (Grob, 1983).

By the start of the twentieth century, a barely nascent psychiatric profession whose tasks centered entirely on the management of insane asylums had won the argument that good science demanded the institutional control of madness via state mental hospitals. However, almost as soon as psychiatry had made this commitment, it began to reconsider this approach to the problem of madness.

The Mad Population Grows by Federal Fiat

The horrors of World War I traumatized humanity and served as the spawning ground for new psychiatric problems such as "shell shock" and "battle fatigue." The phenomena of large numbers of individuals potentially opting out of their forthcoming military responsibilities during wars by claiming to be mad or by once in service developing psychiatric "disabilities" is well-known. "Everyone who served in the United States Army of World War II is familiar with the word 'goldbricking,' which meant, in military slang, malingering" (Eissler, 1951, p. 219). *Malingering* is the term for those who do not want to go and fight in a war or find the violence abhorrent once in the military and fake being ill[3] to avoid participating rather than declaring themselves conscientious objectors and facing close scrutiny and potential public condemnation.

The political problem of explaining large numbers of reluctant military recruits, when the military needs all able-bodied individuals for combat, can be greatly reduced by recasting malingering as diagnosable mental disorders and medically treating or honorably discharging their "victims" rather than court-martialing hundreds, if not thousands, of dissidents. The latest of these war-related diseases is the Vietnam War–related version, posttraumatic stress disorder (PTSD, Young, 1995).

Redefining the feigning of insanity to avoid combat because of fear of killing or being killed as a mental disorder rather than a moral dilemma allowed the "ill" individuals to be "diagnosed" then "treated," followed by either a rapid return to active duty or an exit from the military with an honorable medical discharge instead of being court-martialed. Joseph Heller's famed novel *Catch 22* tells an extended story of such maneuvers. This approach would mostly take care of those already in the military. But what to do about those at-risk individuals who were among the yet undrafted?

The passage of the Selective Service Act of 1917 had created a Division of Neurology and Psychiatry under the War Department to evaluate and reject recruits diagnosed with psychiatric disorders. Psychiatrist Thomas W. Salmon, the medical director of the National Committee for Mental Hygiene, recommended that the military exclude recruits found to be "insane, feeble-minded, psychopathic and neuropathic" (as quoted in Pols & Oak, 2007, p. 2133). His suggestion, which became the justification for military screening of draftees in both world wars, assumed that various war neuroses or mental breakdowns resulted from personal characteristics (i.e., constitution, genetic makeup, temperament, or early childhood experiences) that tended to be invariant within individuals and would undermine their ability to function effectively as soldiers (Pols & Oak, 2007). As a result, 103,000 individuals were excluded or discharged from the military in World War I for neuropsychiatric disorders (Jones, Hyams & Wessely, 2003, p. 41) out of approximately 2.8 million who were drafted (Wikipedia, 2011). This screening process was never evaluated, so we know nothing about its effectiveness or validity. The Division of Neurology and Psychiatry also oversaw "the treatment of mentally ill service personnel" already in the military (Connery, 1968, p. 15).

The federal involvement continued to grow. In 1930 the Veterans Administration was created to provide ongoing health care, including comprehensive mental health treatment, to veterans. The Division on Mental Hygiene was also organized within the Public Health Service around that time. This division's various roles included studying drug addiction, administering some of the associated treatment facilities, providing mental health treatment to federal prisoners, and offering diagnostic services to the federal judiciary (Connery, 1968). This expanded the federal role in mental health to few other client populations beyond the military personnel. The division served as the institutional center of this still-limited federal involvement until the National Institute of Mental Health (NIMH) started its work in 1949. World War II helped make the entire nation's mental health a federal government concern.

During World War II, the massive recruitment of millions of young draftees for the military focused the country's attention on mental health issues as never before. According to the 1945 congressional testimony of General Lewis B. Hershey, then director of the Selective Service System, the rejections for military service based on mental difficulties included "somewhere around . . . 856,000 . . . for mental diseases, and an additional 235,000 . . . as neurological cases. In addition to that there are 676,000 that have been turned down for mental deficiency" (as quoted in Connery, 1968, p. 16), totaling approximately 1.8 million recruits rejected due to neuropsychiatric difficulties out of the 36 million men classified for military service (Flynn, 1993). These numbers aroused broad public concern among average Americans about the extent of mental illness in the United States. General Hershey presented these data as part of his dramatic testimony to Congress supporting the ultimately successful effort to pass the National Mental Health Act of 1946. This act created the previously mentioned NIMH and gave broad authority to the federal government in developing and implementing national mental health policy and programming (Connery, 1968).

The "discovery" of a staggering number of military-age men with psychiatric problems unveiled by General Hershey accomplished its intended political and pragmatic aims. It impressed both politicians and the public of the seriousness of the national menace of "mental illness" and it justified the culling of undesirable individuals from the military for "medical" reasons. The problem, not unlike the issues raised a century earlier by the efforts of Dorothea Dix to convince state governments to fund state mental health hospitals based on exaggerated claims and bad statistics, was that this successful expansion of the federal government's involvement was based on bad methodology. The military's diagnosing of hundreds of thousands of citizens as psychiatrically disturbed was made by understaffed and insufficiently trained personnel, relying on screening procedures and tools lacking any predictive reliability, in ludicrously brief interviews of two minutes or so, all within a social environment tainted by eugenics, racism, and homophobia. Grob (1994b) recounts that

> The military feared in particular that the inadvertent recruitment of homosexual males would have a devastating effect on the armed forces and supported any measures that might exclude them. . . . Screening . . . was arbitrary and capricious; racial and ethnic considerations intruded in the process . . . and personality tests were biased and unreliable. (pp. 192–193)

The screening problems, never resolved, ultimately led to the abandonment of the entire effort under the order of General George C. Marshall in 1944 (Pols & Oak, 2007, p. 2134). These concerns were quickly superseded by the sharp increase of "nervous breakdowns" occurring in the battlefield. The most politically expedient explanation for mental problems that were described earlier as malingering was the impact of the war itself on the personalities of these men. The military psychiatrists argued that "environmental stress, that is, the actual conditions of combat played a major etiological role; predisposition was not a significant factor" (Grob 1994b, p. 193). Here was a pretentious and medical-sounding explanation for the common-sense observation that combat conditions seriously frightened and disabled some people. They recommended first aid psychiatry as the treatment of choice. Treatment was provided directly in the combat zone instead of in some more permanent but remote military medical facility that would have, it was argued, weakened the soldier's ties to his unit and prolonged the sick role. First aid psychiatry included "mild sedation, a night of sound sleep, and warm food . . . brief psychotherapy, rest and relaxation under psychiatric guidance" (Grob, 1994b, p. 194).

The simplicity and apparent success of such treatment under war conditions (most soldiers returned to their units within a week) logically suggested to the psychiatrists returning to their practices after the war that "treatment in civilian life, as in the military, had to be provided in a . . . community setting, rather than in a remote, isolated, and impersonal institution" (p. 195). The emphasis on environmental causes of mental disturbances helped foster theories of preventing mental disorders through the control of environmental factors. These efforts fit well with the already successfully established "scientific" public health model for the prevention and treatment of infectious diseases. Since President Harry Truman's Scientific Research Board had already expressed strong interest in having the federal government support biomedical research and insisted on the need for developing a national health policy, the incorporation of mental health policy into this broader federal health endeavor seemed a natural progression (Grob, 1994b).

The National Mental Health Act of 1946 embodied this commitment. It declared "mental illness" a serious public health problem, authorizing for the first time "extensive research, demonstration projects, training programs, and grant-in-aid to the states for mental health purposes" (Connery, 1968, p. 16). The NIMH, also a result of this act, provided the organizational infrastructure for centralizing federal authority over the nation's mental health policy. The act, building on the arguments of the psychiatrists returning from the Second World War, put the authority of the federal government behind policy efforts to "stimulate a new form of community mental health activity. . . . [T]reating mental illness in the patient's normal environment rather than in a mental hospital" (Connery, 1968, p. 19).

The Shifting Psychiatric Landscape

These developments were aided and abetted by the various exposés of harmful and coercive institutional psychiatric practices published in the early decades of the twentieth century. These provocative accounts further highlighted the problems of institutional care and undermined its optimistic early promise in the eyes of the general public. In the late 1940s, Albert Deutsch described a visit to a psychiatric ward:

> Cots and beds were strewn all over the place to accommodate the 289 mental patients packed into wards intended for 126. Cots lined the corridors, with restless patients often strapped to them. It appeared that about one-third of all patients . . . were under mechanical restraint that night—tied down to their beds by leather thongs, muffs or handcuffs linked to chains. (as quoted in Grob, 1994b, p. 204)

Although according to Grob the actual living conditions of the nation's state mental hospital systems were apparently improving by the 1950s, this was ignored for the most part and the emphasis was on expanding community-focused care. The post-war belief in the primacy of environmental and psychological causes of emotional disturbance supported arguments for early intervention as a way to avoid developing serious "mental illness" and the inevitable hospitalization accompanying it. This belief went well with the federal flow of dollars to community care in the late 1950s and 1960s based on the various federal legislative acts mentioned earlier. There was an intuitive common-sense logic to "curing" through supportive community caring, but it lacked empirical support (Grob, 1994b, pp. 234–236).

Such beliefs reinforced and supported the notion that fragmented state mental health services could only be mended by comprehensive federal planning and funding. These political, philosophical, and practical develop-ments, together with the introduction in the 1950s of psychotropic drugs, which were promoted as having great "scientific" promise of managing or eliminating frightening psychiatric symptoms (and which were functionally understood as increasing socially appropriate behavior without the need for obvious coercive physical restraint), provided the justification for the commit-ment to treat in the community the hundreds of thousands of institutionalized psychiatric inmates. Not only was this seen as an attainable reality but as a significant moral and social good.

Deinstitutionalization, as this approach came to be known, became the focus and the political agenda of those making mental health policy from the late 1950s onward. As the federal government expanded its involve-ment with mental health policy through its legislative activity, the role of state governments diminished and with it the role of state-funded and -run mental hospital systems. The Mental Health Study Act of 1955 provided substantial federal dollars ($1.25 million) to "research . . . and study . . . resources, methods and practices for diagnosing, treating, caring for, and rehabilitating the mentally ill" (Connery, 1968, p. 39). Business involvement with the management of federal mental health policy began almost imme-diately. That year, the Smith, Kline, and French Company, a pharmaceutical powerhouse and distributor of chlorpromazine (Thorazine), the very first antipsychotic ever approved by the FDA in 1954, provided a grant of $10,000 to subsidize the planning of the coordinating committee to organize the Joint Commission on Mental Illness and Health (JCMIH). The commission originally consisted of eighteen key organizations, including representatives from the American Psychiatric Association (APA), the American Medical Association (AMA), the American Psychological Association, and the American Association of Psychiatric Social Workers. The AMA and APA had five representatives each, while all the others had one each (p. 40). The membership was skewed toward the medical perspective, which would strongly influence the commission's development of their recommendations for mental health policy.

The stated commission agenda was to look at "mental illness" in completely new ways. The JCMIH, although instrumental in setting up the Mental Health Study Act of 1955, applied for and was selected to conduct a study authorized under it. This selection highlighted the strong ties already in place between professional interest groups and the government bureaucrats developing federal policy. The study, costing almost $1.5 million dollars, resulted in a report—*Action for Mental Health*. It recommended a massive program to inform and educate the public about mental health problems, and called for a dramatic increase in federal dollars to cover the cost of developing and implementing their recommendations for improved mental health services (we further discuss the commission and its report in chapter 3).

These recommendations called for increasing the authority and power of NIMH by becoming the source of the federal dollars for research on mental illness, by the establishment of academic mental health research centers throughout the country, by increasing the number of jobs available in the mental health professions, and, finally, by increasing federal spending to support mental health treatment. These recommendations helped pave the way for the federal government becoming the principal funder of mental health research and the chief arbiter of the "standards for the quality of care of the mentally ill" in the United States (Connery, 1968, p. 45).

The 1956 amendment to the Public Health Service Act under its Title V continued this effort to centralize mental health policy by authorizing grants for work improving the methods of diagnosis and treatment of mental illness and for funding NIMH to subsidize research efforts on better inpatient management and treatment techniques for state hospitals. The concentrated effort by the leadership of the NIMH to gain control over mental health research and program funding and policy development combined with the political activities of relevant professional lobbies in support of this federal takeover culminated in the passage of the Mental Health Acts of 1963 and 1965. These authorized the creation and staffing of comprehensive community mental health centers throughout the United States with the aim of seamlessly integrating and delivering the necessary mental health services in the communities where patients lived.

Robert Felix, the then-influential director of NIMH, in his pivotal US Senate testimony for the passage of the 1963 act predicted that its effect would be to facilitate "the day when the State mental hospitals as we know them today would no longer exist" (Connery, 1968, p. 51). The act was passed, and his prediction that state mental hospitals would no longer be the same, more or less has been realized. The state hospital inmate populations eventually plummeted, but the hope that community-based care would revolutionize the provision of mental health services and improve the independence and the well-being of the mad has not (Scull, 1981a). In fact, it appears that this effort merely shifted many of these inmates into other "museums of madness," such as nursing homes and jails. Scull tells us, "By the mid-1970s, nursing homes had become 'the largest single place of care for the mentally ill,' [with as many as 900,000 mentally disabled residents] absorbing some $4.3 billion or 29.3% of the direct care costs associated with mental illness" (1981a, p. 747). In 1998 the US Department of Justice's Bureau of Justice Statistics (BJS) estimated that 283,800 "mentally ill" prisoners were being held in the nation's penal institutions (BJS, 1999).

Regardless of the actual long-term outcomes, these activities served as the birthing ground for an "interlocking directorate"—of professional groups, mental health activists/lobbyists, private individual and foundation donors, government bureaucrats, and the pharmaceutical industry—that effectively has come to shape and run the "science" of mental illness and its treatments in the United States:

> As a revolution . . . passage of the mental health legislation of 1963 and 1965 had all the earmarks of a coup d'etat, carefully staged and managed, with the full implications for the country at large to come later, after changing the palace guard. . . . [T]he 1963 Act was but another episode in the continuing story of the expanding activities and influence of the National Institute of Mental Health. From its beginnings in 1949, partly the result of bureaucratic instinct, partly the result of professional dedication, NIMH's aggressiveness in pursuing its own expansion was exceeded only by its success. . . . Strategically placed congressmen, . . . who chaired the relevant appropriations subcommittees were carefully cultivated by Dr. Felix, aided and abetted by interested private groups and individuals. Among the more important of theses surrogates were the American Psychiatric Association, the National Association for Mental Heath and its state affiliates, and—through the good offices of Mike Gorman, executive director of the National Committee Against Mental Illness—Mrs. Mary Lasker, long known for her efforts . . . through the Albert and Mary Lasker Foundation on behalf of medical advances. (Connery, 1968, p. 61)

These developments led to the strong centrally organized political structure for dealing with madness that is currently in place. NIMH has cemented its role as the principal distributor of federal mental health research funding (its research budget has grown from approximately three quarters of a million dollars in 1948 to nearly 1.2 billion dollars in 2006). It is also the agency that closely coordinates the development of mental health policy. This dual role of the federal government in determining mental health policies and doling out the research dollars seeking to validate these policies has deeply politicized psychiatric science. NIMH is committed to biological explanations of madness. Projects relying on that presumption have formal funding priority. Other theoretical perspectives (related to psychological, social, environmental, and personal explanations of mad behavior) are deemed adjunct or irrelevant approaches.

Thomas Insel, the current director of NIMH, declared in one of America's premier academic journals:

> Just as research during the Decade of the Brain (1990–2000) forged the bridge between the mind and the brain, research in the current decade is helping us to understand mental illnesses as brain disorders. As a result, the distinction between disorders of neurology (e.g., Parkinson's and Alzheimer's diseases) and disorders of psychiatry (e.g., schizophrenia and depression) may turn out to be increasingly

subtle. That is, the former may result from focal lesions in the brain, whereas the latter arise from abnormal activity in specific brain circuits in the absence of a detectable lesion. As we become more adept at detecting lesions that lead to abnormal function, it is even possible that the distinction between neurological and psychiatric disorders will vanish, leading to a combined discipline of clinical neuroscience. (Insel, 2007, p. 757)

As we pointed out in the introduction, Insel's rhetoric smacks of propaganda and wishful thinking rather than good science. After all, the claim that the distinctions between neurological disorders and mental disorders "*may* turn out to be increasingly subtle" also means that they *may* turn out to be exactly what they are today, categorically distinct.

This concludes the "factual" history we have gleamed, not being trained historians ourselves, from consulting the works of some of the best-recognized chroniclers of madness. But, before we summarize and conclude what this history may mean, let us take a look at what is often thought to be unnecessary when using assumed objective historical scholarship: evidence for unacknowledged personal perspectives of the prominent madness chroniclers, on whom most people rely for their historical understandings of madness.

The Modern Historical Chroniclers of Madness

These historians are, in alphabetical order, Norman Dain (1964), Gerald Grob (1973; 1983), Roy Porter (1987a; 1987b; 2002), Charles Rosenberg (2007), Andrew Scull (1979; 1993) and Edward Shorter (1997). Professor emeritus at Rutgers University, Norman Dain's major work is *Concepts of Insanity in the United States* (1964), which Gerald Grob (1973) believes is the best academic discussion of early American psychiatric thinking (p. 153), and Andrew Scull (1993) calls one of "the best and most scholarly . . . accounts from this era" (p. 119).

Gerald N. Grob is the Henry E. Sigerist Professor of the History of Medicine (Emeritus) at the Institute for Health, Health Care Policy and Aging Research, Rutgers University. The dean of American psychiatric historians, over a thirty-year period Grob authored five major books (1966; 1973; 1983; 1991; 1994) and dozens of articles detailing the history of American psychiatric care from its colonial beginnings through the dawning of the twenty-first century. He is also a past president of the American Association for the History of Medicine (AAHM).

The late Roy Porter (1946–2002) was a professor at the Wellcome Institute for the History of Medicine in London, who edited or wrote over a hundred books and is probably, because of the rigor and prodigious academic fecundity of his writings, the most cited historian of medicine. Porter has published more than a dozen books on psychiatry and madness alone. That he managed to accomplish all of this before his early death at age fifty-five makes his achievement even more impressive.

Charles E. Rosenberg is a professor of history at Harvard University, a fellow of the American Academy of Arts and Sciences, and a past president of the AAHM and Society for the Social History of Medicine. He has written or edited more than a dozen books and numerous articles on medical and psychiatric issues.

Andrew Scull is a Princeton-educated academic who currently is the chair of the Department of Sociology at University of California, San Diego. He has published many books on the history of madness, is a recipient of the Guggenheim Fellowship, and was the president of the Society for the Social History of Medicine.

Finally, Edward Shorter, a professor of medical history at the University of Toronto, has also written several books on psychiatric history, the best known being the 1997 work, *A History of Psychiatry*. In addition to these principal historians, we will reference other scholars who have contributed to the writing of psychiatric history.

The Problem with Historical Messengers

The field of psychiatric historiography, that is, the history of psychiatric history, is reported to be "passionate, partisan and polemical" (Micale & Porter, 1994, p. 3). Yet, despite this implied diversity of perspectives, we believe that most historians of madness accept that what is contained within the category of madness is best understood as a form of *illness*. That term usually is understood as medical, and some historians fully accept that madness is brain disease. However, because the term *illness* may be vague, its use provides wiggle room for historians who are unsure whether madness is physical disease, but nevertheless feel that "mental illness" is real illness in some sense. This strategic use of the term *illness* biases either weakly or strongly their presentation of the historical "facts" regarding madness. For example, Andrew Scull—in a rebuttal to a psychiatrist's attack that he, Scull, considers madness "merely a literary or a philosophical concept"—responds thus:

> If I am less inclined than Dr. Crammer to concede that the definition of madness as illness is a pre-social, "natural" feature of the universe, and instead regard the boundaries of what constitutes insanity as labile and greatly influenced by social factors, that is not at all the same thing as the assertion that "mental illness" is some sort of literary or philosophical conceit. (Scull, 1995, pp. 387–388)

Scull's viewpoint is based, he writes, on the fact that "like many lay people I . . . unfortunately have first hand experiences of the ravages of mental disorder on those near and dear to me" (p. 387). Scull is an important historian who has through his careful scholarship exposed some of the most egregious acts of terror and coercion in the field of psychiatry. He appears to consider madness an illness but is not ready to declare that such an illness is a "natural feature of the universe," leaving us, his readers, confused. Is madness to be considered a medical disease like any other? If not, how should his general readership think of it? Since most contemporary laypeople (with whom he identifies himself in the second quote) think of mental disorder as a medical problem, his undefined use of *mental illness* and *mental disorder* will resonate medically to many of them.

Some of our historians narrate the history of psychiatry as a triumphal progress through time. In their accounts, primitive ignorance eventually gave way to the development and implementation of a scientific psychiatry through the key "discovery" that troubling and disturbing behaviors are medical diseases (Deutsch, 1967, pp. 517–518). Other historians take a more cautious position, believing that "the history of our responses to madness . . . is . . . far from being a stirring tale of the progress of humanity and science" (Scull, 1993, p. xvii). Finally, perhaps alone among those publishing psychiatric history, Thomas Szasz (1920-2012), a psychiatrist himself although his own psychotherapeutic practice never relied on medical interventions, attempted to delegitimize psychiatry as a medical enterprise. He consistently maintained that psychiatry was not a medical discipline to heal sick people but a unique policing profession. Szasz was often dismissed or excoriated by his psychiatric contemporaries for arguing that the societal response to madness (including the medical management of madness in all its guises) is primarily a political, legal and moral endeavor. His works develop in great detail the notion that the metaphors of medicine served to convert state-supported policing activities of socially disturbing behavior into medical interventions for a public health menace (Szasz, 2007).

These differing accounts of madness and its psychiatric management expose as naïve the idea that psychiatric history proceeds by reporting the cold, hard facts and nothing but. In their book, *Discovering the History of Psychiatry,* Roy Porter and his co-editor Mark Micale write that "both empirically and interpretively, extant histories of psychiatry reveal a vastly greater degree of difference among themselves than historical accounts of any other [medical] discipline" (1994, p. 5). Over time, they argue, organic medicine has demonstrated dramatic scientific advances in its understanding of the nature and etiology of disease, but mental/psychological medicine has failed to provide a similarly unified explanatory framework for its targeted problems (see Micale and Porter, 1994, ch. 1).

Psychiatry is the sole medical specialty lacking physiological validation for *any* of its particular entities, including all the serious and persistent mental disorders (Kupfer et al., 2002). Thus, in our view it remains an open question whether the psychiatric profession is treating medical diseases, such as diabetes or heart failure (entailing impersonal pathophysiological processes), or instead responding to the moral and behavioral anguish of individuals failing in the game of life as Szasz and a few others argue.

The various historical texts referenced in the present chapter, while occasionally documenting this ambiguous ontological understanding of madness, nevertheless routinely employ medically-impregnated language to tell their stories. Expressions such as *lunatic, lunacy, crazy, chronic mental illness, severe and persistent mental illness, mental illness, psychosis, insanity, the insane, psychotics, mental medicine, psychiatry, psychological medicine, mental disorder, disorder, mental disease,* and *disease* are used frequently and interchangeably throughout this literature. The habit of comingling words that are prone to ambiguous interpretations, such as *insane, crazy,* or *illness,* with others that also have more formal medical definitions in contemporary medicine, such as *disease* or *psychosis,* has consequences. As Scull suggests, "The concepts which we use to delimit and discuss any particular segment of reality inevitably colour our perceptions of that reality" (1993, p. 376). We think that the terms that many historians have adopted in their books have a medical bias.

Micale and Porter's own characterization of the medical field's activities toward mad behavior as "mental medicine" exemplifies some of these conceptual difficulties. Regardless of the empirical reasons for using the phrase *mental medicine,* when two distinguished historians matter-of-factly use such terms it affects readers' understanding. Are readers to think that the authors are naming and circumscribing a formal domain of medicine, or is the phrase meant as a literary flourish? If intended formally, do Micale and Porter mean that *mental* medicine should be held to the same scientific criteria and methodology as the other domain they identify as *organic* medicine? If meant metaphorically, should not the metaphorical nature of the expression be pointed out? Their essay does not provide answers to these questions, and the authors also employ expressions such as *psychological* medicine, further adding to the possible confusion.[4] It would help if Micale and Porter had explicated their claim that psychological medicine is "[p]oised precariously between the medical sciences and the human sciences" (1994, p. 5).

Through Metaphors Darkly

As philosopher Murray Turbayne tell us in his important book *The Myth of Metaphor* (1970):

> [w]e tend to forget that there are many subjects that we speak of only in metaphors . . . for example mind and God. The histories of the sciences of psychology and theology record . . . the unending search for the best possible metaphors to illustrate their unobservable subjects. . . .We find later theorists objecting to earlier metaphors that . . . have become obsolete. We find them substituting new metaphors for old ones that are either worn out by over-use or that

present an unappealing picture. But we also find many of these theorists writing as if they were replacing false accounts of these subjects by true accounts, or as if they were replacing metaphorical accounts by literal accounts. (p. 96)

Political scientist Kenneth Minogue argues that certain words and phrases can effectively give the impression that mere opinions possess more empirical certainty and stability then they actually do because of the power of their metaphorical imagery. He identifies these terms as "perceptual metaphors" (1985, p. 141). For example, when watching people, we do not, using our senses, directly *perceive* the complex content suggested by the terms *lunacy, madness, disease,* or *illness*; instead we *see* physical behavior (such as rocking, pacing, screaming, staying immobile) or *hear* reports and complaints of discomfort (claims of feeling light-headed, feeling pain, seeing unseen beings and things, receiving verbal commands to commit harm to self or others) or *view* signs of physiological processes (hot forehead, abscess, swollen abdomen, rash, and so on).

In order to make sense of these observations, we rely on perceptual metaphors such as *disease, madness,* or *illness* to package and mold them. In choosing to attach the word *disease* to a set of perceptions that otherwise would be viewed as disturbing or offensive behavior, we are "implicitly claiming a conclusiveness which has not [necessarily] been demonstrated" (p. 141). And we are also notifying our audience that we expect *them* to perceive disease too. Thus, the use of expressions like "mental disease" or "mental illness" for describing in historical texts certain *ideas or behaviors thought (by some) to be in some way abnormal or disturbing* is not a neutral act. In the absence of an explicit clarifying statement by the author (i.e., "*disease* is here being used metaphorically"), these terms cannot but put their audiences into a medical state of mind or evoke medical conditions because most people have been taught and redundantly reinforced throughout their lives to associate those terms with medicine. If they omit such clarifications, historians may promote a medical interpretation even when striving for neutrality. (The analysis to follow in no way should be seen as a condemnation of these scholars as inept or incompetent. In fact, we have a great deal of professional respect for most of them and their painstaking scholarship, on which we rely in the present book. It is precisely because of their fine work on unearthing the available historical record that we think they should be more cautious in their use of metaphors.)

To make our point more explicit, we would like to further examine some of the work of Andrew Scull. We selected him because we admire his overall analysis of the historical plight of the mad. We use his work to make the point that even the most able and critical psychiatric historians may inadvertently promote a medical perspective. In *The Most Solitary of*

Afflictions, Scull (1993) discusses the sad condition of one group under the purview of the modern mental health care system whom he characterizes as "younger psychotics" (p. 391). Psychosis can be the direct result of organic diseases like dementias, stroke, brain tumors, infections, and chemical overdoses, but the term is also applied to individuals who act quite strangely in the absence of any organic cause. Scull, however, offers no assistance in his text as to how he intends his readers to understand these "younger psychotics." (Should they be considered diseased or distracted?) He writes:

> Psychiatrists and other social control experts . . . negotiate reality on behalf of the rest of society. Theirs is preeminently a moral enterprise . . . I would argue that . . . the boundary between the normal and the pathological remains vague and indeterminate and mental illness . . . an amorphous all-embracing concept. Under such conditions, there exists no finite universe of "crazy" people. (pp. 391–392)

Scull in this passage seems to support the notion that psychiatry arbitrarily constructs mental illness as a way to conceptualize, respond, and control marginalized social dependents, and that the enterprise may have no logical limits, resting on an "all-embracing concept." But in an earlier section of the book, while criticizing Szasz's alleged position, he avers, "I cannot accept . . . that mental alienation is simply the product of arbitrary social labeling or scapegoating, a social construction *tout court*" (Scull, 1993, p. 5). What *does* Scull think mental alienation is the product of? In an earlier article, he includes a long note about the problem of using conventionally available terms that smack of a medical perspective, such as *mental illness*, when trying to write more or less neutrally about madness for a diverse audience. After explaining in some detail why there is no good way out of the dilemma, he concludes that "[f]aced with this problem, I have chosen to refer almost interchangeably to madness, mental illness, mental disturbance and the like" (Scull, 1990, p. 307, note 1).

Ordinarily, this would do. But Scull's note does not just contend that the terms *madness, mental illness, mental disturbance*, and the like do not have generally agreed-upon definitions and thus may be in some sense interchangeable metaphorically. He also asserts that madness itself, despite its ill-defined names, is real. He maintains, "To recognize that, *at the margin*[5], what constitutes madness is fluctuating and ambiguous . . . is very different from accepting the proposition that mental alienation is simply the product of . . . social labeling and scapegoating" (p. 307, note 1, italics added). Moreover, Scull believes that accepting *mental illness* as a socially-constructed reification would be denying the many visible negative outcomes associated with the problematic behaviors the mad engage in. Perhaps he is arguing that, for him, *madness*, when he calls it *mental illness*, is just another term for certain extremely troubling or troubled behavior that has dire consequences both for the person and others close to the person, and not, as often assumed by the laity, a medical problem. (It is hard to know unambiguously what kind of reality *mental illness* is for Scull.) Moreover, perhaps "younger psychotics" is referring not to medically ill individuals but to young people who have been waylaid by life's exigencies and have been the victims of the failure of our social welfare safety net. If that was Scull's intent, it might have been more useful to spell that out rather than resort to terms that have been associated with the medicalization of deviant behavior (on medicalization of deviance, see Conrad & Schneider, 1992) and therefore easily misunderstood as medical. He depicts the mad as the recipients of "the enormity of the human suffering and the devastating character of the losses" (Scull, 1990, note 1) resulting from madness. He suggests that the mad are therefore the "victims of this form of communicative breakdown" (note 1)[6].

A few pages after the explanatory note, he goes on to refer to some of the severely troubled individuals he is concerned with as "chronic schizophrenics" (1990, p. 309). The use of that term usually indicates, at least in psychiatric literature, individuals who are suffering from what is asserted to be a medical disorder, *schizophrenia* (APA, 2000). Scull, in his role of psychiatric historian, is presumably using the term in the same way. His colleague Gerald Grob, based on his reading of Scull, also contends that Scull "accepts the reality of mental disorders" as a medical issue (1994a, p. 274). For our part, we would characterize Scull's view as ambiguous, since as far as we know he has published no explicit statement of his position on the matter, even while continuing to discuss "those afflicted with the most serious of mental ills" in his latest work (Scull, 2011, p. 124).

Even careful scholars who are generally critical thinkers have a tough time maintaining judgmental neutrality when it comes to inexplicable human behavior and use terms in their works that have powerful medical connotations (e.g., chronic psychotics, schizophrenics, disease). This may be done by some authors because the words provide a congenial explanation of mad behavior. By other authors, medical language may be used to avoid implying any deliberate intention or moral agency on part of the "sufferers." Others, on the other hand, may try to uncover a "method to madness," revealing the possible intention, moral purpose, and explicit goals to someone's "mad" behavior. All these efforts involve situating the madman within his context and circumstances, explicating the madman's point of view, and the reactions of those around the madman and *their* points of view. This is historical work *par excellence* and of course has been attempted (Porter, 1987a), but when it has, we think that it makes it extremely difficult to account for psychiatry's development as a profession learning to identify and treat *diseases*. Finally, using medical connotations may be done to ensure that one's work is published without too much difficulty.

One further complication is these historians' reticence to make explicit their own beliefs about madness. According to one younger historian, such reluctance may exist because "autobiography risks functioning as a 'subversive supplement' to the author's scholarship, in that it can expose personal commitments and experiences which undermine professional authority" (Engstrom, 2000, p. 423). The reluctance is completely understandable, but some textual exploration can easily identify the personal biases that, left unexamined and uncontrolled, may slant these histories toward a medical perspective. Let's turn to them next.

Authorial Beliefs

Roy Porter in his *Brief History of Madness* claims that "the . . . historical survey [of madness] which follows . . . rests content with a brief, bold and unbiased account of its *history*" (2002, p. 4, italics in the original). The use of *unbiased* seems calculated to reassure readers that he produces narratives of historical facts as he finds them, with no worrisome distorting assumptions attached. But, in a publication written some twenty years prior, *Mind-Forg'd Manacles*, he admits that he "necessarily" makes assumptions regarding the nature of madness/insanity (1987b, p. 15). Madness, according to him, is best treated "like heart-failure . . . as a physical fact; but . . . interpret[ed] like witchcraft . . . principally as a socially constructed fact" (p. 15). Porter wants us to think of insanity both as a "personal disorder (with a kaleidoscope of causes, ranging from the organic to the psychosocial) and . . . [as] also articulated within a system of sociolinguistic signs and meanings" (p. 16). The labeling of insanity as "personal disorder" is strictly Porter's own invention, and we cannot tell if by it he is referring to an organic disease (he offers no references in the text supporting the substance of his claims) or something else altogether.

Fortunately, we can get some further insight regarding Porter's beliefs in a later, edited work, *A History of Clinical Psychiatry* (1995). He and his co-editor, psychiatrist German Berrios, address the issue of the organic bases of madness in their introductory chapter. They write that psychiatric historians can make useful contributions to clinical psychiatry by "building on the *belief* that mental disorders are complex and distorted reflections of dysfunctional brain sites and states" (Berrios & Porter, 1995, p. xviii, emphasis added) to establish which past socially mediated descriptions of mad behavior can "validly" be mapped to certain abnormal biological processes and which cannot. So Porter does appear to believe that madness has a physical basis and that history can help point out what aspects of past societal labeling of disturbing behavior represents real biological illness and what "'psychiatric phenomena' were noise" (p. xviii). But this belief in the biological underpinnings of mental disease is just that, a belief—as Porter is careful to state. Porter's amalgamated medical definition of madness as a condition resulting from brain and/or psychosocial abnormality and processed through a cultural and semantic filtering system is shared by most of our other historical sources as we shall see.

Albert Deutsch presumes that mad behavior is mental disease, even if early man was lost in myth and magic to explain it. His book, originally published in 1937, *The Mentally Ill in America* (1967) consists of his distillation of much historical material through the medical sifter. As he asserts, "it is safe to assume that mental disease has always existed among mankind" (p. 2), and, "[t]he conquest of schizophrenia . . . will surely rank among the greatest of medical triumphs when it is accomplished" (p. 506). The reality of mental disorder entities is never doubted; he simply equates madness with mental disorder as he tells us that "[i]n early Greece, as in Egypt, mental disorders were looked upon as divine or demoniacal visitations" (p. 5). As the best example of mental disorder in ancient Greek mythology, Deutsch offers the inflicting of madness on Hercules by the goddess Hera. This problem, Deutsch claims, "today would be diagnosed as epileptic furor" (p. 6). Nonetheless, like every other psychiatric historian, Deutsch also admits, despite his commitment to madness as disease, that "[a] mantle of mystery still hangs over a large area of mental disorder [although] . . . researchers . . . are striving manfully to tear apart this mantle, to bring light upon the nature of mental disease" (p. 518).

Another historian, Norman Dain, developed his classic book detailing the evolving historical *Concepts of Insanity in the United States* (1964) while working for three years as the research assistant to Eric T. Carlson, the associate attending psychiatrist at the Payne Whitney Psychiatric Clinic of New York Hospital (Dain, 1964). In it Dain states, "[o]f course even today no one understands the biology and chemistry of mental illness" (p. 207), but he never seems to question the appropriateness of assuming that the human problems he is describing are to be understood as mental illnesses. He regrets that most people still do not see that mad people are really "sick and helpless" (p. xii) and sees his job in *Concepts of Insanity* as explicating "the problems that confronted Americans in their early efforts to discard unscientific and unduly pessimistic attitudes and to place insanity under the aegis of medicine" (p. xii).

More recently, the Canadian historian Edward Shorter, among contemporary psychiatric historians perhaps the most committed believer in psychiatric disorder as brain disease, was asked if he believed that "clinical depression" was an organic illness. He responded: "Yes, I believe depression is caused by some kind of brain process. It's a disease that is in a way just as organic as mumps or liver cancer" (Shorter, n. d.). This belief directs his presentation of historical data. In his often-cited book, *A History of Psychiatry,* Shorter, relying on his academic authority, states unequivocally that "[i]f there is one central intellectual reality at the end of the twentieth century, it is that the biological approach to psychiatry—treating mental illness as a genetically influenced disorder of brain chemistry—has been a smashing success" (1997, p. vii).

His uncritical commitment to the reality of biological causes of psychiatric diseases is illustrated by his discussion in *A History of Psychiatry* concerning the increases in the frequency of certain psychiatric illnesses during the nineteenth century. He names "in particular neurosyphilis, alcohol psychosis and . . . schizophrenia" (Shorter, 1997, p. 49). But the facts are that neither of the first two is a psychiatric disease. Neurosyphilis is a neurological disease with behavioral correlates, a brain infection caused by the bacteria *Treponema pallidum*, if untreated leading to death. Alcohol psychosis is caused by toxic chemical poisoning: either too much alcohol consumption or sudden withdrawal from it. The historical record is clear that both these physiological disease processes, along with a few others, were analogically applied by nineteenth-century mad-doctors to explain the phenomena they came to call schizophrenia (see especially Boyle, 2002). About the latter, some anonymous wit famously said that "unlike neurosyphilis it is a disease where the treating psychiatrists perish before the patients do." Shorter's silence concerning the hard empirical evidence for the reality of the first two entities and the absence of such evidence for schizophrenia (though he lumps all three together as "mental diseases," having been demonstrated as biological diseases) can only be attributed to political calculation, not scientific judgment. What would be needed from him as an honest historical broker are the scientific facts of the matter both pro and contra, from the historical record, regarding schizophrenia. The current *DSM* states explicitly that "no laboratory findings have been identified that are diagnostic of Schizophrenia" (APA, 2000, p. 305). Of course Shorter knows this, as he explains in a later work when he concedes that "so little is understood about the underlying causes of psychiatric illness. Not having a solid 'pathophysiology' or understanding of the mechanisms of disease, psychiatry cannot rigorously delineate disease entities on the basis of anatomical pathology, as other medical fields do" (Shorter, 2005, p. 9).

The previously identified Gerald Grob is possibly the most well-known American psychiatric historian. In an extended footnote found in his 1983 book, *Mental Illness and American Society*, he argues forcefully that the psychiatric definition of *mental illness* is not fundamentally different from the medical definition of *disease* (pp. 35–36). Grob implies that they are both appropriately subject to medical knowledge and medical authority. Yet, in the ultimate paragraph of that footnote he admits candidly:

> In fact, we know relatively little about what is designated as mental illness, and that makes it difficult to prove or disprove its existence. . . . Assertions about the existence or nonexistence of mental illness represent in large measure acts of faith which reflect commitments to a particular course or courses of action. (p. 36)

This fence-sitting allows Grob's early writings to be variably interpreted by his readers, depending on their own individual predilections, while promoting his standing as an objective historian of mental illness.

In his 1998 presidential address delivered to the American Association for the History of Medicine, Grob states that "psychiatrists are compelled to deal with individuals whose pathologies are rarely clear cut and certainly never simple. Severe and persistent mental disorders—like cardiovascular, renal and other chronic degenerative disorders—require a judicious mix of medical and social support programs" (Grob, 1998, p. 213). This address is an apparently nuanced discussion of a type of difficult health problem. One could miss the use of perceptual rhetoric and metaphors (severe and persistent mental disorders—like cardiovascular disorders) to both define and frame his arguments. Although Grob knows that mental disorders are without any of the physiological markers of the biological diseases, he still analogizes the "severe and persistent mental disorders" to biological diseases.

This medical inclination did not necessarily result from Grob's historical research but rather from his personal experiences. As he notes in his *Mental Illness and American Society*, "I would be less than honest if I did not speak of some personal views which undoubtedly influence my understandings of the past" (1983, p. xii). In preparation for the writing of his first psychiatric history, Grob attended Worcester State Hospital's training, provided to its psychiatric residents. This instructional opportunity allowed him to become familiar with clinical cases and institutional life at least as portrayed by those running the institution. He writes that his experience "with severely and chronically mentally ill patients led me to reject many social control and deviance theories and reflexive anti-psychiatric thinking" (Grob, 1994a, p. 270). He admits that receiving instruction from psychiatrists at a mental hospital regarding patients "posed a risk of accepting conventional psychiatric claims at face value" (p. 270), but says that he was able to maintain at least partial distance from these beliefs. This is belied, however, by his use of conventional psychiatric labels to describe the inmates and their problems at Worcester State Hospital. It is worth noting that while Grob used his mental hospital experiences to accept the reality of "severe and persistent mental disorders" and to reject social control and deviance theories that conflict with such an understanding, the sociologist Erving Goffman used similar experiences while conducting ethnographic research within St. Elizabeth's Hospital to develop the very theories that Grob rejected (Goffman, 1961).

In his later work Grob has more explicitly "come out" and committed himself to the mental illness as medical/brain disorder assumption and compromised his scholarly objectivity by getting involved with the highly politicized process of federal health-care policy. A 2006 article on mental health policy coauthored with a prominent academic psychiatrist, Howard Goldman, presumably expressing their joint views, defines *mental illness* according to the US *Surgeon General's Report on Mental Health* (US Department of Health and Human Services, 1999). The article quotes part of that report, as follows: "Mental illness is the term that refers collectively to all diagnosable mental disorders. Mental disorders are health conditions that are characterized by alterations in thinking, mood, or behavior . . . associated with distress and/ or impaired functioning" (p. 738). The surgeon general's report adds that all diagnosable mental disorders are contained in the *Diagnostic and Statistical Manual of Mental Disorders IV* (1994) (*DSM-IV*) and claims that they are all brain disorders even though the report recognizes clearly that no physiological markers are yet identified for any of them (1999, ch. 1).

Finally, Charles E. Rosenberg is an eminent medical historian who generally tends to be judicious in maintaining an agnostic perspective toward "the particularly ambiguous status of hypothetical ailments whose presenting symptoms are behavioral or emotional" (Rosenberg, 2006, p. 408). Nevertheless, in *Our Present Complaint* (2007), he states that "[m]ost of us would agree that there is some somatic mechanism or mechanisms . . . associated with grave and incapacitating psychoses" (p. 39). This statement commits him to a disease model based on biopathological mechanisms for at least these psychoses. He indicates in the quote above, however, that he is skeptical of the more general trend to convert (medicalize) other behavioral deviance (i.e., homosexuality, alcoholism, or hyperactivity—see his chapter 3) into disease entities. He neglects in this otherwise critical, thoughtful, and well-documented book to tell readers why grave and incapacitating psychoses, most probably schizophrenia would be one, should have such mechanisms credited to them, lacking any current evidential support. (See, for example, APA, 2002, pp. xviii–xix, and other discussions throughout this book, especially chapters 5, 6, and 7).

Language is the filter through which public knowledge is communicated. The use of certain key words and not of others by recognized experts lubricates the expectations of audiences about how a social problem may best be understood. The consistent use of medical labels like *mental illness, mental disorder,* and *mental disease* by psychiatric historians as substitutes for the older descriptors *madness* or *insanity* tends to reify the view of madness as medical disease.

Many of these historians' semantic choices seem to be related to their personal belief or inclination that mental illness is a real medical entity or process. That belief confuses replacing an old metaphor by a new one with progressing from unscientific beliefs to scientific facts. Since, at best, the nature of madness is as yet unclear—disease or derangement?—we think it would be better if psychiatric historians would tell their stories by using more ontologically neutral terms, although we recognize the metaphorical nature of language. These terms could include: *aggression, agitation, anguish, behavioral disorderliness, defiance, demoralization, derangement, distraction, hopelessness, sadness, severe emotionally distress, stress.* Historians should more closely endeavor, as some do, of course, to contextualize to the fullest extent possible the phenomena that they are attempting to describe by means of historical records. By using neutral terms in their narratives without prejudging what has been discovered and scientifically established, historians would signal to their audiences that they are also groping, like other informed citizens, though they are giving us information to come to our own deeper understandings.

The use of these neutral words would not and should not prevent historians from presenting accurately and completely the views of all historically important figures, including those who use(d) medical terms and theories to "explain" madness. If any historian believes that madness is mental illness, that historian should reveal that, so the reader may be fairly and properly put on notice, just as a believer in phlogiston should put readers on notice when presenting a history of physics or a believer in the divinity of Jesus should put his readers on notice when presenting a history of Judaism.

The determination of historical facts is always an ambiguous process, depending on a particular historian's personal beliefs, agenda, and decisions regarding what evidence to attend to and to ignore in constructing a narrative. (As authors of this book, this insight also applies to our work and we take up this issue of our own personal or professional biases in the concluding chapter.) As Engstrom suggests, "the conceptual frameworks we have for thinking about mental anguish are (and likely always will be) woefully inadequate. That's what the history of psychiatry has taught me" (E. J. Engstrom, personal communication, October, 9, 2008).

Conclusion

While keeping in mind caveat lector, due to the inevitably fallible nature of our historical facts, we can conclude that our brief historical tour of the phenomena called madness and its overall management has brought us close to where we began. The ontological status of madness remains unsolved in the twenty-first century. Both coercion and concern have periodically animated society's treatment of the mad, sometimes concurrently. Early on in America's history, families took care of their distracted relatives. As the US became a more economically specialized and politically organized society, the need for bureaucratic structures for social management became more pressing. The increasing population and urbanization of America led to a more mobile populace, leaving fewer families intact to take care of mad relatives. These circumstances led to the creation of institutional substitutes to provide care for these dependents. Simultaneously and in response to these developing institutions, a class of professional helpers emerged who claimed special expertise in the management of the mad. These helpers at first were lay managers using more or less authoritarian moral treatment, but over time physicians became interested in the mad trade and offered medicalesque reasonings and medical analogies for why the mad were mad, and society was persuaded. These physicians, however, offered no evidence to confirm their reasonings. By the mid-nineteenth century, state governments were gradually taking charge of mental institutions, which were increasingly medicalized. Government involvement accelerated through the twentieth century with the federal government taking control from the states by the 1950s. Over the next two decades, the federal government, psychiatric professionals, various interest groups, and Big Pharma formed an interlocking directorate that managed, through political action rather than scientifically informed strategy, to shift much of the location of mad treatments from a few very similar, distinct, and clearly identifiable walled institutions to a plethora of dissimilar, diverse, and dispersed institutions in "the community." This well-coordinated enterprise controls the research agenda as well as the policy development in mental health today.

In Shakespeare's time, when it came to understanding madness one could only offer a tautology. *Madness* was defined as being nothing but mad. Today we are left not exactly with a tautology, but with a mystery. The modern term for mad behavior is the medically encapsulated notion of *mental illness*, but that term really refers to many different hypothesized syndromes, most of which the *DSM* calls mental disorders. The term *mental illness* is a black box. The medically-oriented argue that these syndromes are brain diseases, Thomas Insel, the NIMH's director, speculates that "abnormal activity in specific brain circuits" are the causes of mental illnesses. Unfortunately, after a hundred years of these hypotheses, not a single biological marker for a single psychiatric disorder has been identified to validate distress and misbehavior as a medical disease.

Insel and other psychiatric authorities (Andreasen, 1997) reassure the public, despite their continual inability to provide the evidence, that if the public is just patient for a little while longer and holds on to the descriptive *DSM* syndromes, diagnostic lesions underling these syndromes will definitely be identified in the not too distant future, initiating a psychiatric utopia—one in which psychiatric science will deliver specific cures for our behavioral problems. Despite the failed promises, very few people seem to be exploring alternative ways to understand and address madness.

If one accepts philosopher Karl Popper's view that doing good science requires submitting one's most cherished paradigms and viewpoints to rigorous empirical tests and criticism to see if they stand up to such scrutiny (Popper, 1989), then at least one important use of historical knowledge becomes evident. By examining the historical record (even with all its limitations), one can learn about the many "scientific" psychiatric paradigms and treatments that have regularly failed (e.g., the nineteenth-century asylum system, moral treatment, and the government-operated state mental hospital system). These failures suggest that all interested persons should be skeptical of the current conventional wisdom regarding madness because this may, under conceptual and empirical examination, also prove to be mistaken.

Keeping both these cautionary and hopeful concluding thoughts in mind, let us turn to the current best efforts at managing the mad: community treatment.

Notes

1. We tend to agree with Tom Szasz that the better term for the coercive paternalistic approach used by most psychiatrists is the pediatric model, since "(t)ypically physicians treat adults who seek their services. Only pediatricians and psychiatrists treat persons who do not seek their services" (Szasz, 2004, p. 323). But due to its widespread use, we will continue for the sake of expediency to refer in the rest of the book to this unique patronizing model relying on force for servicing mad adults as the "medical model" (to be explicated in more detail in chapter 3).

2. This unchaining is a complete fabrication (see Scull, 1993, p. 377, especially note 4).

3. To clarify what may sound unsympathetic or accusatory: we believe that, when facing difficult or traumatizing life circumstances, wanting to escape is a quintessentially human response. We even have descriptive terms at the ready to identify these possible responses: "heroic" or "cowardly." How one responds to such circumstances is not knowable in advance, and claiming illness is often one of the obvious options to avoid moral condemnation from self and others. Human beings are capable of fooling themselves as easily as others; it is called "self-deception." We suggest that the claims of feeling ill often are genuinely held by the claimants and may be just these sorts of self-deceptions rather than necessarily calculated fraudulent deceptions. Unfortunately, feeling as if we are ill in no way establishes that we have a medical illness. We go to doctors in part to help us clarify whether our felt "symptoms" are manifestations of objective physical pathological processes qualifying as medical disease.

4. This is similar to the term *behavioral health*, whose use in the medical and psychological literature first appeared in the 1970s and dramatically spiked starting in the mid-1990s (see, for example, Google's ngram using this term). This obvious metaphor appears well-suited for its primary purposes, as far as we can discern them at present: to justify both the involvement of psychologists and social workers in the health care arena and the renewed involvement of physicians in changing patients' behaviors.

5. This begs the question of what in madness' "center" as opposed to its margins is invariable and unambiguous.

6. Thomas Szasz would agree but would also add that, as sentient moral agents involved in transactions with others, they are responsible at least in part for the breakdown in communication and their subsequent difficulties. Szasz—who has been described by Micale and Porter in their edited volume *Discovering the History of Psychiatry* (1994) as "offer[ing]

fundamental rereadings of exemplary episodes and topics in the history of mental medicine" (p. 23) worthy of a full chapter in that book—has never asserted what Scull (1993) and many other of his critics claim to be Szasz's position, namely, that mental alienation is merely the result of social labeling and scapegoating and is a myth. Szasz argues that emotional difficulties and tragedies are real, but result from the minor and serious problems that people experience while trying to make a life, rather than the consequence of biological pathology. He suggested that "[t]o regard 'minor' upheavals in living as problems in human relations, learning and so forth—and more 'major' upheavals as due to brain disease, seems to be a rather simple example of wishful thinking" (Szasz, 1961, p. 94). In his first and most often cited but rarely fully understood classic, the *Myth of Mental Illness* (1961), Szasz did not write a polemic full of simplistic claims as Scull asserts (Scull, 2011, p. 100), but rather a detailed and scholarly treatise outlining, as its subtitle states, the "foundations of a theory of personal conduct." Using a combination of semiotic, rule-following, and game-model analysis, Szasz proposes a theory of human behavior applicable to both the "normal" and "deviant."

References

Abbott, A. (1988). *The system of professions: An essay on the division of expert labor.* Chicago: University of Chicago Press.

American Psychiatric Association. (1994). *Diagnostic and statistical manual of mental disorders Fourth edition.* Washington, DC: American Psychiatric Association.

American Psychiatric Association. (2000). *Diagnostic and statistical manual of mental disorders Fourth edition, Text revision.* Washington, DC: American Psychiatric Association.

Andreasen, N. C. (1997). Linking mind and brain in the study of mental illnesses: A project for a scientific psychopathology. *Science, 275,* 1586–1593.

Bauer, P. T. (1981). *Equality, the third world, and economic delusion.* Cambridge, MA: Harvard University Press.

Bentall, R. P. (Ed.) (1990). *Reconstructing schizophrenia.* New York: Routledge.

Berrios, G. & Porter, R. (Eds.). (1995). *A history of clinical psychiatry.* New Brunswick, NJ: Athlone Press.

Boyle M. (2002). *Schizophrenia: A scientific delusion?* New York: Routledge.

Bruner, J. S., Goodnow, J. J. & Austin, G. A. (1986) *A study of thinking.* New Brunswick, NJ: Transaction, Inc.

Bureau of Justice Statistics. (1999). More than a quarter million prison and jail inmates are identified as mentally ill. Retrieved from http://bjs.ojp.usdoj.gov/content/pub/press/MHTIP.PR

Cohen, S. & Scull, A. (Eds.) (1983). *Social control and the state.* New York: St. Martin's Press.

Connery, R. H. (1968). *The politics of mental health.* New York: Columbia University Press.

Conrad, P. & Schneider, J. W. (1992). *Deviance and medicalization: From badness to sickness.* Philadelphia, PA: Temple University Press.

Dain, N. (1964). *Concepts of insanity.* New Brunswick, NJ: Rutgers University Press.

Deutsch, A. (1967). *The mentally ill in America.* New York: Columbia University Press.

Eissler, K. R. (1951). Malingering. In G. B. Wilbur & W. Muensterberger (Eds.), *Psychoanalysis and culture* (pp. 218–253). New York: International Universities Press, Inc.

Engstrom, E. J. (2000). Zeitgeschichte as disciplinary history: On professional identity, self-reflexive narratives, and discipline-building in contemporary German history. *Tel Aviver Jahrbuch für deutsche Geschichte 29,* 399–425.

Engstrom, E. J. (2003). *Clinical psychiatry in imperial Germany: A history of psychiatric practice.* Cornell, NY: Cornell University Press.

Engstrom, E. J. (2008). Personal communication, October, 9, 2008.

Flynn, G. Q. (1993). *The draft, 1940–1973.* Lawrence, Kansas: University of Kansas Press.

Goffman, E. (1961). *Asylums: Essays on the social situations of mental patients and other inmates.* Oxford, England: Doubleday.

Gollaher, D. (1995). *Voice for the mad: The life of Dorothea Dix.* New York: Free Press.

Goldman, H. H., & Grob, G. N. (2006). Defining "mental illness" in mental health policy. *Health Affairs, 25,* 737–749.

Grob, G. (1966). *The state and the mentally ill: A history of Worcester State Hospital in Massachusetts.* Chapel Hill, NC: University of North Carolina Press.

Grob, G. N. (1973). *Mental institutions in America: Social policy to 1875.* New York: Free Press.

Grob, G. N. (1983). *Mental illness and American society: 1875–1940.* Princeton, NJ: Princeton University Press.

Grob, G. N. (1991). *From asylum to community: Mental health policy in modern America.* Princeton, NJ: Princeton University Press.

Grob, G. N. (1994a). The history of the asylum revisited: Personal reflections. In M. S. Micale & R. Porter (Eds.), *Discovering the history of psychiatry* (pp. 260–281). New York: Oxford University Press.

Grob, G. N. (1994b). *The mad among us: A history of the care of America's mentally ill.* Cambridge, MA: Harvard University Press.

Grob, G. N. (1998). Psychiatry's holy grail: The search for the mechanisms of mental diseases. *Bulletin of the History of Medicine, 72,* 189–219.

Insel, T. (2007). Neuroscience: Shining light on depression. *Science, 317,* 757–758.

James, W. (1890/1981). *The principles of psychology.* Cambridge, MA: Harvard University Press.

Jones, E., Hyams, K. C., & Wessely, S. (2003). Screening for vulnerability to psychological disorders in the military: An historical survey. *Journal of Medical Screening, 10,* 40–46.

Kessler, R. C., Chiu, W. T., Demler, O., Merikangas, K. R., & Walters, E. E. (2005). Prevalence, severity, and comorbidity of 12-month DSM-IV disorders in the national comorbidity survey replication. *Archives of General Psychiatry, 62,* 617–627.

Kupfer, D. J., First, M., & Regier, D. A. (Eds.). (2002). *A research agenda for DSM-V.* Washington, DC: American Psychiatric Association.

Leiby, J. (1978). *A history of social welfare and social work in the United States, 1815–1972.* New York: Columbia University Press.

Micale, M. S., & Porter, R. (Eds.). (1994). *Discovering the history of psychiatry.* New York: Oxford University Press.

Minogue, K. (1985). *Alien powers: The pure theory of ideology.* London: Palgrave Macmillan.

Ozarin, L. (2006). From N.Y. Lunatic Asylum to New York Hospital's Westchester division. *Psychiatric News, 41,* 29.

Pinel, P. (1962). *A treatise on insanity.* New York: Hafner Publishing Company.

Pols, H. (2006). Waking up to shell shock: Psychiatry in the US military during World War II. *Endeavour, 30,* 144–149.

Pols, H. & Oak, S. (2007). War & military mental health: The US psychiatric response in the 20th century. *American Journal of Public Health, 97,* 2132–2142.

Popper, K. R. (1989). *Conjectures and refutations.* London: Routledge.

Popper, K. R. (1998). *The world of Parmenides: Essays on the pre-Socratic enlightenment.* New York: Routledge.

Porter, R. (1987a). *A social history of madness.* New York: Weidenfeld & Nicolson.

Porter, R. (1987b). *Mind-forg'd manacles: A history of madness in England from the Restoration to the Regency.* Cambridge, MA: Harvard University Press.

Porter, R. (1997). *The greatest benefit to mankind: A medical history of humanity from antiquity to the present.* London: HarperCollins.

Porter, R. (2002). *Madness: A brief history.* New York: Oxford University Press.

Read, J., Mosher, L. R., & Bentall, R. P. (Eds.). (2004). *Models of madness.* New York: Brunner-Routledge.

Rosenberg, C. (2006). Contested boundaries: Psychiatry, disease and diagnosis. *Perspectives in Biology and Medicine, 49*(3), 407-424.

Rosenberg, C. E. (2007). *Our present complaint: American medicine, then and now.* Baltimore: John Hopkins University Press.

Rothman, D. J. (1990). *The discovery of the asylum: Social order and disorder in the new republic.* Boston: Little, Brown.

Rush, B. (1812). *Medical inquiries and observations upon the diseases of the mind.* Philadelphia: Kimber & Richardson.

Scull, A. (1979). *Museums of madness: The social organization of insanity in nineteenth century England.* New York: St. Martin's Press.

Scull, A. (1981). *Madhouses, mad doctors, and madmen.* Philadelphia: University of Pennsylvania Press.

Scull, A. (1981a). A new trade in lunacy: The recommodification of the mental patient. *American Behavioral Scientist, 24,* 741–754.

Scull, A. (1985). Madness and seregative control: The rise of the insane asylum. In P. Brown (Ed.), *Mental health care and social policy* (pp. 17–40). Boston: Routledge & Kegan Paul plc.

Scull, A. (1990). Deinstitutionalization: Cycles of despair. *Journal of Mind and Behavior, 11,* 301–312.

Scull, A. (1993). *The most solitary of afflictions.* New Haven, CT: Yale University Press.

Scull, A. (1995). Psychiatrists and historical "facts" part two: Re-writing the history of asylumdom. *History of Psychiatry, 6,* 387–394.

Scull, A. (2011). *Madness: A very short introduction.* New York: Oxford University Press, Inc.

Shorter, E. (1997). *A history of psychiatry.* New York: John Wiley & Sons Inc.

Shorter, E. (n. d.) *Interview.* Retrieved from http://www.ibiblio.org/pub/electronic-publications/stay-free/archives/21/edward_shorter.html

Shorter, E. (2005). *A historical dictionary of psychiatry.* New York: Oxford University Press, Inc.

Szasz, T. (1961). *The myth of mental illness.* New York: Hoeber.

Szasz, T. (1994). *Cruel compassion: Psychiatric control of society's unwanted.* New York: John Wiley & Sons, Inc.

Szasz, T. (2007). *Coercion as cure: A critical history of psychiatry.* Somerset, NJ: Transactions Publishers.

Turbayne, C. M. (1970). *The myth of metaphor.* Columbia, SC: University of South Carolina Press.

U.S. Department of Health and Human Services. (1999). *Mental Health: A report of the surgeon general.* Rockville, MD: U.S. Department of Health and Human Services, Substance Abuse and Mental Health Services Administration, Center for Mental Health Services, National Institutes of Health, National Institute of Mental Health.

Viets, H. (1935). Some features of the history of medicine in Massachusetts during the colonial period (1620–1770). *Isis, 23,* 389–405.

Whitaker, R. (2002). *Mad in America: Bad science, bad medicine and the enduring mistreatment of the mentally ill.* New York: Perseus Publishing.

Wikipedia: The Free Encyclopedia, s.v. "Conscription in the United States." Retrieved October 25, 2011, from http://en.wikipedia.org/wiki/Conscription_in_the_United_States#World_War_I

Young, A. (1995). *The harmony of illusions: Inventing post-traumatic stress disorder.* Princeton, NJ: Princeton University Press.

3

The "Therapeutic" Coercion of the Mad in the Community

For more than 200 years now the doctrine has been increasingly held that there is such a thing as mental illness, that it is a sickness like any other, and that those who suffer from it should be dealt with medically: they should be treated by doctors, if necessary in a hospital, and not blamed for what has befallen them. This belief has social uses. Were there no such notion, we would probably have to invent it.

Erving Goffman, 1970

To allow every maniac liberty consistent with safety; to proportion the degree of coercion to the . . . extravagance of behavior; . . . that bland art of conciliation, or the tone of irresistible authority pronouncing an irreversible mandate . . . are laws of fundamental importance . . . to the . . . successful management of all lunatic institutions.

Phillippe Pinel, 1806

Introduction

This chapter addresses the community-based management and treatment, by public or state-controlled psychiatric agencies, of those judged to be mad in America. The employment of coercion (force or its threat, not requested or wanted) enabled the emergence of nineteenth-century American asylums with their state-granted legal authority that allowed mad-doctors to incarcerate people involuntarily with considerable discretion and little oversight. Today, the legal grounds for involuntary hospitalization have narrowed to include those who are deemed to be at immediate risk for harm to self or others as a result of a mental illness. Psychiatric coercion, however, has expanded to include coercing people outside hospital walls, in the community. Coercion made the emergence of public psychiatry possible. We argue in this chapter that coercion sustains its existence even today.

We believe it essential to differentiate, on the one hand, state supported involuntary psychiatry (the twenty-first century grandchild of "institutional psychiatry") based on coercion from, on the other hand, contractual or voluntary psychiatry. In the second enterprise, the person seeking help and the psychiatrist or mental health practitioner offering it mutually agree to work together to address the intrapersonal or interpersonal difficulties identified by the help seeker. The relationship, which can be terminated by either person at any time, is based initially on mutual respect or neutrality, and usually involves persuasive discussion with no coercion imposed by the practitioner (to the extent that the practitioner shares what he or she knows about the treatments). This sort of practice occurs more frequently with the "worried well" and those who are more likely to be able to afford to pay for someone to work with them on their life difficulties.

By arguing that coercion sustains the existence of public psychiatry even today, we are not making the point that psychiatrists are more malevolent, mean, sadistic, or less caring than other people. Rather, we are making the simpler point that coercion applied with sufficient force and regularity works—if by working we mean obtaining people's behavioral compliance. Coercion, we argue, has always been an essential method for managing the complexities of human misbehavior. Psychiatry, a profession specializing in managing complex human behaviors, has not only unfailingly chosen to employ coercion in this endeavor, but has unfailingly claimed that coercion was in the best interests of those coerced.

Getting caught by the police for speeding usually results in an immediate penalty of a steep fine on the driver. For most folks this penalty "works," in that at least for a while after receiving the ticket they may not speed or will keep a sharper eye out for the enforcers. They are quite likely to alter their driving behavior to avoid further coercion or punishment. But do drivers learn as a result that speeding is fundamentally wrong and dangerous? We doubt it, if the continuing high rate of traffic citations is any indication (see, for example, Florida, 2010).

Yet few would suggest that what the police do to enforce driving codes is a therapeutic enterprise. No one would mistake this police activity for the treatment of a medical condition called automobile speeding disorder. The job of the police is to detect and punish drivers who breech socially and legally expected behavior: in this case, conformity with the traffic laws that manage potentially lethal activity (driving powerful vehicles). Society expects that punishment will alter the speeder's behavior and reduce accidents. Similarly, psychiatry, the government-certified profession for maintaining "normal" behavioral order, is expected to detect and manage people who manifestly violate intrapersonal and interpersonal norms, codes, or rules. Psychiatry is also authorized to use force to gain the compliance of recalcitrant individuals.

Ultimately, force may be needed to ensure that people conform to the rules of normal life. The question is: Is the psychiatric use of force a scientifically derived therapeutic endeavor and is psychiatric coercion any different from other versions of institutional coercion in society? That is, is it to be considered treatment rather than punishment?

A Brief Overview

We begin this chapter by examining some of the findings of the 1961 report of the *Joint Commission on Mental Illness and Health* (JCMIH), the first federal commission ever created to review society's formal governance of mad Americans and to propose a comprehensive national plan to "provide more humane care for the mentally ill" (p. xxix). We first describe the commission's view of what mental illness is and then discuss briefly its findings on the historical role of force and coercion in the psychiatric treatment of mad Americans. Next, we describe how coercion operates in psychiatry, including its foundational role in the creation of public psychiatry, and review the contemporary literature to describe some of its current manifestations in community treatment. We also attempt (given the scarcity of national data) to estimate the prevalence of coercive practices in current psychiatry in America. We then briefly explore how and why the employment of coercion has become a leading area for academic research, especially regarding its "clinical effectiveness." To frame that discussion, we found it necessary to examine the notion of evidence-based practice (EBP), which has gained immense popularity among mental health authorities and academics over the past decade and which we believe is used to justify the continuation of coercive practices in public psychiatry. We conclude this chapter by examining one of the most promoted and researched EBPs for those diagnosed with serious mental illness, assertive community treatment (ACT), exposing its use of administrative and clinical coercion to produce "successful" outcomes in the treatment of its recipients.

A Commission on a Failed Mission

A Vacuous Definition of Mental Illness

As America moved into the mid-twentieth century, the *Joint Commission on Mental Illness and Health* (JCMIH, 1961) was created under the auspices of the Mental Health Study Act of 1955 to review how mad people were previously managed in the United States. Its findings were expected to "make recommendations for combating mental illness in the United States" (p. v). Led by Jack R. Ewalt, chairman of the Department of Psychiatry at Harvard Medical School, the commissioners included notable mental health authorities like Kenneth Appel, a former president of the American Psychiatric Association; Ernest M. Gruenberg, an expert on the epidemiology and chairman of the Department of Mental Hygiene at the Johns Hopkins School of

Hygiene and Public Health; and Mike Gorman, the executive director of the National Mental Health Committee (JCMIH, 1961). The commission's ultimate advice to the federal government was to fully embrace the medical model of psychiatry and invest in a national mental health program. Although the commission members subscribed to the medical illness model of disordered behavior, they admitted that "[m]ental illness is different from physical illness," being "a disorder with psychological as well as physiological, emotional as well as organic, social as well as individual causes and effects" (p. xviii) that are "so closely intertwined that so far science has been unable to unravel the causes and establish their relative importance" (p. 86).

This mid-twentieth-century effort to define or describe *mental illness* is a perfect example of a panchreston. Dictionary.com (2011) defines *panchreston* as "a proposed explanation intended to address a complex problem by trying to account for all possible contingencies but typically proving to be too broadly conceived and therefore oversimplified to be of any practical use." To claim, as the commission does, that madness is a medical illness and that it occurs as a result of the impact of human physiology, sociology, biology, and psychology or any possible combinations of them (JCMIH, 1961, p. v), is merely making a vacuous statement.

Coercion as the Prime Tool of Public Psychiatric Practice

In contrast to its definition of *mental illness*, the commission's historical research on how the mad were managed displayed no ambiguity whatsoever. It argued that the mad—for centuries, both here and in Europe—have been subjected to "a superstitious and retaliatory approach . . . The instrument of this approach is punishment" (JCMIH, 1961, p. 25). The commission recognized that this was attenuated by periodic efforts to employ less directly coercive approaches (i.e., moral treatment) but which rather quickly were abandoned and replaced by more forceful and outright coercive manipulation and management. An entire section in chapter two of the commission's report, "Punishment as Treatment" (pp. 25–28), is devoted to a discussion of its routine employment. The chapter quotes Benjamin Rush, a signer of the Declaration of Independence, whose visage adorns the official emblem of the American Psychiatric Association: "Terror acts powerfully . . . and should be employed in the cure of madness" (p. 27).

The report traces how the religiously inspired notion that sinful behavior causes disease justified interventions by the medical and occasional lay superintendents running America's nineteenth-century's madhouses. These interventions included "a wide assortment of shock techniques" (JCMIH, 1961, p. 28), such as bleeding to the point of fainting, near drowning, rapid spinning, forced vomiting, and applying an early form of electric shock to the body. The commission members acknowledged that all of these techniques forced on unwilling mad people were based on "fallacious medical rationales"

(p. 28), implying either that some genuine medical rationales could today justify the employment of coercion on the mad, or else, as we shall see in other statements in the report, rejecting the use of any medical rationale for coercion and rejecting coercion tout court. In looking at some justifications for coercion and torture proposed by leading alienists of eighteenth- and nineteenth-century America, it is difficult to tell whether those who employed it did so because they thought it helped to "cure" or because it produced immediate behavior change, or both. Benjamin Rush designed a "tranquilizing" chair that he described as follows in a letter to his son:

> I have contrived a chair and introduced it to our [Pennsylvania] Hospital to assist in curing madness. It binds and confines every part of the body. By keeping the trunk erect, it lessens the impetus of blood toward the brain. By preventing the muscles from acting, it reduces the force and frequency of the pulse, and by the position of the head and feet favors the easy application of cold water or ice to the former and warm water to the latter. Its effects have been truly delightful to me. It acts as a sedative to the tongue and temper as well as to the blood vessels. In 24, 12, six, and in some cases in four hours, the most refractory patients have been composed. I have called it a Tranquilizer. (cited in Scull, 1993, p. 73, footnote no. 104)

Another section of the JCMIH report, "The Tranquilized Hospital," discussed contemporaneous treatments for the mad, namely, some chemical agents which the commission believed had "revolutionized the management of psychotic patients in American mental hospitals" (1961, p. 39). The authors described the effects of these "major tranquilizers" (known as antipsychotics or neuroleptics today): "tranquilizing patients who are hyperactive, unmanageable, excited, highly disturbed, or highly disturbing . . . [with] the most noticeable effect of the drugs . . . [being] to reduce the hospital ward noise level" (p. 39). They did not discuss whether the drugs were ever voluntarily requested or consumed by psychiatric patients. As we note later in this chapter, many of the coercive psychiatric techniques employed today have the principal aim of forcing patients to take their medications, which they abandon in large numbers as soon as they are given the opportunity. For example, a recent, major federally sponsored study on the effectiveness of antipsychotics in the treatment of schizophrenia found that 74 percent of those enrolled quit taking their assigned drug before the study's completion due to the lack of drug efficacy, accompanied by many unpleasant and dangerous adverse effects they experienced (Lieberman et al., 2005, discussed in chapter 6).

The principal purpose of these chemicals was to make highly disturbing individuals "more appealing to all those who must work with [them]" (JCMIH, 1961, p. 53). These chemicals, contrary to current widely held beliefs that they target specific psychotic disorders, suppress the central nervous system activity of anyone—normal or diagnosed—taking them (Healy & Farquhar, 1998). By blunting emotions and dramatically curtailing physical activity, including the disturbing and violent dramatic behavior often attributed to diagnosed psychotics, they are touted as remarkable medical breakthroughs, rather than less conspicuous methods of restraint than were used previously for controlling problematic behavior in the asylum. The JCMIH report acknowledged that many professionals understood the pragmatic purpose of these drugs, having "dubbed them chemical straight jackets" (1961, p. 39). In its enthusiasm for the use of these new drugs, the commission neglected to discuss—given the long history and experience of psychiatry with aversive and shock treatments—what sort of morbidity these chemicals, which rapidly produced stupor and physical immobility, would have in the longer term on their recipients (for a fuller story see Gelman, 1999 and chapters 6 and 7 in the present book).

In sum, the commission's overall review of America's policy toward the mad from colonial times to the mid-twentieth century found that the policy had been to confine the mad in institutions against their will and subject them to various physically and emotionally brutal treatments. The commission went further, proposing that institutional confinement (the systematic employment of coercion) without any other effective means of treatment had "shown beyond question that much of the aggressive, disturbed, suicidal and regressive behavior of the mentally ill . . . is very largely an artificial product of the way of life imposed on them" (JCMIH. 1961, p. 47), and that "[t]o be rejected by one's family, removed by the police, and placed behind locked doors can only be interpreted, sanely, as punishment and imprisonment, rather than hospitalization" (p. 53). The commission's point was unmistakable: America's approach to madness for the previous two hundred years, whether by a physician or by a policeman, relied on the use of coercion.

Psychiatry has carefully used medical rhetoric to reinforce its medical image and justify its coercive authority, without necessarily matching it with humane, effective interventions. This is not merely a feature of our distant past. Assertive community treatment was invented in Madison, Wisconsin, in an institution that began its life in 1860 as the Mendota Asylum for the Insane. Renamed in 1935 as Mendota State Hospital, it emerged in 1974 as Mendota Mental Health Institute. These name changes appear to reflect the changing functions of the institution over 150 years, moving from a place of involuntary custodial "asylum" care to a venue for conducting scientific research and treatment as a "mental health institute." Yet the institution does today exactly what it has always done: manage involuntarily detained mad people. As explained in 2011 on the State of Wisconsin's website, "Mendota's Civil Program provides services to adults who are in need of psychiatric treatment. All admissions are involuntary" (Mendota Mental Health Institute, 2011).

Decommissioning Institutional Care

Regardless of what they were named, insane asylums and their often inhumane practices had by the early decades of the twentieth century drawn a
great deal of negative attention from the media and advocates. This resulted
in the commission's recommendations that state mental hospitals be dramatically deemphasized in a public system of care and that the mad be managed principally in the general community within a system of "integrated
community service[s]" (JCMIH, 1961, p. 289). The community was, after
all, where the mad were always expected to return after being released from
confinement. The recommendation to move the inmates of state hospitals
back to the community for treatment simply confirmed a visible, numerical shift that had slowly begun in 1955 (Scull, 1976). We often hear, and
the commission report suggested, that the shift was due primarily to the
introduction of major tranquilizers. A body of research and analysis since
then, however, has established that this shift was more importantly due to
the imposition of administrative policies "to prevent the accumulation of
long-stay institutionalized patients" (Scull, 1976, p. 178). The beginnings
of this administrative shift could be noted in some hospitals in the United
States as well as in England, especially those which adopted a policy of "early
discharge, or the avoidance of admissions altogether beg[u]n . . . well before
the national swing was noticed in 1955" (p. 178). The initial modest decline
in hospital populations began before psychoactive chemicals were routinely
employed[1]. Gronfein (1985) notes in his analysis of psychotropic drugs
and deinstitutionalization that "discharge rates were increasing before the
advent of the drugs" (p. 448) and further demonstrates that the larger-scale
transfer of patients truly began in the mid-1960s, more than a decade after
the introduction of these drugs (see chapter 7).

The community was assumed to be, albeit with no real scientific evidence
(Grob, 1994, Scull, 1976), a more supportive environment for enhancing the
personal autonomy and freedom of the mad, conditions which it was further
assumed would increase the likelihood of cooperation between mental health
providers and their charges. This hypothesized, enhanced therapeutic alliance,
aided by the use of the newly introduced major tranquilizers, was expected to
reduce the need for institutional coercion while at the same time attenuating
the problematic behaviors of the mad.

According to Scull (1992), the commission report was "[l]argely written by
a specialist in public relations" (p. 568). This would account for its optimistic
tone and its vaguely articulated and surprisingly nonspecific bureaucratic
content. The optimism no doubt reflected attitudes in a country that had
recently been victorious in a world war and was brimming over with enthusiasm and the can-do attitude. America had recently demonstrated its ability
to alleviate the physical human suffering that resulted from war. Following

the carnage and destruction that lay waste to the European continent during World War II, America successfully developed and implemented a European recovery and reconstruction strategy, the Marshall Plan. So it was not a great stretch, when turning to address another troubling area of human conduct arising at home, madness, that a new, concerted effort was expected to yield rapid success through energetic central organizing and planning by the federal bureaucracy. For a variety of reasons, however, detailed by Grob (1991), the commission's plan failed to be "a precise blueprint that could serve as the basis for legislative action" (p. 209). Ultimately, it lost some of its credibility among powerful government bureaucrats: it was considered, for example, by the NIMH's Philip Sapir, chief of that agency's Research and Fellowship Branch, to be "pedestrian, platitudinous, rehashes of previous statements ... so incredibly bad that there seems almost no point in making specific criticisms" (quoted in Grob, 1991, p. 217). Nonetheless, in some roundabout way, several basic proposals in the report did find their way into federal mental health policy.

Some ten months after its publication, a special Governors' Conference of Mental Health endorsed its general findings and stated "that Federal, State, and local governments as well as private and voluntary efforts must be combined to achieve the goals we seek" (Connery, 1968, p. 46). This endorsement added impetus to President Kennedy's appointing a cabinet-level committee on these issues, which then "developed proposals for action which accepted most of the Joint Commission's findings and many of its recommendations, including its urgent pleas for extensive federal participation in combating mental illness" (p. 47). The Joint Commission findings were echoed by President Kennedy in his "Message on Mental Illness and Mental Retardation" to the US Congress in 1963, recommending a brand-new, community-focused approach to the problem which, as he stated, was "designed in large measure, to use Federal resources to stimulate State, local, and private action" (p. 48). We've cited the remarks from President Kennedy and the Governors' Conference on Mental Health to illustrate, not their particular concern with coercion, but the redirecting of federal financing efforts toward new social goals identified under the "mental health" rubric.

Despite President Kennedy's congressional message and the subsequent congressional activity (discussed in chapter 2), the grim psychiatric reality was that by the mid-1960s the mad, who were previously managed through total institutions and involuntary confinement, were now being discharged to mostly unwelcoming rather than accepting communities whose "residents ... fought hard to ensure that ... patients ... released ... are not released into *their* neighborhoods" (Scull, 1976, p. 197). This new wave of hospital discharges was due principally to changing patterns of funding for state mental hospitals and the rising hope about the psychotropic drugs (Gronfein, 1985) induced in decision-makers and others. This posed a number of professional problems for psychiatry and the mental health professions.

First, the publicly dependent mad constituted a heterogeneous mix of individuals (e.g., elderly, senile, physically disabled, abandoned, destitute, deviant) confined together mostly to keep them from disturbing others and also to remove them from the public's consciousness (out of sight, out of mind). But the aggregation of such different individuals and their different problems under the presumption that they were all suffering from medically treatable illnesses was not supported by the research conducted in or outside institutions (Scull, 1976).

Second, there was no indication that those discharged from the state institutions would voluntarily seek psychiatric help, and yet state legislatures, beginning in the late 1960s, were tightening criteria for involuntary institutionalization. Third, short of chemical sedation for subduing and managing agitated behavior (Davis, 1965), no effective treatments existed to bring people to conform or act normally. In addition, the drugs had a host of debilitating effects (Crane, 1973). And, finally, the psychiatrists actively promoted the belief that they had a handle on the "medical" problem of madness and that the public mental health system could be responsible for helping the former asylum inmates to be better off in the community.

In short, psychiatry had to devise a community-based approach of managing their mad patients that appeared to be medical, noncoercive, humane, and effective. It did this in part by creating a new pseudo-medical rubric for the mad—the severely mentally ill (SMI)—and concocting new forms of coercion usable in the new settings.

The Role of Coercion in Institutional Psychiatry

The profession of psychiatry or mad-doctoring emerged in the eighteenth century in parallel with the decision to construct a few specialized buildings especially for the mad in order to confine and manage them involuntarily. (The first involuntary admission in America occurred in the City of Brotherly Love, Philadelphia, in 1752 [Anfang & Appelbaum, 2006].) This fortuitous development allowed for "unparalleled scrutiny of lunatics under controlled conditions, particularly while interacting with keepers, [to form] the matrix for the practical (experimental) discipline of managing the mad" (Porter, 1987b, pp. 174–175). Many of these keepers turned out to be medical men looking for stable employment. This early, loosely organized, fledgling economic enterprise for managing the mad had been institutionalized by the middle of the nineteenth century (see Rothman, 1990, chapter 5), with mad folk "incarcerated in a specialized, bureaucratically organized, state-supported asylum system which isolated them both physically and symbolically from the larger society . . . [a]nd . . . now recognized [madness] as one of the major varieties of deviance . . . a uniquely and essentially medical problem" (Scull, 1993 pp. 1–2). This state-sanctioned confinement gave free reign to mad doctors to experiment on their charges and claim

that these approaches were prima facie scientific medical techniques to control the behaviors of this group and, coincidentally, confirm the doctors'
authority. These assertions gave credence to psychiatrists' claim to be doing
effective medical treatment when actually they were constructing a "new
apparatus for the social control of the mad" (Scull, 1993, p. 3).

The singular authority granted to psychiatry to imprison mad individuals
for treatment in specialized facilities, whether called asylums, mental hospitals, or community-based mental health clinics, is the key to its professional
importance. The undisputed historical fact of psychiatry's authority to employ
coercion, however, has not been adequately recognized for what it has meant
for mental health practice: police authority makes truly voluntary psychiatric
treatment in the current public mental health field a near-impossibility.[2] All
the relevant "stakeholders" (the mad, their families, their friends, the psychiatrists that treat them, and society at large) are on notice that involuntary commitment and the use of force are ready to be deployed on any diagnosed mad
person refusing to follow prescribed psychiatric treatment. That knowledge
shapes the behavior of all the parties to the psychiatric encounter as surely
as the knowledge that one's parent regularly but inconsistently uses physical
punishment shapes the behavior of a child. The uncertainty of not knowing
when punishment will be employed makes compliance by the victim more
likely. So voluntary medical treatment, in the sense that most people think
of it when they consult their physician for a physical health problem, is less
likely to occur in public psychiatric practice.

Those who can afford medical care or purchase health insurance go to
their personal physician by choice, whether for an annual checkup or over
a concern about some possible ailment. Regardless of the doctor's recommendation, they can choose to follow it entirely, partly, or reject it all together
because the power imbalance between a medical patient and the doctor is
only marginally in favor of the doctor. It is based on the doctor's presumed
better informed opinion about the problem, attributed to her because of her
specialized education, training, and experience—the particular reasons a
patient would seek a physician's advice in the first place. But once informed
about his medical condition and having received advice or even exhortation
from the physician, the patient retains full control over his course of action
from that moment onward. This is true even if the health problem diagnosed
by the doctor, if left untreated, will lead to death shortly. (Our physicians
cannot force us to take statins for our coronary heart disease or involuntarily
inject insulin into our bodies to control our runaway diabetes.)

In contrast, if the diagnosed mad person resists "emergency" psychiatric
treatment (in which the person is deemed to be at risk for harm to self
or others), she knows that she can be rapidly involuntarily hospitalized
in a locked facility and treated against her active protests and physical
resistance. This knowledge colors and shapes all engagements between

mental health patients and mental health professionals. No true voluntary treatment can ever occur, because no mad person can freely walk away from the recommended treatment if there is a serious disagreement between the psychiatric professional and that patient. It is true that the problematic behavior of the patient must be judged to place the patient or others at risk for harm in order to involuntarily commit and treat, but only if this behavior is *judged to result from a mental illness* (e.g., Evel Knievel's undoubtedly dangerous, death-defying motorized leaps never earned him the unwanted attention of psychiatrists). Since this judgment is a "clinical decision" (a statutorily authorized personal judgment of the professional), this is not a difficult standard to meet. In involuntary psychiatric treatment, psychiatric decisions and legal power intertwine to become virtually indistinguishable.

Psychiatric Coercion in Contemporary America

Madness Counts

In 1961, when the JCMIH published its report, 527,500 people were inmates in state and county mental hospitals in the United States (Scull, 1976, p. 176), and fewer than one million people in total were diagnosed mental patients using services in community mental health clinics and state and county mental hospitals (Grob, 1994, p. 248). Today, the NIMH (2011) declares that "[m]ental disorders are common in the United States . . . An estimated 26.2 percent of Americans ages 18 and older . . . suffer from a diagnosable mental disorder in a given year . . . this figure translates to 57.7 million people." The NIMH further specifies that about 6 percent of those individuals are diagnosable with a major mental illness (3.5 million people). Assuming that these figures are accurate, and considering that we have almost doubled our population since 1961 to about 310 million in 2010, we are left to contemplate the meaning of having 3.5 million adult American citizens—equivalent to the population of the State of Connecticut—diagnosed as having a "major mental illness" or being "seriously mentally ill" (SMI)[3], terms used interchangeably in the academic literature.

Financing Madness

This amazing epidemiological uptick in psychiatric diagnoses (problems regarding the validity of psychiatric diagnoses are addressed in chapters 4 and 5), especially the functional diagnosis of SMI, has occurred despite the huge increase in the number of mental health professionals, treatment centers, and funds devoted to preventing or treating mental illness. In 2010 the NIMH budget was $1.5 billion, most of it earmarked for research on SMIs and their treatments. Almost a third of the funding, about $400 million, was spent on brain and basic behavioral research (NIMH, 2011), designed to verify NIMH's institutional assumption that mental illnesses are brain diseases. The federal government has increased its funding for NIMH (2011) from $288 million in 1986 to $1.5 billion in 2010, making that agency the seventh highest funded of the twenty-seven institutes and centers that comprise the National Institutes of Health (NIH).

To estimate the total spent by both private and public funding sources annually on behavioral research and services, we use the data from 2005 (the latest comprehensive national figures available for mental health service expenditures). NIMH research funding that year was approximately $1.4 billion (NIMH, 2011), while the total national private and public expenditures for mental health services totaled roughly $113 billion—about 60 percent of it coming from tax revenues (Garfield, 2011). The huge increase in mental disorder diagnoses in the last few decades suggests that we have failed to effectively treat the problem despite the substantial dollars spent annually on research and services to develop effective treatments. NIMH director Thomas Insel proclaimed to an audience of researchers attending the 2006 NIMH Alliance for Research Progress meeting that "[w]e know a lot about evidence-based treatments" (NIMH, 2006, p. 1). If this is true, what actually is being done with the mad may be surprising.

The Numbers of Mad Coerced

In Hospitals. The threat of involuntary hospitalization and the use of coercion is no idle one. Given how the American tradition and political system conceive of the loss of liberty, one might expect such loss under any state-sanctioned circumstances to be meticulously documented, as it is in connection with criminal arrests and incarcerations. Nonetheless, there currently exist no national data regarding involuntary hospitalization or even unduplicated counts of the number of individuals hospitalized psychiatrically in a single year. Thus, one is forced to rely on extrapolations from state and local data for any such estimates. In an earlier publication (Gomory et al., 2011), based on the data released by two large states (California and Florida), we conservatively estimated that around 1.37 million American adults are the subjects of involuntary hospitalization each year. This number makes up about 62 percent of those hospitalized for any psychiatric reason but does not include the unknown proportion of those deemed to be "voluntarily" hospitalized but who are aware that they might or will be forced into hospitalization if they do not submit (Sorgaard, 2007). Our own guess is that the large majority of psychiatric hospitalizations, perhaps all, are involuntary.

In Prisons. Another group of involuntarily confined mad people are those currently confined in US jails. The data are not based on actual national counts, since no such comprehensive data exist and must be estimated from studies conducted on subsamples of this population. Recent research (Steadman, Osher, Robbins et al., 2009) suggests that the average prevalence of serious mental illness among the approximately 2.1 million people incarcerated in US jails, prisons, and penitentiaries is 14.5 percent for men and 31.0 percent for women. Conservatively, these percentages convert to roughly 330,000 mad people confined in our penal institutions as a result of having been found guilty of criminal offenses.

In the Community. New developments in the application of force and coercion on the mad have emerged from the community, where the mad mostly live and are treated today. Not surprisingly, here too no national prevalence data exist, but again, by reviewing some of the most recent studies on community-specific psychiatric coercion, one can make educated guesses. One study conducted in five US cities (Swartz, Swanson, Kim et al., 2006) found that 44 to 59 percent of the sampled individuals reported having been subjected to at least one of four coercive measures (the researchers call them "tools," p. 38) while in outpatient community treatment.

In Toto. Using the above information, our tentative, evidence-informed guess is that at least 50 percent of the mad in the above three settings are the regular recipients of at least one form of psychiatric coercion. We can put numbers to this percentage by using the latest data available from the federal government on "patient care episodes" (the odd name the federal government uses for the count of the total number of persons under psychiatric care[4] in any one year in the United States). We find that there were 9.5 million patient care episodes in 2002 (Manderscheid, & Berry, 2006, p. 209), translating at a minimum to 3 to 4 millions of our mad citizens subjected to coercion in the name of mental health in any single year.

"Tools" of Community Coercion

Community-based mechanisms of coercion are deployed by the judicial and the public welfare systems—the two major institutions outside the mental health system in which the mad are located (Monahan, 2008). The judicial system employs several coercive civil mechanisms on noncriminal mad persons to keep them out of hospitals and force them into community treatment, by far the cheaper option (Swartz, Swanson, Kim et al., 2006). The most well-known of these is court-ordered outpatient commitment, and it usually comes in three forms: first, conditional release from involuntary hospitalization if the person is willing to submit to mandated community treatment; second, as a substitute for involuntary hospitalization for those meeting commitment criteria; and third, as a form of preventive detention for those who are not legally committable but are considered to be "at risk."

Mad individuals who are adjudicated of a minor or nonviolent crime are further subjected to mental health courts, such as so-called "drug courts." These courts use judges' recently expanded extralegal role to force some mad criminals into psychiatric treatment by "play[ing] a hands-on, therapeutically oriented, and directive role at the center of the treatment process"

(Monahan, Bonnie, Appelbaum et al., 2001, p. 1200). The research indicates that such courts appear to have at best a moderate effect in reducing criminal recidivism among those who complete their programs (a high dropout rate is common). However, because the participants are often selected by judges "based on personal knowledge of an individual's history" as those "most likely to succeed," even this outcome is not generalizable (Sarteschi, Vaughn, & Kim, 2011, p. 14).

The social welfare system uses two prominent coercive measures to gain behavioral compliance. One is by controlling any funds to which the mad may be entitled. This is done by appointing for recalcitrant individuals payees, who control the patient's access to public disability benefits, predicated on the patient's level of cooperation with psychiatric treatment. The second measure is by providing access to subsidized housing only to those who comply with treatment, an effective mechanism of subjugation because most of the public mental health patients cannot afford to pay fair market rents from their monthly disability checks. These coercive tactics are today ordinarily called "leverage" by academics (Monahan, Redlich, Swanson et al., 2005). John Monahan, the dean of psychiatric coercion scholars, goes as far as to argue "that framing the legal debate on mandatory community treatment primarily in terms of coercion has become counter productive . . . [and it is] unhelpful and [a] misleading assumption that all types of leverage necessarily amount to coercion" (2008, p. 284). Apparently he forgets that "mandated community treatment" means, if it means anything, treatment not voluntarily sought but forced on the patient. The scientific work of some eminent scholars of coercion might be summed up in one phrase: Coercion by any other name is not coercion.

To illustrate how reputable researchers and mental health professionals can come to such judgments, we devote the next section to examining some of the purportedly scientific bases for the acceptance and dissemination of coercive practical interventions designed to change the behavior of mad people who reside in the community. This involves looking first at the evidence-based practice movement and its progenitor, evidence-based medicine.

The Limits of Evidence-Based Medicine

The relatively recent phenomena of evidence based practices (EBPs) proliferating currently in all of the helping professions are derived from the dramatic growth and legitimation of their parent movement, evidence-based medicine (EBM). The latter emerged during the 1990s when its advocates promoted it as a "new paradigm" for selecting the best options among available medical treatments (Haynes, 2002) and governments saw in it a method to control expenditures on medical care. Looking at the Medline bibliographic database shows that prior to 1990, zero publications were indexed with the terms *evidence-based medicine, evidence-based treatment,* or their abbreviations. For the 2000–2005 period, however, 13,989 hits for EBM and 1,331 hits for EBP or EBT were recorded (Flaum, 2007). These data indicate the suddenly increased popularity of this new terminology among academics and clinicians. The terminology is new, but EBM methodology is not.[5]

EBM is defined by its developers as:

> [T]he conscientious, explicit and judicious use of current best evidence in making decisions about the care of individual patients. The practice of evidence based medicine means integrating individual clinical expertise with the best available external clinical evidence from systematic research. By individual clinical expertise we mean the proficiency and judgment that individual clinicians acquire through clinical experience and clinical practice. Increased expertise is reflected in many ways, but especially in more effective and efficient diagnosis and in the more thoughtful identification and compassionate use of individual patients' predicaments, rights, and preferences in making clinical decisions about their care. By best available external clinical evidence we mean clinically relevant research, often from the basic sciences of medicine, but especially from patient centered clinical research into the accuracy and precision of diagnostic tests (including the clinical examination), the power of prognostic markers, and the efficacy and safety of therapeutic, rehabilitative, and preventive regimens. (Sackett, Rosenberg, Gray, Haynes, & Richardson, 1996, pp. 71–72)

It is extremely difficult to resist the allure of a protocol that proposes (1) combining the best objectively derived evidence of treatment effectiveness, with (2) the application of caring and sensitive clinical expertise of individual clinicians, to (3) choose those specific treatments that mesh with particular patients' "predicaments, rights and preferences" while simultaneously (4) ameliorating specific patient illnesses. Perhaps the popularity of the EBM idea is due to this seductive linguistic combination of all that scientific medicine aims to accomplish as a healing enterprise and for suggesting that such a utopian research program is actualizable. Clinical epidemiologist Alvan Feinstein and a colleague warned about EBM in 1997: "[h]ardly anyone can disagree with the goal of getting clinicians to make 'conscientious, explicit, and judicious use of current best evidence' for decisions in patient care" (p. 529). The devil is in the details.

Despite its popularity, EBM has come under serious criticism. Here are the most problematic issues. First, the randomized controlled trial (RCT) that EBM identifies as the gold standard for determining effective outcomes uses *group aggregated averages* in the data analysis and cannot as a result provide useful information on how to select an effective treatment for any particular individual, the goal of all clinical practice. Alvan Feinstein, credited by EBM developer and epidemiologist David Sackett (2002) with putting clinical epidemiology on the scientific map, notes that "randomized trials were not intended to answer questions about the treatment of individual patients" (Feinstein & Horwitz, 1997, p. 532).

Second, in order for RCTs to be used validly, the sample of patients must be a random sample selected from a population, all having the same underlying disease. This proves well nigh impossible in psychiatric samples (as we will discuss in the next two chapters) since psychiatric diagnoses are neither reliable (Kirk & Kutchins, 1992) nor valid (Boyle, 2002), and therefore cannot be used as a method to identify a sample of people with the same mental disorder (Wolf, 2000, p. 101). As the *DSM* states, "In the DSM-IV there is no assumption that each category of mental disorder is a . . . discrete entity . . . dividing it from other mental disorders or from no mental disorder. . . . [T]herefore . . . individuals sharing a diagnosis are likely to be heterogeneous even in regard to the defining features of the diagnosis" (APA, 2000, p. xxxi). We understand that our assertion of unreliability and invalidity may strike some readers as unduly harsh, yet even prominent *DSM* architects acknowledge it, as we discuss in chapters 4 and 5.

Third, although RCTs may be useful in deciding if an active drug is better than a placebo (i.e., a nonactive pill or process also known to influence the outcome being researched) to treat, say, an infection, they may not be the best way to evaluate the effectiveness of socially complex bundles of services usually provided by public social welfare and mental health systems. These services include various components, such as case management, psychiatric medication monitoring, cognitive-behavioral treatment, employment training, activities in daily living, and budgeting classes. Depending on a particular agency's philosophy and funding requirements, each service package and each component therein may be organized and implemented differently across agencies, and even within a single agency. The resulting "lack of precision makes it difficult to model the causal pathways of interventions, which is central to the RCT model" (Wolf, 2000, p. 101). To further complicate the portrait: if attempts are made to test the various components' separate effects on the patients, that is, to *unbundle* bundled services, the strong possibility exists that some important elements of the *bundled* intervention will be overlooked because they are hard to measure or so idiosyncratic that they cannot be standardized and transferred uniformly to another setting. For example, it may be that the most "highly effective aspects of the intervention are those unmeasured aspects that are associated with highly stylized characteristics of the staff, say their interactional style or level of motivation" (p. 101).

Fourth, comprehensive evaluations of treatment outcomes from multiple studies carried out by combining data from all the studies have their own limitations. Such systematic pooling of study results, known as a meta-analysis, has come to be seen in EBM as the gold standard for deciding on an intervention's effectiveness. Meta-analyses now number in the thousands in the psychiatric outcome literature alone. Yet the limitations of meta-analyses need closer scrutiny. One such limitation is that meta-analyses often take the information given in individual RCT studies as factually accurate. As many scholars have pointed out, those who conduct meta-analyses do not necessarily assess independently how well each individual RCT was implemented or evaluate the impact of potentially bad implementations on the quality of the data gathered (Bailar, 1995; Feinstein 1995; Feinstein & Horwitz, 1997; Oakes, 1986; Rothman, Greenland, & Lash, 2008, p. 682; Williams & Garner, 2002). In addition, no meta-analysis considers the impact of the administrative organization of an intervention program and its rules and regulations on the success of the intervention. As we argue later for ACT, these rules and regulations, not its hypothesized clinical[6] interventions (the foci of analysis for such systematic reviews), are often responsible for reported successes. The American statisticians Richard Berk and David A. Freedman go further and advise:

> [W]ith respect to meta-analysis, our recommendation is simple: just say no. The suggested alternate is equally simple: read the papers, think about them, and summarize them. Try our alternative. Trust us: you will like it. And if you can't sort the papers into meaningful categories, neither can the meta-analysts. (2001, p. 21)

In fact, an editorial in January 2012 in the *BMJ* (formerly known as the *British Medical Journal*, and perhaps the staunchest proponent of EBM in the world) introducing a series of articles on missing clinical data and their impact on the methodology of EBM, noted the flaws of quantitative findings in systematic reviews of clinical trials:

> These articles confirm . . . that a large proportion of evidence from human trials is unreported, and much of what is reported is done so inadequately. . . . What is clear from the linked studies is that past failures to ensure proper regulation and registration of clinical trials, and a current culture of haphazard publication and incomplete data disclosure, make the proper analysis of the harms and benefits of common interventions almost impossible for systematic reviewers. (Lehman & Loder, 2012)

A fifth issue regards what kind of evidence is best for determining if the treatment is effective. Should we rely strictly on statistical analyses of numerical data as EBM advocates urge, or should we more broadly incorporate other systematically reviewed empirical evidence currently disallowed under EBM?

Some doctors argue that "the general priority given to empirical evidence derived from clinical research is not epistemologically tenable" (Tonelli, 2006, p. 248) but should only be considered as one source along with others. These other sources could be evidence obtained from well-conducted observational and naturalistic studies, gathering of individual case studies into a searchable database (sometimes referred to as experience-based evidence), studies on human and animal physiology, as well as evaluations of patient goals, values, and specific features of the delivery system relevant to practice (Tanenbaum, 2006; Tonelli, 2006). Even if expanded sources of evidence were considered, how should different forms of evidence be weighed and in what order in distinguishing better from worse interventions? These methodological conundrums may have no resolution since each form of evidence may derive from different and irreconcilable theoretical perspectives.

Sixth, the part of the EBM definition urging the need to consider clinical judgment (i.e., the subjective calculation of the helping professional regarding the problem), as well as the patient's personal wishes when choosing the proper EBM treatment, greatly appeals to common sense. EBM proponents, however, have consistently admitted that they have not a clue as to how to incorporate these two subjective elements into the protocol of EBM (Cohen, Stavri, & Hersh, 2004, Haynes, 2002). Without a procedure for selecting, organizing, and integrating the best research evidence, best clinical judgment, and patients' preferences, the EBM approach for choosing an effective treatment for a given individual presenting with a given illness is no more "scientific" than the approach used by ethical clinicians in the past. These clinicians carefully weighed the best information available to them from multiple sources in order to choose the best care based on their education, training, experience, and positive therapeutic alliance with their patients (Feinstein & Horwitz, 1997). Feinstein and Horwitz note that "most good clinicians have regularly assembled evidence when they reviewed their own experience, developed clinical judgment, read the medical literature, attended medical meetings, and had discussions with one another. This activity seems entirely compatible with the . . . practice of EBM" (1997, p. 529).

A seventh crucial issue is that deciding what constitutes EBM requires experts "certified" as authorities in the subject. Such an EBM certification must be done by authorities who themselves were certified in such expertise by prior certified authorities, and so on. So, rather than dramatically reducing or eliminating arbitrary or authority-based individual medical decision making or substituting an objective for a subjective decision-making process in choosing best practices as some have argued (Gambrill, 1999), EBM has turned out to represent merely another form of expertly justified *authority*. The subjective judgment of individual clinicians now becomes the subjective judgment of the authorized EBM evaluators[7] who are expected to come to consensus regarding which studies meet the consensus protocol for systematically evaluating RCTs (see especially, Fenstein & Horwitz, 1997; Gupta, 2003), leading to a new "orthodoxy" promoted now as scientifically objective (Williams & Garner, 2002). To illustrate this reliance on inside experts, examine how the authors of one of these "rigorous" systematic reviews (in this case, of intensive case management), explain their approach:

> The authors of this review do include an active pioneer of develop-
> ing and implementing the experimental intervention model across
> the scientific community and clinical world [Dr. Marshall] and one
> included study is his (Marshall-UK). As a team we have tried to
> ensure that decisions are made by rational consensus and not to
> have an expert in the team would have been an inadvisable omis-
> sion. In some cases protocol rules were not clear enough and need
> for subsequent clarification arose and post hoc decisions had to be
> taken. (Dieterich, Irving, Park & Marshall, 2011, p. 50)

They appear to rely on "expert" authority and group consensus in their meta-analysis, precisely the sort of contamination by authority figures that EBM was supposed to combat.

Finally, and perhaps most problematically, the effectiveness of EBM itself has never been tested according to its own principles. Do clinicians who prac-tice EBM achieve better outcomes then those who do not? Nobody knows. That question has never been put to an EBM-favored test, for example, by conducting a controlled trial of evidence-based-medicine–trained clinicians versus those not trained to assess an ability to select and implement effective treatment to help their patients. Thus, the optimistic claims of EBM effec-tiveness are not themselves evidence-based (Cohen, Stavri & Hersh, 2004). The whole EBM project is untested, even though it has been promoted and marketed for over twenty years. Such uncertainty regarding the validity of EBM would suggest caution in marketing its wholesale adoption. Unfortu-nately, there is little doubt that it has been heavily marketed with resounding success, judging from its adoption as an organizing, pedagogical, and practice principle in Western medicine and the helping professions.

These criticisms have not gone unnoticed, and recent warnings have come directly from some EBM developers. Haynes (2002) wrote that "accelerating the transfer of [EBM] research findings into clinical practice is often based on incomplete evidence from selected groups of people, who experience marginal benefits . . . raising questions of the generalizability of the findings" (p. 1) and that at best it should be "an adjunct to healthcare decisions" (p. 6). The EBM developers have also concluded that "EBM has long since evolved beyond its initial (mis)conception that EBM might replace traditional medicine. EBM is now [instead] *attempting* to augment rather than replace individual clini-cal experience" (p. 1, emphasis added). This is a more modest stance by the EBM creators, demoting it to an "adjunct" role in medical decision making, and a withdrawal from their original claims that EBM represents "[a] NEW paradigm for medical practice" (The Evidence-Based Medicine Working Group, 1992, p. 2420). Nevertheless, other helping professions continue to view EBM as a research and training panacea.

Evidence-Based Practice in Mental Health

EBM and its methodology is now the "best practice" approach used in the broad field of mental health, albeit under a slightly altered name, evidence-based practice (EBP). American researchers working with the SMI explain:

> Over the past two decades, we have witnessed amazing strides in the development of effective service models for people with SMI . . . in 1998 . . . a national consensus panel identified six practices . . . attaining the status of EBP.

> . . . EBP in mental health is part of a larger evidence-based medicine movement which quickly has become a dominating influence in medicine . . . Following the model of evidence-based medicine, EBPs are founded on the meta-principles of (1) using the best available evidence, (2) individualization, (3) incorporating patients' preferences and (4) expanding clinical expertise. (Bond, Salyers, Rollins, Rapp, & Zipple, 2004, pp. 576–577)

Relying on the professionals' and perhaps the general public's resonance to the simplicity and seductiveness of the idea of EBM, implementations of evidence-based mental health practices for the SMI have been moving full steam ahead, its promoters ignoring the deep questions raised concerning the construct and the application of EBM.

The supporters of evidence-based medicine have developed a sophisticated research infrastructure, including prominently the Cochrane Collaboration. This enterprise uses volunteer medical professionals and academics who constitute work groups, conducting systematic rankings and reviews of the numerous randomized controlled trials of treatments available for many physiological problems, some psychiatric problems, and more general behavioral issues, such as the effectiveness of smoking-cessation programs. These systematic reviews, used to determine which treatments should be designated as evidence-based, are stored in Cochrane's researchable electronic database available by paid subscription and in virtually all medical libraries. The evidence base for mental health interventions that is subjected to these procedures is far more limited and generally lacks the kind of consistent methodological scrutiny that physiological medical interventions have usually undergone (Drake at al., 2001).

A further fundamental difference characterizes how EBM and mental health EBP determine their recommended interventions. EBPs, specifically the ones receiving support from American psychiatric science's key politi-cal patron, the NIMH, are selected through expert *consensus* rather than by formal protocols as recommended by EBM: "[strict] rules for designating a practice as an EBP . . . were not imposed in the Implementing EBPs Project; rather panels of research scientists were asked to review controlled studies" (Mueser et al., 2003, p. 389). Perhaps to minimize the reaction to such a major alteration of EBM protocol, the participating researchers promised to disclose their method of arriving at consensus, along with their findings, by publishing them during 2001 in one of the leading mental health journals, *Psychiatric Services* (Mueser et al., 2003, p. 389). In reviewing that journal, we could find no such content regarding what is probably the highest-profile community intervention EBP for the severely mentally ill: assertive community treatment.

Usually, in reaching consensus, a group, regardless of its purpose or membership, must get all members to agree to one expressed, or explicit, understanding. This is not a scientific but rather a social and political pro-cess. Unless explicit procedural and methodological criteria of the process are agreed to before starting, consensus reaching is arbitrary and may be captured by those in the group who are most persuasive rhetorically rather than scientifically. How the expert consensus agreement for the EBPs was reached is not described in the published literature, but it is noteworthy that this process was carried out with the sanction of NIMH under the auspices of the Robert Wood Johnson Foundation (Mueser et al. 2003, p. 388), funded by the family fortune derived from Johnson & Johnson, the eighth largest pharmaceutical company in the world (five former executives of which sit on the foundation's board of trustees as of this writing).

Since the identification of EBPs is meant to reduce clinicians' uncertainty in choosing effective treatments, the certification of treatments as EBPs by a consensus vote of approved experts should be based on consistently demon-strated success of the intervention. If, however, the evidence used to make the certification is weak, faulty, or ambiguous, then the certification can have the unintended consequence of institutionalizing coercive, ineffective, or even harmful treatments with almost no possibility of reversing those decisions. Statistician Kenneth J. Rothman observes:

> Many of the commonly used modes of causal inference are fallacious . . . one such method of inference, the method of "consensus," has been embraced, presumably for political reasons, by the National Institutes of Health. . . . The National Institutes of Health regularly convenes Consensus Development Conferences to address specific questions and draw inferences. . . . Were consensus a correct basis for inference, then a once flat earth must have become spherical . . . Consensus itself requires no further justification, and may be based on shared beliefs that are irrational. (Rothman, 1988, p. 6)

This difficulty is illustrated by the fact that among the consensus, some certified mental health EBPs are considered more valid than others: "[A] mong EBPs identified by the RWJ conference . . . three practices (supported employment, ACT [Assertive Community Treatment], and family psychoeducation) have strong and convincing evidence for effectiveness whereas the evidence is weaker for the remaining three" (Bond et al., 2004, p. 580). Unfortunately, whether based on strong or weaker evidence, once an intervention is labeled an EBP, its authority has immeasurably increased and rarely if ever will it be reevaluated.

The distortion of the original EBM approach in American mental health practice can be seen by the rhetorical turn taken in two articles published five years apart with the same lead author, psychologist Gary Bond, a leading replicator/evaluator/promoter of assertive community treatment. As we have earlier noted, Bond et al. stated in 2004 that mental health EBPs were founded explicitly on the EBM process and its key "meta-principles of (1) using the best available evidence, (2) individualization, (3) incorporating patients' preferences and (4) expanding clinical expertise" (Bond, Salyers, Rollins, Rapp, & Zipple, 2004, pp. 576–577). In 2009, however, Bond and his colleagues declared that those explicit principles were unnecessary for mental health EBPs:

> *Evidence-based medicine* sometimes refers to a process—the judicious use of the best scientific evidence, combined with clinical expertise and consumer preferences in making decisions in health care . . . The term EBP, has been used similarly in the mental health field . . . The term EBPs also refers to specific evidence-based (or empirically supported) interventions . . . (usually randomized controlled trials). Thus the acronym, EBP, is used throughout this article to refer to *specific interventions* and not to the *process* of clinical decision making. (Bond, Drake, McHugo et al., 2009, pp. 569–570)

Providing two distinct and independent definitions of EBP in mental health—one as a specific intervention to be used preferentially because it has been deemed to be effective and the other definition as a process of clinical decision making identical to the definition of EBM—allows Bond and his colleagues to change the scientific rules of the game for mental health EBPs. Talking about mental health EBPs in the first sense as "effective" interventions gives the impression that they are identical to EBPs identified for physiological medical problems through the EBM protocol (using systematic reviews) and have the same scientific credibility as the EBM-identified interventions (weak though they may be to informed observers). But the reality is that these mental health EBPs are not identified through the same procedures (systematic reviews of RCTs, but instead through expert consensus) and cannot be considered as analogs to EBM-derived treatments.

The various problems regarding mental health EBP that we have discussed here have not been adequately addressed or solved by the EBP experts. These experts are well aware of most of the problems, an awareness that prompted at least one meeting to gather and summarize the concerns regarding EBPs "voiced by members of diverse stakeholder groups; consumers, family members, policy makers, administrators and researchers" (Essock et al., 2003, p. 920). The resultant report was authored by fourteen of the self-styled leaders of the EBP mental health movement who magnanimously state that they in "the spirit of science being transparent and welcoming a public discussion . . . offer this collection of concerns [regarding EBPs] . . . hop[ing] that these summaries will be useful to others" (p. 921).

Their report is a confirmation that the criticisms we have raised are shared by many who are affected by EBPs. But this sort of mea culpa exercise seems to be geared for public relations more than anything else, since, after admitting that many problems exist with EBPs, the authors do not suggest revisiting the procedures and methods used to name EBPs or reevaluate their selections. Instead, they praise their original choices, saying that the "National Evidence-Based Practice Project study groups identified six EBPs for community mental health treatment of persons with severe mental illness . . . [which] provide a strong foundation for defining minimal services for people with severe mental disorders" (p. 932). Further, they insist that these EBPs are characterized by "sensitivity to individual differences, by attention to choices and preferences, by client centeredness, by empowerment, by diversity of methods, and by reliance on clinical skills and judgment" (p. 937). *Evidence-based practice* apparently means "trust us."

Assertive Community Treatment: Psychiatric Coercion as EBP

Earlier in this chapter we traced the relentless use of coercion to control the mad in America for four centuries, with each iteration marketed, not as the use of force to manage a disobedient and troubling group, but rather as the application of better and more progressive treatments to aid a group suffering from a serious medical condition. These treatments are presented as having been developed through the latest and most advanced science available in any particular era and progressively building upon previous work to create increasingly more effective treatments that now have arrived in full scientific glory as EBP. We think these claims were bogus in the eighteenth century and we believe they are bogus in the twenty-first century, as we will demonstrate in our review of the most "validated" of the EBPs for serious mental illness, ACT.

ACT History

The common claim is that assertive community treatment is "widely recognized as an evidence-based practice for adults with severe mental illness"

(Bond, Drake, Mueser, and Latimer, 2001, p. 155). ACT appears to be well-credentialed, having built its credibility more than a decade ago on "a research base includ[ing] 25 well-controlled studies" (p. 155). The National Alliance on Mental Illness states that ACT is the most widely replicated and frequently used community treatment for SMIs throughout the world. Only five states in the United States do not have ACT teams, while forty-three states make their Medicaid funds available for its reimbursement (Aron, Honberg, Duckworth et al., 2009). ACT is without question the leading community treatment for SMIs:

> Since the deinstitutionalization era began nearly 50 years ago, several models of community-based care for persons with severe mental illnesses have been developed. Of these models, the assertive community treatment (ACT) program has by far the strongest empirical support. (Essock et al., 1998, p. 176)

We will now scrutinize the veracity of these claims and the allegedly convincing evidence for its effectiveness. Originally called training in community living (TCL), ACT was one of those mental health programs developed during the late 1960s and early 1970s to respond to the federal mandate for shifting the locus of care and control of psychiatric patients from isolated institutions into the community (Stein & Test, 1985). It was considered to be an immediate success: soon after its first randomized controlled study (Marx, Test, and Stein, 1973), ACT received the Gold Achievement Award in 1974 from the American Psychiatric Association. Its developers stated that ACT fit closely the prevailing psychiatric disease model and its concomitant reliance on psychiatric drugs: "Congruent with our conceptual model, we tell our patients that indeed we believe they are ill, otherwise we would not be prescribing medication for them" (Stein & Diamond, 1985, p. 272).

The Origins of ACT's Methods

ACT originated at Mendota State Hospital in Madison, Wisconsin, in the 1960s and 1970s. Key protagonists in the hospital at the time were: (1) psychiatrist Arnold M. Ludwig, the hospital's director of research and education; (2) the creators of ACT, psychiatrists Arnold J. Marx, Leonard I. Stein, and psychologist and Professor of Social Work Mary Ann Test; and (3) less directly, clinical social worker Frank Farrelly and psychologist Jeff Brandsma. Farrelly and Brandsma together fashioned and tested at Mendota State a therapeutic approach they called "provocative therapy" (Farrelly & Brandsma, 1974) and influenced the treatment approaches of those involved with ACT.

In 1985 Stein and Test edited a book reporting on the first ten years of the TCL/ACT effort, *The Training in Community Living Model: A Decade of Experience.* They describe the development of their professional thinking this way:

> Ideas rarely arise de novo; they are generally formed from the building blocks of prior knowledge and experience. To become lasting, they must be nourished in an environment that is willing to set aside the accepted attitudes and practices that resist new concepts. . . . In the mid 1960's . . . several psychiatrists [Marx and Stein] who had just finished their residency joined the hospital staff. These psychiatrists were imbued with the therapeutic zeal frequently found in young, uninitiated physicians. In addition, Arnold Ludwig joined the staff as director of research and education. His first two projects involved many members of the hospital staff. The projects represented . . . an effort to transform the hospital . . . into an institute whose primary goals were research, demonstration, consultation and training. (pp. 7–9)

This quote identifies most of the key TCL/ACT players and describes their intimate involvement in the research conducted at Mendota State after the appointment of Ludwig as director of research and education and suggests that what they learned from these projects informed their understanding and treatment of patients.

Patient Descriptions

The Mendota State researchers, despite their view that their patients are medically ill (a perspective that ordinarily does not hold the patient responsible for the consequences deemed to flow from having an illness), appeared to have entertained if not hostile, at least negative attitudes toward patients. Patients in a locked ward (the STU) at Mendota State Hospital are not described in medical terms but as adversaries:

> Professionals have overlooked the rather naive possibility that schizophrenic patients become "chronic" simply because they choose to do so . . . If he so desires, he can defecate when or where he chooses, masturbate publicly, lash out aggressively, expose himself, remain inert and unproductive or violate any social taboo with the assurance that staff are forced to "understand" rather than punish behavior. (Ludwig & Farrelly, 1967, p. 737–741)

These two authors wrote an earlier article (in 1966) which is entitled "The Code of Chronicity." The code, according to them, is employed by the mad, along with other "weapons of crazyness" (p. 565). They concluded that these patients were:

> Obviously . . . not . . . a group of fragile, broken-spirited persons but rather . . . tough, formidable adversaries who were "pros" and who

had successfully contended with many different staffs on various wards in defending their title of "chronic schizophrenic." (Ludwig & Farrelly, 1966, p. 566)

As a result, Ludwig and Farrelly felt that the only medical cure was to coerce the patients to mimic the "sane" behavior of the staff:

> To become well patients would have to think, feel, and behave . . . similar to staff. The concept of normality and sanity as therapeutic goals . . . would have to [be] deliberately concretize[d] . . . by insisting that patients employ staff persons as models for behavior. . . . Furthermore, we would *not* play at democracy in therapeutic community meetings; not the majority, but health and sanity, *as defined by staff*, would rule. (1966, pp. 566–567, emphasis added)

The psychiatric commitment to use coercion to cure, exhibited throughout the profession's history, could not be better illustrated than by these experts' efforts to force their inmates to conform in order "to become well." The similarity to the later ACT approach, as described by ACT insider, psychiatrist Ronald J. Diamond, is uncanny:

> Paternalism was to a large extent accepted with little question. . . . *Staff were assumed to know what the patient "needed."* Even the goal of getting patients paid employment *was a staff-driven value* that was at times at odds with the patient's own preferences. Current assertive treatment programs continue to be influenced by traditions . . . from this . . . history. Paternalism continues to be reinforced by mandates from the community to "control" the behavior of otherwise disruptive patients. (Diamond, 1996, p. 53)

Punishment as Treatment

Leonard Stein, after replacing Arnold Ludwig as the director of research and education at Mendota State Hospital, coauthored a study with "provocative therapy" advocate Brandsma, entitled "The Use of Punishment as a Treatment Modality: A Case Report" (Brandsma & Stein, 1973). The study examined the value of using involuntary electric shock to reduce the "unprovoked" assaultive behavior of a "retarded, adult, organically damaged" (p. 30) twenty-four-year-old woman. This publication appeared during the time that TCL/ACT community research was already well on its way (see Marx, Test, & Stein, 1973) and was apparently part of a line of research focused on force and violence as treatment, begun earlier at Mendota State. Ludwig, Marx, Hill, and Browning (1969) had previously published a single-case study on a paranoid schizophrenic patient, entitled "The Control of Violent Behavior through Faradic Shock." The authors justified this study by its "uniqueness," because "this procedure was administered *against the express will* of the patient" (p. 624, emphasis added). They used an electric cattle prod as the "aversive conditioning agent," because it was "an excellent device for providing a potent, noxious stimulus . . . capable of producing a faradic shock spike of approximately 1400 volts at 0.5 milliamperes, the resulting pain lasting . . . as long as the current was permitted to flow" (p. 627).

The methodology of Brandsma and Stein's experiment reveals what can only be termed sadism. To obtain a "baseline" measure (a requirement of single-subject design research) of this patient's assaultive behavior, she was baited and ridiculed so she would respond aggressively:

> The patient was required to sit in an armchair throughout. . . .
> During the base rate week the staff quickly developed a consistent provocative approach in order to ensure a high frequency of behavior from the patient . . . This consistently involved: 1) ignoring the patient in conversation; 2) refusing to give the patient candy or snacks when others were eating them; 3) denying all requests, for example, during the session if she asked if she would be able to go for a walk that afternoon, she was immediately told, "No you can't."; 4) refusing to accept her apologies or believe her promises of good behavior; 5) The . . . female sitting next to her often leading the provocation; 6) using provocative labels for her behavior, i.e., "animalistic, low grade"; 7) discussing family related frustrations, i.e., her mother's refusal to write or visit, how her dead grandmother would be displeased with her present behavior if she were alive. It should be noted that throughout the program the patient was kept in a seclusion room at all times except when involved in a baseline or treatment session. (Brandsma & Stein, 1973, pp. 32–33)

Brandsma and Stein's research exemplifies mad science at its worst, by daring to torture an imprisoned, nonconsenting subject and by publishing an article full of scientific misinformation and distortion. Brandsma and Stein cited the classic behavioral study by Azrin and Holz (1966) to support their use of punishment, stating that "our clinical reports back up the more controlled animal studies on punishment. For example . . . Azrin and Holz . . ." (Brandsma & Stein, 1973 p. 36). In fact, the Azrin and Holz had argued that punishment is *ineffective* as a method of behavioral change, especially for human subjects, listing its primary disadvantages as follows:

> The principal disadvantages of using punishment seem to be that when the punishment is administered by an individual, 1) the punished individual is driven away from the punishing agent, thereby destroying the social relationship; 2) the punished individual may engage in operant aggression directed toward the punishing agent;

and 3) even when the punishment is delivered by physical means rather than by another organism, elicited aggression can be expected against nearby individuals who were not responsible for the punishment. (Azrin & Holz, 1966, p. 441)

Despite this clear refutation of their brand of behavioral treatment that Brandsma and Stein cited to support their own therapeutic use of an electric cattle prod, they falsely concluded that "the extant literature now supports the assertion that 'punishment therapy' is a useful tool to modify certain behaviors" (Brandsma & Stein, 1973, p. 37). Their research demonstrated that "punishment therapy" was not effective. As they report about their subject, "[u]nfortunately the intensity of her now low frequency, occasional attacks was still sufficient to relegate her to a life of relative social isolation" (p. 36) and even a year after the intervention "the punishment contingency continues . . . in seclusion with only a few hours out per day when accompanied by a male aide" (p. 35). The patient was not better off after the coercive treatment and was relegated to permanent solitary confinement.

What is noteworthy in this publication is how easily actions like baiting, punishment, and torture could be applied to a difficult patient by "doctors" and be described as scientific research on "treatment." The early transformations of control and punishment as treatment at Mendota State appear to have influenced research on ACT over the next several decades.

What Is ACT?

According to Test (1992), ACT has four essential characteristics:

Core Services Team [made up of 3-5 members, with at least a primary case manager, psychiatrist, and backup case manager per patient]: The team's function is to see that all the patient's needs are addressed in a timely fashion. . . . Having one team provide most of these services minimizes the . . . fragmentation of . . . care systems and allows for integrated clinical management. . . .

Assertive Outreach and In Vivo Treatment: An essential ingredient . . . is the use of assertive outreach . . . [staff] reaches out and takes both biological and psychological services to the patient[in the community]. . . .

Individualized Treatment: Because persons with serious mental illnesses . . . are greatly heterogeneous and both person and disorder are constantly changing over time, treatment . . . must be highly individualized. . . .

> Ongoing Treatment and Support: . . . even very intensive community treatment models do not provide a cure for severe mental illness, but . . . a support system within which persons with persistent vulnerabilities can live in the community and grow. It appears these supports must be ongoing rather than time limited. (1992, pp. 154–156)

Treatment Effect or Administrative Coercion?

A 2001 article in the journal *Psychiatric Services* claimed that ACT was to be deemed an EBP because it had shown superiority over alternate treatments:

> Research has shown that assertive community treatment is . . . more satisfactory to consumers and their families. Reviews of the research consistently conclude that compared with other treatments under controlled conditions, such as brokered case management or clinical case management, assertive community treatment results in a greater reduction in *psychiatric hospitalization and a higher level of housing stability.* (Phillips, Burns, Edgar et al., 2001, p. 771, emphasis added)

The clinical effectiveness of any treatment is usually measured in symptom reduction, reduced disability, better functioning, or improvements in behavior, self- or other-rated. What is noteworthy about the quote above is that keeping people out of a hospital or in a community residence is used as the markers of success. It might come as a surprise then that an award-winning "treatment" program made few claims that it improved patients' clinical condition. In fact, Philips et al. admit that "[t]he effects of assertive community treatment on *quality of life, symptoms, and social functioning* are similar to those produced by these other treatments" (p. 771, emphasis added). In other words, ACT does not reduce the mad behavior or improve the functioning of the severely mentally ill any more than any other approach. Decades earlier the ACT inventors admitted: "a change in the site of treatment [from the hospital to the community] says nothing about whether the patient's clinical status or functioning has improved. Some would argue that only the place of a person's suffering has changed" (Test & Stein, 1978, p. 360).

Nonetheless, ACT aspired to do more. In 1992 Mary Ann Test indicated that they always "target[ed] goals for the model . . . going far beyond the reduction of time in hospitals. Additionally, improvements in patients' psychosocial functioning and quality of life are sought" (Test, 1992, 164). But over time, the ACT model failed to achieve these clinical outcomes that would be routinely expected of any treatment in medicine. If traditional clinical effectiveness was not achieved by ACT, what was the basis for its purported success? Let's examine five core claims of success.

ACT's "Successes"

Claim #1. ACT significantly reduces hospitalization when compared to alternate treatments.

Evidence. Reduced hospitalization and inpatient treatment costs are the only consistent outcomes found across studies. On the surface, reducing hospitalization rates can be mistaken as reducing symptomatic behaviors and therefore the need for hospitalization. But, in fact, ACT methods have no direct bearing on reducing symptoms or the need for hospitalization. They simply reduced hospital stays by using a fairly strict *administrative* rule not to admit or readmit any ACT patients for hospitalization, regardless of the psychiatric symptoms, but to carry out all treatment in the community. The comparison group of troubled patients at the same time could be freely readmitted.

Test and Stein (1978) provided an early clue to the importance of program control over hospitalization and discharge: "Community treatment results in less time spent in the hospital. This finding is certainly not surprising since experimental patients were usually not admitted to hospitals initially and there were subsequent concentrated efforts to keep them out" (p. 354). Many ACT articles acknowledge that reduced hospitalization in ACT is the result of administrative rules, not clinical treatment. Scott and Dixon (1995), examining the impact of case management and ACT programs, observe that "the effectiveness of ACT models in reducing hospitalization may be a function of their capacity to control hospital admissions, length of stay, and discharge" (p. 659). Several studies have noted that the length of hospital stay returned to pre-intervention levels when ACT team . . . control of discharge was blocked by hospital authorities" (Craig & Pathare, 1997, pp. 111–112). Finally, Minghella, Gauntlett, and Ford (2002), discussing the failure of some assertive outreach teams in England to reduce hospitalization, write that "[w]hile the teams partly adhered to the ACT model, there were major areas of deviation. The teams had little influence over admissions and discharge" (p. 27).

In short, if one does not allow particular people to be hospitalized, they won't be. A crucial point to be made here is that the identical type of psychiatric administrative activity is used either to force people into hospitals for treatment (involuntary civil commitment), to prevent them from entering hospitals, or to force people out of them into the community for treatment (ACT). All these approaches are coercive: they do not consider whether any of the patients being forced into the hospital want out or whether those being kept out want in. Client choice is not an option.

Claim #2. ACT is more cost effective than standard interventions.

Evidence. Since hospitalization is by far the more costly treatment, the cost savings are not dependent on specific ACT clinical interventions but on keeping people away from hospitals, which, as we have just reviewed, is a byproduct of the ACT administrative coercion. Cost reduction could occur with any other treatment rigorously pursuing the same objective.

Claim #3. ACT provides significantly greater patient satisfaction.

Evidence. Most people prize their freedom; few prefer to be confined in hospitals. ACT's clients are the same, but patient satisfaction appears to be independent of distinct ACT activity. The greater autonomy provided by *any* community treatment (as compared to a locked hospital ward), not the particular interventions of ACT, would explain increased satisfaction. In the Australian study previously mentioned, the patients were surveyed at a twelve-month follow-up: "The majority (80%) of experimental group patients who were not admitted to the hospital were pleased and grateful about it; only 30% of control group patients were pleased and grateful about being admitted to hospital, whereas 39% were upset and angry" (Hoult, 1986, p. 142). Stated differently, "Treatment preference was explored by asking *all* patients whether they prefer admission to Macquarie Hospital or treatment at home by a community team. The majority of the project (87%) and control (61%) patients preferred community treatment" (Hoult et al., 1983, p. 163, emphasis added). A majority (61 percent) of the group that *did not* experience the ACT treatment still preferred community treatment rather than incarceration in an institution. In fact, the experimental group reported that the most important elements of the ACT treatment were the availability of staff for frequent caring; supportive, personal contact; and the enhanced freedom—therapeutic elements not specific to ACT (p. 163).

Lending further support, a survey of "patient perspectives" on ACT "ingredients" (McGrew, Wilson, & Bond, 1996) identified in order of preference: "helping relationship, attributes of therapist, availability of staff, and non-specific assistance" as what patients liked most (p. 16, table 1). These attributes are not ACT specific; they apply to all forms of "helping." The least liked of the twenty-five elements associated with ACT was "intensity of service"—the component most representative of ACT-intrusive philosophy. The survey's authors, themselves longtime ACT experts, admit, "Somewhat surprisingly, non-specific features of the helping relationship emerged as the aspects of [ACT] most frequently mentioned as helpful" (McGrew et al., 1996, p. 190).

Claim #4. ACT increases [independent community] housing stability (Bond et al., 2001, p. 149).

Evidence. We conclude, in agreement with most other reviews, that the evidence supports this claim. ACT patients, but *not* control group patients, are more likely to find rooms and apartments in the community, rather than using many specialized residential settings (Test, Knoedler, Allness, Kameshima et al, 1994, p. 4). But just as ACT patients are not allowed to be hospitalized, ACT patients are administratively directed only to "independent" housing. So what is achieved is not a clinical treatment success, as much as an assertive administrative rule to help patients find independent-living settings.

Finally and most importantly:

Claim #5. "The assertive community treatment approach never was, and is not now, based on coercion" (Test & Stein, 2001, p. 1396).

Evidence. One of the rationales which the ACT inventors cited to explain the shift from psychiatric institutional care to community care was the reduction of coercive management and the promotion of autonomy to improve the social functioning of the SMI (Marx et al., 1973). Another was the desire to reduce the harmful effects of institutional living. Test and Stein's unequivocal rejection of accusations that ACT is coercive (as quoted above) was in response to an article in APA's community psychiatry journal, *Psychiatric Services*.

The historical record suggests that the Test and Stein denial is open to debate. For example, here is how Stein (1990) describes the role of the ACT team:

> [S]erves as a fixed point of responsibility . . . and is concerned with *all* aspects of . . . the patients' lives that influence their functioning, including psychological health, physical health, living situation, finances, socialization, vocational activities, and recreational activities. The team sets no time limits for their involvement with patients, is assertive in keeping patients involved . . . In addition to the day work . . . the team is available 24 hours a day, seven days a week. (p. 650, emphasis added)

This methodology appears highly intrusive. ACT activities may include such coercive moves as becoming the representative "financial payee" of the patient, providing opportunities to blackmail the patients by enforcing medication compliance or threatening to withhold monies belonging to the patient (Stein & Test, 1985, pp. 88–89). This appears to be forcing treatment on ACT patients who do not want it (pp. 91–92). Even bribery may be appropriate ACT treatment: "it might be necessary to pay a socially withdrawn patient for going to the movies in addition to buying his ticket" (Test & Stein, 1976, p. 78).

To validate the use of assertive outreach and treatment, the original ACT researchers rely on two studies, one of which is their own (Test, 1981, p. 80). The other study is by Beard, Malamud and Rossman (1978), who describe their Fountain House outreach program as follows: "Phone calls, letters, and home and hospital visits [were] made by both staff and members. Through such contacts, subjects who dropped out were provided with further information. . . . In those . . . instances when an individual requested that no further contacts be made, his wishes, of course, were respected"

(p. 624). Respect for the wishes of people who choose not to be involved in the Fountain House program contrasts with the coercive methods used by Test and Stein (1976):

> A staff person attempting to assist an ambivalent patient to a sheltered workshop in the morning is likely to receive a verbal and behavioral "no." . . . If . . . the staff member approaches the patient with a firm, "It's time for you to go to work; I'll wait here while you get dressed," the likelihood of compliance increases. The latter method allows less room for the patient to "choose" passivity. (p. 77)

Two questions come to mind: why is the patient described as ambivalent, when the patient's reported behavior indicates a resolute opposition to going to work? Second, why is the patient's active refusal redefined as "passivity"? The disregard of patients' expressed wishes and the reinterpretation of their behavior to justify programmatic interventions appear to be characteristics of ACT—in fact it appears to give meaning to "assertive" treatment. The Fountain House model, by contrast, discontinues patient outreach efforts if asked.

Coercion and control, despite Test and Stein's denial, appear to be integral parts of the ACT model when it appears to be effective. According to the candid admission of Diamond (1996), a close associate of the original ACT group in Madison:

> Paternalism has been a part of assertive community treatment from its very beginning . . . Paternalism continues to be reinforced by mandates from the community to "control" the behavior of otherwise disruptive patients. . . . A significant number of patients in community support programs . . . have been assigned a financial payee . . . This kind of coercion can be extremely effective.

> . . . Obtaining spending money can be made . . . dependent on participating in other parts of treatment. A patient can then be pressured by staff to take prescribed medication. . . . [T]he pressure to take medication . . . can be enormous. . . . While control of housing and control of money are the most common . . . methods of coercion in the community, [and] other kinds of control are also possible. This pressure can be almost as coercive as the hospital but with fewer safeguards. (pp. 53–58)

The fact is that discussion of ACT coercion is routinely found throughout the psychiatric literature. A large body of literature now addresses the "therapeutic" value of community-based coercion of mental health patients, an ongoing discussion that can be tied directly to the existence of ACT.

A 1996 edited book legitimated the study and use of such coercion with the title specifically identifying ACT and its coercive approach: *Coercion and Aggressive Community Treatment: A New Frontier in Mental Health Law* (Dennis & Monahan, 1996). More recently, the importance of conventional psychiatric coercion research has been further validated by a major new book published in 2011, also coedited by John Monahan, *Coercive Treatment in Psychiatry: Clinical, Legal and Ethical Aspects*. While some psychiatric experts are busy asking "Is Assertive Community Treatment Coercive?" (Appelbaum & LeMelle, 2007), ACT experts acknowledge that "assertive engagement" or "assertive outreach" is a core element of ACT. These concepts are included in the most popular scale for evaluating ACT program replications' fidelity to the original Madison model, the Dartmouth Assertive Community Treatment Scale (DACTS). Assertive engagement is measured (in DACTS) primarily by counting the frequency of formal coercive legal mechanisms (i.e., mandated outpatient treatment or appointed financial payees). Its developers state transparently that "[i]t should be noted that the criterion for assertive engagement was operationalized in such a way that it emphasized use of legal mechanisms" (Teague, Bond, & Drake, 1998, p. 229). Davis (2002) has suggested that "[c]oercion in assertive community treatment may take formal or explicit form, such as the enforcement of conditions of a treatment order. Usually, however, coercion is less obvious and by extension more difficult for workers to come to terms with" (pp. 245–246). A report prepared in 2000 for the Federal Health Care and Financing Administration and the Substance Abuse and Mental Health Services Administration devotes a whole section to ACT coercion. The report notes that "[w]ithin the context of ACT programs, coercion can include a range of behaviors including, friendly persuasion, interpersonal pressure, control of resources and the use of force. . . . Research generally suggests that coercion may be harmful to the consumer" (LewinGroup, 2000, p. 43). It is noteworthy that "friendly persuasion" is included as an example of "coercion" in a federal report on psychiatric treatment. This appears like a simple error. Or is it in fact part of a strategic effort to broaden the meaning of coercion? Is the inclusion of noncoercive interpersonal activity (friendly persuasion appears to us as an essential ingredient of *voluntary* talk therapy) in the preceding list of coercive activities an effort to domesticate externally imposed force as treatment? Similar strategic inclusions have occurred in psychiatry before. The most common examples of this are the linguistic efforts to authenticate "mental illnesses" as physical diseases by lumping together problems such as depression and schizophrenia within lists of common neurological disorders or "brain-based disorders" that have identifiable neurological signs, such as Parkinson's disease or Alzheimer's disease, though neither depression nor schizophrenia have any such signs.

ACT appears merely as a recent manifestation, adapted to the exigencies of life beyond hospital walls, of the longstanding, coercive strain that has characterized psychiatric interventions with mad persons to this day and that duplicitously assumes the cloak of scientific activity and scientific progress.

Conclusion

Psychiatric practice, by our reading, appears to have lost even the semblance of moral rectitude regarding the employment of coercion. It used to pretend that when men and women of science, motivated by the desire to heal, forced mad persons to submit to their ministrations, this was not coercion but medical treatment. Today such a pretense no longer seems necessary. A thriving body of research, supported among others by the NIMH and the MacArthur Foundation (Dennis & Monahan, 1996, p. 15), fully explores the therapeutic value of coercion. The deprivation of autonomy and freedom is increasingly being redefined as a therapeutic tool rather than a violation of human rights.

When we searched the Medline database up to and including 2007 for indexed articles about psychiatric coercion (using *coercion, outpatient commitment,* and *civil commitment* as independent key words), we identified 796 articles. Only 22 articles were published before 1970, in contrast to 665 articles between 1991 and 2007 (39 articles a year). The first noticeable spike in publications occurred in 1971, around the time community treatment became a focus of research. In the abstracts, we note only a handful of voices dissenting from the general view that coercion, though "controversial," is ultimately just another therapeutic mechanism deserving examination.

Indeed, some eminent psychiatric scholars have recently unabashedly defended the use of psychiatric coercion, without any pretense that it is somehow a form of medicine. It *is* just plain coercion. Jeffrey Geller (2012), professor of psychiatry and director of public sector psychiatry at the University of Massachusetts Medical School, asserts that "the psychiatrist's *option* to employ coercion is an integral component of functioning in this recovery oriented paradigm . . ." (p. 493, italics added). Geller is candid about the level and forms of coercion in outpatient treatment:

> Coercive interventions, with little or no review by anyone other than a physician or a treatment team or administrator, are rampant in entitlement programs; they include leveraged housing (for example, "If you want to live in this residence, you have to take your medication as prescribed and go to a day program"); representative payeeships; "bargained" psychopharmacologic regimens (for example, "You take your antipsychotic and you can have a benzodiazepine"); waiver of civic responsibility (for example, jury duty); treatment "contracts" through Individual Service Plans; and threats of emergency detention (for example, civil commitment). (p. 494)

Geller proposes that *regardless* of psychiatric status, individuals routinely get coerced in the community, which he finds equivalent to "prevention and treatment":

> A person who repeatedly gets stopped for speeding loses his or her license and must attend classes to get it back (treatment). . . . Someone who disrupts a public event is removed from the venue (treatment, behavior modification). If you park illegally, the car is towed and you get fined . . . (treatment and prevention). (p. 495)

After medicalizing drivers' education, Geller feels he must now demedicalize forced treatment by medical doctors: "If a person behaves in a way that is dangerous to others, and the danger can be mitigated by psychiatric treatment, the person gets treatment. . . . It is coercion in the same way that others in the community are subjected to coercion. It is not coercion because of 'psychiatric status': it is an intervention to address behavior. Just as we all experience" (p. 495).

But Geller is clearly mistaken here. He confuses public laws that all citizens must obey to avoid punishment with coercion that only the mad endure precisely because they are deemed mad by psychiatrists. Society does not enact special laws to coerce speeding drivers on the basis that they suffer from a mental illness that is responsible for their speeding. But society coerces dangerous people into psychiatric treatment *only* on the basis of special laws that require a diagnostic evaluation by a psychiatrist. Actually, Geller is on to something, but not what he intended. Geller repeats that coercion occurs everywhere in society, not just in psychiatry, because he wants to make psychiatric coercion palatable. But as he makes this argument, he is forced to recognize that *no existing psychiatric treatment can compete with coercion*: "the notion that we can eliminate all coercive interventions by using our current array of psychopharmacologic agents, psychotherapies, and rehabilitation interventions is without precedent" (p. 494). Undoubtedly, Geller is admitting that psychiatry relies on a foundation of coercion.

Another eminent psychiatric scholar, Allen Frances (2012), best known as the Chair of the *DSM-IV* Task Force and whose views on diagnosis we discuss in chapters 4 and 5, goes even further than Geller in acknowledging the nature of coercion in psychiatry and, probably unintentionally, deals a fatal blow to the claim that coercion has *anything* to do with medical treatment.

In a reply to an article by psychologist Jeffrey Schaler (2012), Frances writes: "I agree completely with Schaler and Szasz that mental disorders are not diseases and that treating them as such can sometimes have noxious legal consequences." He singles out "schizophrenia": ". . . mental disorders are constructs, nothing more but also nothing less. Schizophrenia is certainly not a disease; but equally it is not a myth. As a construct, schizophrenia is useful for purposes of communication and helpful in prediction and decisionmaking—

even if . . . the term has only descriptive, and not explanatory, power" (p. 1). If schizophrenia is "not a disease," as psychiatry has long claimed, Frances must come to terms squarely with the nature of psychiatric coercion: "I have evaluated [patients who 'desperately needed to be protected from hurting themselves or others'] many hundreds of times. While it is never comfortable to coerce someone into treatment, it is sometimes the only safe and responsible thing to do, and occasionally it is life saving. . . . Coercive psychiatry, however unpleasant, must be available as a necessary last resort when nothing else will do" (p. 2). Frances' makes the simple case *for* psychiatric coercion, namely, that the functioning of society requires force when the intermediary social control functions of persuasion and seduction fail (Peckham, 1979). Normally, the imposition of force or violence is entrusted to soldiers and policemen. When psychiatrists or mental health professionals defend and engage in coercion, they are essentially police posing as doctors or therapists.

The use of coercion to control the mad in America for four centuries has continually been marketed not as the use of force to manage a disobedient and troubling group, but as the application of better and more progressive treatments to aid a group suffering from a serious medical infirmity. The presumed treatments are presented as having been developed through advanced scientific techniques and building on previous work to create increasingly more effective interventions. Over the last couple of decades, many of these interventions have been anointed as "evidence-based practices" (EBPs), as we have discussed in this chapter.

It is apparent that coercion is increasingly seen in psychiatry and in other mental health professions and the legal profession as an acceptable form of treatment needing no critical scrutiny beyond meeting the technical criterion of effectiveness. "Psychiatric scientific authority" has transformed coercion into a routine intervention, leaving the average psychiatric researcher to focus on the technical details of the issue (i.e., how well does coercion "work" to produce this or that outcome?) and to lose sight of larger moral issues regarding human freedom, dignity, and autonomy (Cherry, 2010); of the perspectives of those subject to coercion (Oaks, 2011; Olofsson & Jacobson, 2001); and even of the narrower issues of whether coercion should ever be used as a "tool" of helping professionals, free of the safeguards that surround its uses outside of the mental health system.

As we have suggested in this chapter, the two roles of psychiatry—that of social management (involuntary psychiatry) and therapeutic helping (voluntary psychiatry) of the mad—are irreconcilable. In order for one to work the other cannot. Effective social management may require a coercive social technology (ultimately, incarceration) to enforce compliance if social seduction (i.e., friendly persuasive rhetoric or incentives) fails. The availability of psychiatric coercion greatly constrains the choices the mad have about their treatment. Police are not therapists, even when they act to deescalate anger

111

and potentially violent behavior. But psychiatrists, rhetorically equipped by medicine—doctor, mental illness, diagnosis, treatment—can use police-like coercion over the mad. To us, force is force, regardless of how it is labeled. The intentions of those who wield force may be benevolent, but force hurts equally—whether we call it punishment or "punishment therapy."

We believe that a voluntary psychiatry and an involuntary psychiatry cannot both be the same enterprise, evaluated by the same criteria, scientific or otherwise. The small number of dissenting voices concerning the legitimacy of psychiatric coercion does not indicate the rightness of the approach, only the numbing of moral and critical faculties. The historical role of punishment of the mad has conveniently been imbedded in the medical model because of the ways in which control and coercion easily slip into the benevolent rubric of treatment for the relatively powerless and vulnerable. Outside hospital walls, control and coercion have been embraced by various professionals and institutions in society, justifying it as a relatively small price to pay to ensure proper "medical" treatment of distress and misbehavior. The next two chapters scrutinize the evolution of one "scientific" tool of psychiatry that converts personal turmoil into disease and the socially misbehaving into medical patients—the expanding dictionary of psychiatry, *the Diagnostic and Statistical Manual of Mental Disorders.*

Notes

1. The famous study by Erving Goffman described in his 1961 book *Asylums* discusses the toxic effects of being confined in "total institutions." Based on Goffman's field observations of ward behavior at St. Elizabeth's Hospital in Washington, DC in 1955–1956, it makes not a single allusion to the use of major tranquilizers. The first of these drugs, Thorazine was commercially released in the United States less than a year before, in mid-1954. St. Elizabeth's is best known today for detaining the infamous John Hinckley Jr., who attempted to assassinate President Ronald Reagan in 1981.
2. Think of the payment of income taxes. Because the Internal Revenue Service is able to enforce the tax code through criminal and civil sanctions, it would be naïve to conclude that people pay taxes "voluntarily."
3. The rubric of seriously mentally ill or having a serious mental illness (SMI) (sometimes also referred to as "major mental illness" or "serious and persistent mental illness") has been formalized by the federal government. It began to be used in the 1990s. The government definition of SMI "includes all [DSM] diagnoses, substantial disability, and no required duration (some estimates show this [label] as encompassing 5–7% of the U.S. population ages 18+ [about 3.3 million adults])" (Kuntz, 1995, p. 6). What individuals placed in this category share as a group, despite their differing DSM diagnoses, is their "substantial disability," which justifies psychiatric intervention. A "substantial disability" could be physical, such as being blind or having a chronic physical disease such as diabetes or severe coronary disease that may limit full social participation. In this instance, however, "substantial disability" means lacking skills that cause serious and "specific limitations

in work, school, personal care, social functioning, concentrating, or coping with day-today [*sic*] stress" (p. 6). Most SMIs are unemployed and may show little ability in maintaining traditional relationships. They depend on others to take care of them because they appear unable to do basic life chores such as manage their funds, use public transportation, launder their clothes, cook, or dress conventionally (Test & Stein, 1978). As psychiatric epidemiologists Ronald C. Kessler and Shanyang Zhao explain, "Epidemiologic information about the prevalence of individual disorders is much less important than . . . the prevalence of functional impairment, comorbidity, and chronicity" (1999, p. 77). The terms *comorbidity* and *chronicity* mean having several personal difficulties that have lasted for a long time.

4.   The counting of patient care episodes tracked by the federal government since 1955 is a duplicate count, since a person may be admitted to more than one type of service or can receive the same service more than once in any one year. The number of individuals who receive multiple service episodes is unknown, so we are unable to have a total unduplicated count of the number of persons under care in any one year.

5.   EBM is clinical epidemiology on steroids. David Sackett, EBM's most well known developer explains: "Clinical epidemiology has played a central or major role in five recent evolutions (some say revolutions) in healthcare: in evidence generation, its rapid critical appraisal, its efficient storage and retrieval, evidence-based medicine, and evidence synthesis. As more and more clinicians, armed with the strategies and tactics of clinical epidemiology, cared for more and more patients, they began to evolve the final, vital link between evidence and direct patient care. Building on the prior evolutions, and manifest in clinically useful measures and often incorporating the patient's own values and expectations, the *revolution of Evidence-Based Medicine* was introduced by Gordon Guyatt. Since its first mention in 1992, its ideas about the use (rather than just critical appraisal) of evidence in patient care and in health professional education have spread worldwide, and have been adopted not only by a broad array of clinical disciplines but also by health care planners and evaluators" (2002, p. 1164).

6.   *Clinical treatment effect* is defined as some specified non-administrative clinical/biological/behavioral component(s) of a treatment program that can motivate or cause internalized/volitional change, or the "acquisition of coping skills" by clients, which leads to clients' improved functioning that results in reduced hospital stays and greater "independent" community tenure in a community mental health program such as ACT.

7.   The Cochrane Collaboration is the leading organization carrying out and maintaining a database of EBM systematic reviews. It does this through voluntary work groups whose members apparently are only cursorily checked for expertise before joining. As their website informs the curious:

NOTE: Membership of a Cochrane group is not based on formal qualifications. There are no membership fees. The key requirements are that you:

• have suitable skills (and willingness to learn new ones);
• can volunteer some of your time over an extended period;

- work as part of a team;
- support the aims of the Collaboration; and
- share the Collaboration's spirit of goodwill. (Cochrane Collaboration, n. d. Retrieved from www.cochrane.org).

References

Abbott, A. (1988). *The system of professions: An essay on the division of expert labor.* Chicago: University of Chicago Press.

American Psychiatric Association. (2000). *Diagnostic and statistical manual of mental disorders, Fourth edition, Text revision.* Washington, DC: Author.

Andreasen, N. C. (1999). A unitary model of schizophrenia. *Archives of General Psychiatry, 56,* 781–787.

Anfang, S. A., & Appelbaum, P. S. (2006). Civil commitment: The American experience. *Israel Journal of Psychiatry & Related Sciences, 43,* 209–218.

Appelbaum, P., & LeMalle, S. (2007). Is assertive community treatment coercive? *BMC Psychiatry, 7(suppl 1).* doi:10.1186/1471-244X-7-S1-S29

Aron, L., Honberg, R., Duckworth, K., et al. (2009). *Grading the states 2009: A report on America's health care system for adults with serious mental illness.* Arlington, VA: National Alliance on Mental Illness.

Azrin, N. H., & Holz, W. C. (1966). Punishment. In W. K. Honing (Ed.), *Operant behavior: Areas of research and application* (pp. 380–447). New York: Appleton-Century-Crofts.

Bailar, J. C. (1995). The practice of meta-analysis. *Journal of Clinical Epidemiology, 48,* 149–157.

Beard, J. H., Malamud, T. J., & Rossman E. (1978). Psychiatric rehabilitation and long-term rehospitalization rates: The findings of two research studies. *Schizophrenia Bulletin, 4*(4), 622–635.

Berk, R., & Freedman, D. A. (2001). *Statistical assumptions as empirical commitments.* Retrieved August 7, 2011, from University of California, eScholarship website: http://escholarship.org/uc/item/0zj8s368?query=statistical%20assumptions%20as%20empirical%20commitments

Bond, G. R., Drake, R. E., McHugo, G. J., Rapp, C. A., & Whitley, R. (2009). Strategies for improving fidelity in the national evidence-based practices project. *Research on Social Work Practice, 19,* 569–581.

Bond, G. R., Drake, R. E., Mueser, K. T., & Latimer, E. (2001). Assertive community treatment for people with severe mental illness: Critical ingredients and impact on patients. *Disease Management & Health Outcomes, 9,* 141–159.

Bond, G. R., Salyers, M. P., Rollins, A. L., Rapp, C. A., & Zipple, A. M. (2004). How evidence-based practices contribute to community integration. *Community Mental Health Journal, 40,* 569–588.

Boyle, M. (2002). *Schizophrenia: A scientific delusion?* (2nd ed.). London: Routledge.

Brandsma, J. M., & Stein, L. I. (1973). The use of punishment as a treatment modality: A case report. *Journal of Nervous and Mental Disease, 156,* 30–37.

Cherry, M. J. (2010, Winter). Non consensual treatment is (nearly always) morally impermissible. *Journal of Law, Medicine, and Ethics,* pp. 789–798.

Cohen, A. M., Stavri, P. Z., & Hersh, W. R. (2004). A categorization and analysis of the criticisms of evidence-based medicine. *International Journal of Medical Informatics, 73,* 35–43.

Connery, R. H. (1968). *The politics of mental health.* New York: Columbia University Press.

Cochrane Collaboration (n. d.). Retrieved September 30, 2011, from http://www.cochrane.org/about-us/get-involved#REG

Craig, T., & Pathare, S. (1997). Assertive community treatment for the severely mentally ill in West Lambeth. *Advances in Psychiatric Treatment, 3,* 111–118.

Crane, G. E. (1973). Clinical psychopharmacology in its 20th year. *Science, 181,* 124–128.

Davis, J. M. (1965). Efficacy of tranquilizing and antidepressant drugs. *Archives of General Psychiatry, 13,* 552–572.

Dennis, D. L., & Monahan, J. (Eds.). (1996). *Coercion and aggressive community treatment.* New York: Plenum Press.

Diamond, R. J. (1996). Coercion and tenacious treatment in the community. In D. L. Dennis & J. Monahan (Eds.), *Coercion and aggressive community treatment* (pp. 51–72). New York: Plenum Press.

Dictionary.Com (2011). Retrieved October 11, 2011, from http://dictionary.reference.com/browse/panchreston

Dieterich, M., Irving, C. B., Park, B. & Marshall, M. (2011). Intensive case management for severe mental illness (Review). *The Cochrane Library, 2,* 1–243.

Drake, R. E., Goldman, H.H., Leff, H.S., Lehman, A.F., Dixon, L., Mueser, K. T., & Torrey, W. C. (2001). Implementing evidence-based practices in routine mental health service settings. *Psychiatric Services, 52,* 179–182.

Essock, S. M., Drake, R. E., & Burns, B. J. (1998). A research network to evaluate assertive community treatment: Introduction. *American Journal of Orthopsychiatry, 68* (2), 176–178.

Essock, S. M., Goldman, H. H., Van Tosh, L., Anthony, W. A., Appell, C. R., Bond, G. R., Dixon, L. B., Dunakin, L. K., Ganju, V., Gorman, P. G., Ralph, R. O., Rapp, C. A., Teague, G. B., & Drake, R. E. (2003). Evidence-based practices: Setting the context and responding to concerns. *Psychiatric Clinics of North America, 26,* 919–938.

Farrelly, F., & Brandsma, J. (1974). *Provocative therapy.* Cupertino, CA: Meta Publications, Inc.

Feinstein, A. R. (1995). Meta-analysis: Statistical alchemy for the 21st century. *Journal of Clinical Epidemiology, 48,* 71–79.

Feinstein, A. R., & Horwitz, R. I. (1997). Problems in the "evidence" of "evidence-based medicine." *American Journal of Medicine, 103,* 529–535.

Flaum, M. (2007). Update on evidence-based practices in Iowa's public mental health system. Iowa: The Iowa Consortium for Mental Health.

Florida. (2010). Retrieved September 15, 2011, from http://www.flhsmv.gov/reports/2010UTCStats/UTCStats.html

Frances, A. (2012, August 8) A clinical reality check. Retrieved October 15, 2012, from http://www.cato-unbound.org/2012/08/08/allen-frances/a-clinical-reality-check/

Gambrill, E. (1999). Evidence-based practice: An alternative to authority-based practice. *Families in Society, 80,* 341–350.

Garfield, R. L. (2011). *Mental health financing in the United States: A primer.* Washington, DC: Kaiser Commission on Medicaid and the Uninsured.

Geller, J. L. (2012) Patient-centered, recovery-oriented psychiatric care and treatment are not always voluntary. *Psychiatric Services, 63*(5), 493–495.

Gelman, S. (1999). *Medicating schizophrenia: A history.* New Brunswick, NJ: Rutgers University Press.

Goffman, E. (1961). *Asylums: Essays on the social situation of mental patients and other inmates.* Garden City, NY: Doubleday & Company, Inc.

Gomory, T., Wong, S. E., Cohen, D., & Lacasse, J. R. (2011). Clinical social work and the biomedical industrial complex. *Journal of Sociology & Social Welfare, 38,* 135–166.

Grob, G. N. (1991). *From asylum to community: Mental health policy in modern America.* Princeton, NJ: Princeton University Press.

Grob, G. N. (1994). *The mad among us: A history of the care of America's mentally ill.* Cambridge, MA: Harvard University Press.

Gronfein, W. (1985). Psychotropic drugs and the origins of deinstitutionalization. *Social Problems, 32,* 437–454.

Gupta, M. (2003). A critical appraisal of evidence-based medicine: Some ethical considerations. *Journal of Evaluation in Clinical Practice, 9,* 111–121.

Haynes, R. B. (2002). What kind of evidence is it that evidence-based medicine advocates want health care providers and consumers to pay attention to? *BMC Health Services Research, 2,* 1–7.

Healy, D., & Farquahr, G. (1998). Immediate effects of droperidol. *Human Psychopharmacology: Clinical and Experimental, 13,* 113–120.

Hoult, J. (1986). Community care of the acutely mentally ill. *British Journal of Psychiatry, 149,* 137–144.

Hoult, J., Reynolds, I., Charbonneau-Powis, M., Weekes, P., & Briggs, J. (1983). Psychiatric hospital versus community treatment: The result of a randomized trial. *Australian and New Zealand Journal of Psychiatry, 17,* 160–167.

Joint Commission on Mental Illness and Health. (1961). *Action for mental health.* New York: Basic Books.

Kallert, T. W., Mezzich, J. E., & Monahan, J. (Eds.). (2011). *Coercive treatment in psychiatry: Clinical, legal and ethical aspects.* New York: John Wiley & Sons.

Kessler, R. C., & Zhao, S. (1999). The prevalence of mental illness. In A. V. Horwitz & T. L. Scheid (Eds.), *A handbook for the study of mental health: Social contexts, theories, and systems* (pp. 58–78). Cambridge, UK: Cambridge University Press.

Kirk, S. A., & Kutchins, H. (1992). *The selling of DSM.* New York: Aldine De Gruyter.

Kuntz, C. (1995). *Persons with severe mental illness: How do they fit into long-term care?* Rockville, MD: US Department of Health and Human Services.

Lehman, R., & Loder, E. (2012). Missing clinical data: A threat to the integrity of evidence based medicine. *BMJ, 344,* d8158.

LewinGroup. (2000). *Assertive community treatment literature review.* Falls Church, VA: Lewin Group.

Lieberman, J. A., Stroup, T. S., McEvoy, J. P., Swartz, M. S., Rosenheck, R. A., Perkins, D. O., et al. (2005). Effectiveness of antipsychotic drugs in patients with chronic schizophrenia. *New England Journal of Medicine, 353,* 1209–1223.

Ludwig, A. M., & Farrelly, F. (1966). The code of chronicity. *Archives of General Psychiatry, 15,* 562–568.

Ludwig, A. M., & Farrelly, F. (1967). The weapons of insanity. *American Journal of Psychotherapy, 21,* 737–749.

Ludwig, A. M., Marx, A. J., Hill, P. A., & Browning, R. M. (1969). The control of violent behavior through faradic shock. *Journal of Nervous and Mental Disease, 148,* 624–637.

Manderscheid, R.W., & Berry, J.T. (Eds.). (2006). *Mental health, United States, 2004.* Rockville, MD: Substance Abuse and Mental Health Services Administration.

Marx, A. J., Test, M. A., & Stein, L. I. (1973). Extrahospital management of severe mental illness. *Archives of General Psychiatry, 29,* 505–511.

McGrew, J. H., Wilson, R. G., & Bond, G. R. (1996). Client perspectives on helpful ingredients of assertive community treatment. *Psychiatric Rehabilitation Journal, 19,* 13–21.

Mendota State Mental Health Institute. (2011). Retrieved August 20, 2011, from http://www.dhs.wisconsin.gov/MH_Mendota/Programs/civil/Civil.htm

Minghella, E., Gauntlett, N., & Ford, R. (2002). Assertive outreach: Does it reach expectations? *Journal of Mental Health, 11,* 27–42.

Monahan, J. (2008). Mandated community treatment: Applying leverage to achieve adherence. *Journal of the American Academy of Psychiatry and the Law, 36,* 282–285.

Monahan, J., Redlich, A. D., Swanson, J., Robbins, P. C., Appelbaum, P. S., Petrila, J., Steadman, H. J., Swartz, M., Angell, B., & McNeil, D. E. (2005). Use of leverage to improve adherence to psychiatric treatment in the community. *Psychiatric Services, 56,* 37–44.

Monahan, J., Bonnie, R. J., Appelbaum, P. S., Hyde, P. S., Steadman, H. J., & Swartz, M. S. (2001). Mandated community treatment: Beyond outpatient commitment. *Psychiatric Services, 52,* 1198–1205.

Mueser, K. T., Torrey, W. C., Lynde, D., Singer, P., Drake, R. E. (2003). Implementing evidence-based practices for people with severe mental illness. *Behavior Modification, 27,* 387–411.

National Institute of Mental Health. (2006). *National Institute of Mental Health Alliance for Research Progress July 14, 2006.* Bethesda, MD: Author.

National Institute of Mental Health. (n. d.). Retrieved August 12, 2011, from http://www.nimh.nih.gov/health/publications/the-numbers-count-mental-disorders-in-america/index.shtml#Intro

National Institute of Mental Health. (n.d.). Retrieved August 12, 2011, from http://www.nimh.nih.gov/about/budget/cj2010.shtml#BudAct

National Institute of Mental Health. (n. d.). Retrieved September 11-2011, from http://mentalhealth.gov/about/budget/nimh_approp_history.pdf)

Oakes, M. W. (1987). *Statistical inference: A commentary for the social and behavioural sciences.* New York: John Wiley & Sons.

Oaks, D. W. (2011). The moral imperative for dialogue with organizations of survivors of coerced psychiatric human rights violations. In T. W. Kallert, J. E. Mezzich, & J. Monahan (eds.), *Coercive treatment in psychiatry: Clinical, legal and ethical aspects.* New York: John Wiley and Sons.

Olofsson, B., & Jacobson, L. (2001). A plea for respect: Involuntarily hospitalized psychiatric patients' narratives about being subjected to coercion. *Journal of Psychiatric Mental Health Nursing, 8*(4), 357–366.

Peckham, M. (1979). *Explanation and power: The control of human behavior.* New York: Seabury Press.

Phillips, S. D., Burns, B. J., Edgar, E. R., Mueser, K., Linkins, K. W., Rosenheck, R. A., Drake, R. E., & McDonel Herr, E. C. (2001). Moving assertive community treatment into standard practice. *Psychiatric Services, 52,* 771–779.

Porter, R. (1987b). *Mind-forg'd manacles: A history of madness in England from the Restoration to the Regency.* Cambridge, MA: Harvard University Press.

Rothman, D. J. (1990). *The discovery of the asylum: Social order and disorder in the new republic* (rev. ed.). Boston: Little, Brown.

Rothman, K. J. (Ed.). (1988). *Causal inference.* Chestnut Hill, MA: Epidemiology Resources.

Rothman, K. J., Greenland, S., & Lash, T. L. (2008). *Modern epidemiology* (3rd ed.). New York: Lippincott Williams & Wilkins.

Sackett, D. L. (2002). Clinical epidemiology: What, who and whither. *Journal of Clinical Epidemiology, 55,* 1161–1166.

Sackett, D. L., Rosenberg, W. M. C., Gray, J. A. M., Haynes, R. B., & Richardson, W. S. (1996). Evidence based medicine: What it is and what it isn't. *BMJ, 312,* 71–72.

Sarteschi, C. M., Vaughn, M. G., & Kim, K. (2011). Assessing the effectiveness of mental health courts: A quantitative review. *Journal of Criminal Justice, 39,* 12–20.

Schaler, J. A. (2012, August 6). Strategies of psychiatric coercion. Retrieved October 15, 2012, from http://www.cato-unbound.org/2012/08/06/jeffrey-a-schaler/strategies-of-psychiatric-coercion/

Scott, J. E. & Dixon, L. B. (1995). Assertive case management for schizophrenia, *Schizophrenia Bulletin, 21,* 657–668.

Scull, A. (1976). The decarceration of the mentally ill: A critical view. *Politics & Society, 6,* 173–212.

Scull, A. (1992). Book review: Mental health policy in modern America. *The Milbank Quarterly, 70,* 557–579.

Scull, A. (1993). *The most solitary of afflictions.* New Haven, CT: Yale University Press.

Sorgaard, K. W. (2007). Satisfaction and coercion among voluntary, persuaded/pressured and committed patients in acute psychiatric treatment. *Scandinavian Journal of Caring Sciences, 21,* 214–219.

Steadman, H. J., Osher, F. C., Robbins, P. C., Case, B., & Samuels, S. (2009). Prevalence of serious mental illness among jail inmates. *Psychiatric Services, 60,* 761–765.

Stein, L. I. (1990). Comments by Leonard Stein. *Hospital and Community Psychiatry, 41,* 649–651.

Stein, L. I., & Diamond, R. J. (1985). The chronic mentally ill and the criminal justice system: When to call the police. *Hospital and Community Psychiatry, 36,* 271–274.

Stein, L. I., & Test, M. A. (1985). *The training in community living model: A decade of experience.* San Francisco: Jossey–Bass.

Swartz, M. S., Swanson, J. W., Kim, M., & Petrila, J. (2006). Use of outpatient commitment or related civil court treatment order in five U.S. communities. *Psychiatric Services, 57,* 343–349.

Tanenbaum, S. J. (2006). Evidence by any other name. Commentary on Tonelli (2006) integrating evidence into clinical practice: An alternative to evidence-based approaches. *Journal of Evaluation in Clinical Practice, 12,* 248–256.

Teague, G. B., Bond, G. R., & Drake, R. E. (1998). Program fidelity in assertive treatment: Development and use of a measure. *American Journal of Ortho-psychiatry, 68,* 216–233.

Test, M. A. (1981). Effective community treatment of the chronically mentally ill: What is necessary? *Journal of Social Issues, 37*(3), 71–86.

Test, M. A. (1992). Training in community living. In R. P. Liberman (Ed.), *Handbook of psychiatric rehabilitation* (pp. 153–170). New York: Macmillan Publishing.

Test, M. A., & Stein, L. I. (1976). Practical guidelines for the community treatment of markedly impaired patients. *Community Mental Health Journal, 12,* 72–82.

Test, M. A., & Stein, L. I. (1978). Community treatment of the chronic patient: Research overview. *Schizophrenia Bulletin, 4,* 350–364.

Test, M. A., & Stein, L. I. (2001). A critique of the effectiveness of assertive community treatment: A reply. *Psychiatric Services, 52* (10), 1396.

Test, M. A., Knoedler, W. H., Allness, D. J., Kameshima, S., Burke, S. S., & Rounds, L. (1994, May). *Long-term care of schizophrenia: Seven year results.* Paper presented at the Annual Meeting of the American Psychiatric Association, Philadelphia, PA.

The Evidence-Based Medicine Working Group. (1992). Evidence-based medicine. A new approach to teaching the practice of medicine. *JAMA, 268*(17), 2420–2425.

Tonelli, M. R. (2006). Integrating evidence into clinical practice: An alternative to evidence-based approaches. *Journal of Evaluation in Clinical Practice, 12,* 248–256.

Williams, D. D. R., & Garner, J. (2002). The case against 'the evidence': A different perspective on evidence-based medicine. *British Journal of Psychiatry, 180,* 8–12.

Wolf, N. (2000). Using randomized controlled trials to evaluate socially complex services: Problems, challenges and recommendations. *Journal of Mental Health Policy and Economics, 3,* 97–109.

4

And *DSM* Said: Let There Be Disorder

DSM-III exemplified the antiscientific and irrational approach to perfection; it does not discuss or argue, but lays down the law as if it were dealing with a paradigm which no rational person could quarrel with. The fact that such an approach and such an empty, atheoretical, and antiexperimental system can find acceptance in psychiatry says more about the nature of modern psychiatry than any critic, however hostile, might be able to say.

Eysenck, 1986, p. 95

Introduction

The *Diagnostic and Statistical Manual of Mental Disorders,* also known as the *DSM*, is owned and published by the American Psychiatric Association, the APA. For sixty years, the manual has been the classification system of mental illness in the United States. It is revised every fifteen years or so by a committee of psychiatrists appointed by the APA.

From 1952 until 1980, the *DSM* never merited serious attention. The manual was a slim, eighty-page, spiral-bound, administrative codebook. Its primary use was to provide code numbers for the diagnoses that patients received in treatment institutions. It was based on the common-sense judgments of a small group of appointed psychiatrists. There was no pretense that *DSM*'s usefulness extended beyond administrative convenience. It was not a textbook used to train mental health professionals, not a guide for research, not a tool to decide who would receive services for personal problems, not an instrument of corporate or public bureaucracies, not the subject of controversy, and certainly not a document whose authors or overseers claimed as a scientific achievement.

That all changed dramatically in 1980 with the publication of the third edition, *DSM-III*. In this chapter and the next one, we will examine that transformation, its scientific claims, its social consequences, and how the manual's weaknesses are being exploited as the controversial fifth edition is being readied for publication in 2013.

The current controversies encompass a concern about the meaning, nature, and boundaries of madness. As described in chapters 1 and 2, even the terms most people use—which do not have satisfying definitions—are controversial: *insanity, mental disease, brain disease, brain-based disorder, psychopathology, mental illness*, and *mental disorder*. These terms refer to some presumed, ill-defined pathological internal condition in individuals that causes personal or social concern. We will continue to use these terms interchangeably, as all of them remain in play in discussions of madness.

The story in this and the next chapter will center on the evolution of the *DSM*, which represents psychiatry's answer to questions about the meaning of madness. Rather than recounting scientific progress in recognizing and fighting disease, as the NIMH and the leaders of the psychiatric establishment might suggest, the story is a multilayered tale of competing interests, professional politics, commercial interests, and pseudoscientific claims. It is also an account of cultural transformation: how a widening array of human anguish, misbehavior, and travail has come to be viewed as the result of brain disease.

Psychiatrists, although they constitute a minority of mental health workers, literally "own" the contemporary meaning of madness.[1] That ownership is the cornerstone of their profession: its area of responsibility and control. As such, psychiatry must maintain firm control over the meaning of *madness* and ensure that it is shared among experts who recognize it as legitimate and that it remains accepted by the public. In the last forty years, psychiatry periodically has had serious trouble maintaining agreements about the meaning of *madness* and the methods for recognizing it. The common site for those troubles has been the *DSM*. Some historical context will help.

In politics and our personal lives, we tolerate vague language and concepts held together by no more than tacit agreements in order to facilitate social cohesion and avoid potentially interminable disagreements. Scientific inquiry, however, requires that concepts meet higher standards than those expected of political slogans or marketing pitches. Scientific ideas must be subject to systematic, rigorous, and independent scrutiny, verifying that they have a good correspondence with the real world. Psychiatry is the leading mental health profession, and, as in medicine in general, the meaning of the core concept of disease and illness must be broadly shared, specific in content, and have a consistent and verifiable basis in reality. Psychiatrists must establish that they know what mental illness is and are able to recognize people who are mentally ill and those who are not.

In the language of science, having a firm grip on the meaning and recognition of madness requires that any classification of mental illnesses, such as the *DSM*, must possess both reliability and validity. We examine these different but related requirements in this and the following chapter. For now, suffice it to say that the validity of psychiatric diagnoses refers to whether the definition and meaning of *mental illness* can be objectively shown to refer to something that is factually true. The reliability of diagnoses involves establishing whether mental health professionals can independently agree on which diagnosis applies to people evaluated. Agreement among observers, however, does not guarantee truth, because people could agree on something that is factually incorrect. But if people couldn't agree, for example, on who should be diagnosed as bipolar, it makes it very difficult to establish the meaning and nature of that disorder (i.e., the validity of that diagnosis). Reliability should be much easier to establish than validity.

Who Is Mad?

Let us begin with a news story that is typical of how madness is commonly represented in the media. In June 2005, the *New York Times* reported, based on a recently published study (Kessler et al., 1994), that psychiatric researchers had estimated half the American population has had or will have a mental disorder at some time in their life and that more than one quarter of the population had at least one mental disorder in any given year (Carey, 2005). The thrust of the story, and that of many other news reports, is that madness is even more widespread than previously thought, that many people do not recognize their illnesses, and that many of those who are ill are not getting the proper treatment. The striking claim in this instance is the remarkably high proportion of mentally ill that the researchers claimed to have discovered. As described in chapter 2, several generations ago, less than one fifth of one percent of the American population was described as mentally ill—primarily those in state asylums.

The numbers pointing to this epidemic of madness came from a telephone survey of the general population, one of the most influential surveys ever undertaken by psychiatry. Certainly, we are familiar with telephone polls of our political opinions and expected votes in elections, during which our answers are recorded. These polls are usually surprisingly accurate, because people understand the questions and candidly reveal how they intend to vote. The *New York Times* article, however, is addressing a much more complex foundational claim by psychiatry and the NIMH (which sponsored the research); namely, that researchers can ask people a few questions, actually identify if they are mad, and distinguish one form of madness from another.

Psychiatric telephone interviews, such as the one reported, do not ask respondents if they think that they are mentally ill or about which mental illnesses they have had in the past. Instead, telephone interviewers asked randomly selected adults a series of structured questions about rather common behaviors, derived from long lists of behaviors and emotions that are listed as symptoms of mental disorder in the *DSM*. Computers then counted the responses of those interviewed to determine whether the answers matched the *DSM* criteria to qualify for a mental disorder.

Whether this sort of counting is science or propaganda depends entirely on whether the concept of mental illness represented by *DSM* can withstand scrutiny and whether there is persuasive empirical evidence that the diagnoses of mental illnesses in *DSM* and the criteria that define them are credible and can be used consistently. Thus, the *DSM* with its list of disorders and symptoms is the foundational *scientific* cornerstone on which psychiatry stands.

When public health officials want to check the prevalence of a disease, they typically have some reliable method of determining who has and who does not have the disease. For example, populations are screened, not by asking people questions about their feelings, but by using blood or other biological tests to determine the prevalence of HIV/AIDS, H1N1 influenza, pneumonia, cancer, and many other diseases. That is because the presence of diseases is identified by examining living cells. Not so with the "diseases" of madness. There are no biological tests, markers, or pathophysiology for any of the diagnoses listed in *DSM*.

Even in the twenty-first century, little is known about the presumptive causes of mental disorders in *DSM*. Although the psychiatric establishment increasingly claims that mental disorders have some biological causes and has had considerable success in making the public think that this assertion has been scientifically proven, there is little evidence for this. This particular sleight of hand can be seen in the evolution of *DSM*. In the 1980 and prior editions of *DSM*, the manual set aside a section for "organic mental disorders" (with known etiology, e.g., delirium caused by alcohol withdrawal or dementia caused by a cerebrovascular accident). *DSM* claimed that these disorders were associated with "transient or permanent dysfunction of the brain (APA, 1980, p. 101).

In the most recent edition, the approach is different. The term *organic mental disorder* has been expunged: "The term *organic mental disorder* is no longer used in DSM-IV because it incorrectly implies that 'nonorganic' mental disorders do not have a biological basis" (APA, 2000, p. 135). Little more is said, as if somehow science had established in the intervening twenty years the biological basis for all mental disorders. In one sentence, *DSM* appears to disguise ignorance of the etiology for what it calls mental disorders as firm knowledge of their biological basis. The false implication by the APA is that knowledge of some pathophysiology of neurological diseases such Alzheimer's or observations that some people become physiologically dependent on various drugs are analogous to knowledge of the "biological basis" of all mental disorders listed in *DSM*. We shall have more to say on this issue in this and the chapters that follow.

Who is counted as mentally ill depends entirely on the frequently changing list of disorders and an incredibly long checklist of behaviors, mood states or feelings, and verbalizations that *DSM* considers as symptoms of mental disorder. We and many other scholars (Carlat, 2010; Frances, 2010b;

Greenberg, 2010; Horwitz, 2002; 2010, Horwitz & Wakefield, 2012) argue that there are now higher estimates of mental disorders in the United States because the APA keeps adding new disorders and more behaviors to the diagnostic manual. These are some of the new disorders that have been added to *DSM* since 1979: panic disorder, generalized anxiety disorder, posttraumatic stress disorder, social phobia, borderline personality disorder, substance use disorders, gender identity disorder, eating disorders, conduct disorder, oppositional defiant disorder, identity disorder, acute stress disorder, sleep disorders, nightmare disorder, rumination disorder, and sexual disorders, including inhibited sexual desire disorder, premature ejaculation disorder, male erectile disorder, and female sexual arousal disorder.

Each new and old disorder comes with a list of "diagnostic criteria," the behavioral checklists that constitute the heart of *DSM*. As any reader would quickly recognize, these are not lists of strange, bizarre, or inexplicable behaviors. Rather, they appear to describe behavior and traits frequently self-reported or observed in everyday life. In the *DSM*, however, just about any behavior can qualify as a "symptom." Here is a selection from hundreds of behaviors listed in the *DSM* as criteria of mental illnesses: restlessness, irritability, sleeping too much or too little, eating too much or too little, difficulty concentrating, increasing goal-directed activity, fear of social situations, feeling morose, indecisiveness, impulsivity, self-dramatization, using physical appearance to draw attention to self, being inappropriately sexually seductive or provocative, requiring excessive admiration, having a sense of entitlement, lacking empathy, being envious of others, arrogance, being afraid of being criticized in public, feeling personally inept, being afraid of rejection or disapproval, finding it hard to express disagreement, being excessively devoted to work and productivity, and being preoccupied with details, rules, and lists.

For children, signs of disorder occur when kids are deceitful, break rules, can't sit still or wait in lines, have trouble with math, don't pay attention to details, don't listen, don't do homework, lose their school assignments or pencils, or speak out of turn. Granted, one momentary feeling or behavior is not expected to qualify you officially for a *DSM* mental disorder; it requires small clusters of them, usually for several weeks, accompanied by some claimed serious discomfort to you or those around you. Nevertheless, these additional criteria are regularly ignored when there are perceived short-term benefits to be gained from diagnosing someone with a mental disorder.

These new illnesses and extensive lists of behaviors are part of the reason why almost everyone has by now noted that there appears to be an epidemic of mental disorders in the United States (Whitaker, 2010). But the manufactured epidemic is about to spread even further. In the early draft of *DSM-5* (February 2010) are proposals to broaden the definition of *mental disorder*, lower the thresholds for many disorder categories, and create even more illnesses—though a few existing disorders are also slated for termination.

We will have more to say about these matters later in this and the next chapter. Such expansion has its skeptics, who are suspicious of the motivations of the APA and the drug companies, who view the expanding sweep of mental disorders like a lumber company lusts for redwood forests. But unlike typical challenges to the physical or political environment, in the mental health arena there are no legions of watchdogs challenging this medicalization of human foibles. The public's acquiescence in accepting brain disease as an explanation for personal troubles is a puzzle that we will address later. For now, we should review how a small, largely ignored administrative codebook became a massive compendium of human troubles that reshaped psychiatry, mental health services, and the public culture. Although the psychiatric enterprise claimed that this transformation was based on science, we will see that, again, the scientific evidence is elusive.

A Short History of Psychiatric Diagnosis

During the middle of the twentieth century, American psychiatry was heavily influenced by psychoanalysis and paid little attention to official classifications of mental disorders. Diagnostic categories were of minor importance, useful more for administrative counting purposes, first in state asylums and later in clinics (e.g., see *DSM-I* and *DSM-II*). Diagnostic labels (such as Hysterical Personality or Depressive Neurosis, from *DSM-II*) were not emphasized in treatment, research, or training in any of the mental health professions. Diagnoses were uninteresting and banal, except as administrative shorthand or as a way to discuss the more interesting psychological dynamics in a patient's biography and, most importantly, were never claimed to be scientifically valid.

In an ethnographic study of the training of psychiatrists, the anthropologist T. M. Luhrmann (2000) captures the mind-set of those learning to be psychodynamic psychotherapists. Such a psychiatrist

> . . . learns to construct complex accounts of his patients' loves. He thinks in terms of the way his patients are with other people and in terms of the emotions and unconscious motivations that lead his patients to hurt themselves. Here there is no clear-cut line between health and illness. What is wrong with a patient is that his interactions with other people go or have gone awry, and being a good psychiatrist involves understanding how and why. (p. 83)

By contrast, Luhrmann observed that the biomedical, post-*DSM-III* psychiatrist in training

> . . . learns to memorize patterns and starts to use them in a rough-and-ready way. He learns to think in terms of disease and to see those diseases as quickly and as convincingly as a bird-watcher

> identifies different birds. For him, what is wrong with a patient is that the patient has a disease, and being a good psychiatrist involves seeing the patient in terms of the disease. For him there is a clear-cut difference between illness and health. (p. 83)

Until 1980 mental disorders were defined as whatever a committee of psychiatrists listed in the *DSM*. No definition of *mental illness* or *mental disorder* was offered in the manual, and few people were troubled by the absence. The public seemed content to leave the matter to the discretion of psychiatrists. Even without a definition and only vague descriptions in the manual, troubled people were referred to mental health providers, patients received diagnoses and were treated, students were recruited and trained to offer therapies, and research about madness continued to receive funding. In fact, as we describe in chapter 2, the size and scope of the psychiatric enterprise grew briskly following World War II without much clarity about what constituted mental illness or how to distinguish it from a vast array of other problems in living—or even whether it was necessary to make such distinctions.

Developing a definition of madness as mental illness/disorder or establishing its validity, when so little was known scientifically about it, was a conceptual and practical morass. As long as no one demanded clarity, ambiguity had advantages that precision of thought might lose. For example, without any scientific or conceptual guidance, the early editions of the *DSM* published in 1952 (*DSM-I*) and 1968 (*DSM-II*) were at liberty to list all manner of mental disorder categories, such as Inadequate Personality, Gross Stress Reaction, Group Delinquent Reaction of Childhood, and Homosexuality. The manuals were silent on what principles were followed in deciding to include these or any categories. Madness was whatever psychiatrists listed in *DSM*, whether diagnosis with some type of neurosis, psychosis, affective or personality disorder, or one of the "transient situational disturbances," most of which came with only several sentences of description. Notably, there was little public or professional concern regarding psychiatry's singular authority over these matters.

Psychiatric diagnosis is a form of classification, an attempt to group human behaviors that may be disturbing or unwanted into categories of disease that appear to or actually share essential features (a conjunctive category, as discussed in chapter 2). Classification is essential for all science. There could be many bases of classification of diseases in medicine and psychiatry, but the most profound categorizations are grounded in an understanding of the causes of disease (their etiology), because such categories may suggest effective approaches to prevent or treat what is obviously undesirable. Developing a classification of mental disorders based on causes, however, has been impossible for several reasons. First, we don't know what madness is, whether it exists as an entity, whether what are labeled as mental illnesses are "illnesses" in any medically valid sense, or whether the concept itself is a semantic trash bin for all that is behaviorally inexplicable (a disjunctive category, as also discussed in chapter 2). Second, one can't discover causes for something one can't define or identify. Third, one might classify according to the essential *features* or characteristics of the disorders, but there has been virtually no agreement throughout history and even in the modern age, about what these essential features might be—as the changing diagnostic criteria themselves of the *DSM*s over only the past thirty years testify. Nonetheless, as we have seen in chapter 2, putative classifications of madness have existed since ancient times (Zilboorg, 1941). During the twentieth century, two dominant approaches to diagnosis coexisted, each spawned by men born in 1856: Emil Kraepelin and Sigmund Freud.

Creating a Disease

Emil Kraepelin (1856–1926) was a German physician who developed the hypothetical construct of dementia praecox, from which the construct of schizophrenia is derived. Kraepelin postulated the existence of dementia praecox as some kind of metabolic disorder as he went about studying patients in his asylum whom he thought suffered from the disorder (Boyle, 2002, pp. 3ff). The asylum inmates were a heterogeneous population of imprisoned people with a variety of problems who exhibited a diversity of behaviors. Kraepelin's general approach was to observe the inmates' behaviors to find similarities in the way the behaviors changed over time. He wanted to study the whole course of the presumed disease in order to discover distinctive patterns, natural groupings, or entities. He believed that the behavioral patterns he hoped to find would later be discovered to have distinctive biological antecedents and cerebral pathology, as well as a similar onset, course, and outcome (Boyle, 2002, p. 11).[2] In this particular ambition, he failed. But what he succeeded in accomplishing was the creation of an illness label—dementia praecox—which he and other interested physicians presumed to represent a discrete disorder with some underlying biological cause modeled in part on another presumed mental illness, general paresis, which later was found to be a late stage of the brain disease neurosyphilis. His observations and descriptions of those he assumed had dementia praecox did not constitute scientific evidence that dementia praecox existed as a discrete entity. Its existence was presumed a priori (Boyle, 2002, p. 49). This tactic has been used with all subsequent psychiatric diagnoses, none of which were grounded on any convincing evidence of ontological reality.

Kraepelin's approach allowed a fundamental confusion to occur, blurring the difference between, on the one hand, establishing scientifically the existence of a disease by noting within the general population a previously unobserved and non-randomly occurring discrete grouping of physical signs (a syndrome), and on the other hand, assuming the existence of a disease and then describing various odd and disturbing social behaviors as symptomatic of this construction. This confusion provided a platform in the 1970s for the emergence of the expansion of psychiatric diagnosis. As we will see, Kraepelin (and those later referred to as neo-Kraepelinians) labeled selected troublesome or unusual behaviors the symptoms of hypothetical diseases and then took these symptoms as evidence of the existence of the disease, leaving for later the discovery of the hypothesized causative connections between these "symptoms" and the disease. Making these huge leaps possible is the expectation that at some future point the physical evidence of these diseases will be known, as occurred in the past when new technologies or methods, such as autopsies, provided ways of peering into the body itself and uncovered evidence for physical pathology or brain lesions. Indeed, throughout the twentieth century, new technologies were being developed. The discovery of microorganisms by Pasteur, Koch, and others led to the delineation of many clinical diseases and their prevention. Later with X-rays, biochemical tests, and diagnostic radiology, the biological confirmation of the correlations between pathological processes and clinical symptoms could be established. Specific biological tests, such as the Wassermann Test for syphilis, were then developed as the definitive methods of documenting internal pathology (Klerman, 1986, pp. 11–12). Kraepelin's approach to classification was through detailed description of the *behaviors* constituting presumed diseases, the existence of which was left for future medical researchers to document scientifically. His process was to assume that some particular disease existed, identify people who presumably had the disease, then describe their unusual or problematic behaviors and their evolution. We will discuss the contemporary counterpart of this approach shortly.

Making Madness Normal

A contemporary of Kraepelin, Sigmund Freud (1856–1939) was a neurologist also interested in bizarre behaviors. Unlike Kraepelin, however, Freud's work would make him a household word and cultural icon by the middle of the twentieth century. His work not only influenced psychiatric theory and the mental health professions, but culture, art, and literature around the world, whereas Kraepelin remained known only to a few psychiatric scholars.

Unlike Kraepelin, however, Freud's clinical work was not among patients in asylums, but among individual outpatients with less severe problems, in the sense that these problems rarely brought them into open conflicts with authorities. More important, Freud's adult patients could hire and pay him directly and be free to reject his diagnoses or advice if they so wished— something none of Kraepelin's patients/inmates could possibly do. Freud had little interest in classification or the detailed description of symptom patterns. The studies were intensive, in-depth, conversational explorations of what Freud speculated were the intrapsychic worlds of patients. By means of his case studies and conversations, which he later renamed psychoanalysis, Freud explored the presumed psychological and cultural dynamics of human behavior, in particular how hypothesized instinctive, biological urges of humans interacted with the demands of civilization to shape human character. Whereas Kraepelin was a describer and classifier of bizarre, stigmatized, and unwanted behaviors, Freud was a theoretician of the human condition itself. Whereas Kraepelin was interested in the madness and degenerative brain diseases affecting people sent to insane asylums, Freud attempted to explain the psychodynamics of everyday life and civilization.

Freud asserted that curious, strange, or seemingly harmless behavior was potentially an expression of psychopathology. Even though his theories of mind and psychopathology have fallen out of fashion in most countries, a devoted core of his followers, with modified psychodynamic approaches, remains and in certain places thrives, and his work continues to have a lasting impact on psychiatric diagnosis. There are three main elements to his contemporary influence.

First was his ability to make us suspicious about the meaning of behavior. Nothing was what it seemed. Ostensibly loving behaviors could mask aggression; fastidiousness could cover impending disorderliness; a slip of the tongue could harbor clues to unconscious, perverted desires. Using the invented notions of unconscious desires and psychic conflicts; the tug-of-war of id, ego, and superego; and the control functions of defense mechanisms, he argued that what we consciously espouse and how we behave is unconsciously connected to the same psychological dynamics that cause more obvious and severe problems. Psychopathology, he suggested, could be lying just beneath the surface of our most mundane behaviors and feelings. Every behavior might be a possible symptom of latent mental illness.

The second element to his contemporary influence is related to the first. If any behavior might be a symptom, then potentially everyone might be a little mad. In suggesting that psychopathology was part of the bargain of being human, Freud, in *Civilization and Its Discontents,* explained madness as an expected and inevitable part of life. The psychic energy and unconscious conflicts that were required to repress our most primitive urges so that human society was possible, he conjectured, affected our cognitive and emotional lives in ways that could produce anxieties, emotional turmoil, and troublesome or inexplicable behaviors. To resolve these dysfunctional conflicts and subdue the troubling symptoms, Freud and his followers proposed, required in-depth psychoanalysis. The popularity of psychoanalysis grew into a burgeoning potpourri of therapies by the 1970s, not only for the "worried well" and middle class, but for those exhibiting bizarre behaviors. Although the evidence for the "effectiveness" of these therapies or their comparative advantages remained scientifically thin, seeing common behaviors as psychopathology grew in popularity. (In chapter 6 we will see that this is similar to the later popularity of drugs: abundant but thin scientific evidence and growing popularity.)

The third way in which Freud transformed how we viewed disturbing behavior was to further medicalize it. As a neurologist, Freud relied on the language and methods of medicine to understand and describe human behaviors. The medical language of "psychopathology" largely supplanted other forms of discourse about human troubles (e.g., the moral, the spiritual, the legal). Undesirable behaviors, such as excessive elation, sexual interest in children, aggressiveness, or heavy drinking, instead of being viewed as unwise, immoral, criminal, or sinful—the product of poor upbringing, weak character, or willful deviance—were transformed into expressions of illnesses of the psyche (or the more familiar reification, mind). Using the idiom of medicine, Freud may have surmised, allowed for seemingly simple explanations that would deeply resonate with people. Conveniently, Freud offered a remedy—his own style of treatment. Patients had illnesses which were not entirely controllable on their own. Those afflicted were not fully responsible for their actions, being based on activity in the "unconscious." Their behaviors were not willed, any more than getting pneumonia or polio makes a person culpable. People with troubles should seek treatment. Freud's later insight (Freud, 1969, p. 92), that the work of the psychoanalyst was like that of "secular pastoral work," has often been repeated but was drowned by the more powerful mythic image of the physician manipulating unconscious material and restoring the helpless patient to healthy functioning.

In different ways Kraepelin and Freud prepared American culture for the great transformation in psychiatric diagnoses that began in the 1970s and fully bloomed after the publication of *DSM-III* in 1980. What they both contributed was a way to classify hypothesized mental disorders by minute descriptions of the behaviors of those thought to be afflicted, a large list of labels for presumed illnesses, the use of medical and medical-sounding language to describe hypothesized groupings of common behaviors as *psychopathology*, and the notion that countless forms of psychopathology—mental illnesses—were ubiquitous among the populace, lying beneath the surface and requiring medical detection and treatment.

The Vulnerabilities of Mid-Century Psychiatry

By the mid-1950s, with the help of Kraepelin and Freud, American psychiatry had acquired a vast territory of behaviors as its appropriate domain. By 1960 mental disorders had entered the mainstream of American life, under the jurisdiction of the newly established National Institute of Mental Health and the subject of a major report (Joint Commission, 1961) of a presidential commission appointed by Dwight Eisenhower and President Kennedy's mental health initiatives on establishing community mental health centers across the nation. There were troubling currents, however, within this recognition and expansion of psychiatry.

American psychiatry was always a peculiar profession, whose members initially were the managers of state insane asylums. Within medicine, psychiatry was situated at the bottom of the totem pole of medical specialties. For the general US public, which typically venerate physicians and accord them power and status much higher than physicians have enjoyed in other industrial countries, psychiatrists—shrinks—were frequently the butt of jokes and were depicted in movies and television as impish inquisitors quick to make wild and seemingly nutty inferences about the underlying motivations of everyday troubles but also willing to use coercion and brutality (see, for example, the 1948 movie, *The Snake Pit*). This occasional disparagement reflected an ambivalent acceptance of the expanded domain of psychiatry and psychoanalysis and recognition of the overt coercive functions of psychiatrists.

Even Freud's success in influencing American psychiatry was a two-edged sword. On the one hand, problems labeled as mental illness gained more national attention. On the other hand, the methods of treatment proposed by psychoanalysts looked like one-sided, unstructured, nonmedical conversations. For example, psychoanalytic treatment involved no physical examination, no stethoscope or other medical instruments, no probes of the body or laboratory tests to determine the nature of the ailment or its disappearance. Instead, the therapy required that the patient merely lie on a couch and talk to the analyst, who would occasionally make a comment or ask a question. The invention of this sort of "talking therapy" was a creative attempt to reframe interpersonal help giving. Talking to others about personal problems, however, was hardly novel. It was a universal behavior used by troubled people in soliciting help from family, friends, clergy, and counselors of all kinds. As we described in chapter 2, psychoanalysis and its psychotherapy offshoots had the challenge of reinventing talking and discussion as an instrument of medical treatment.

Although Freud was a physician, offering talking therapy did not require the therapist to have the skills of medical doctors, and even Freud, as we mentioned, thought that it was akin to pastoral counseling. The expansion of outpatient, office-based psychotherapy made psychiatric treatment more accessible for many people, but it also attracted the involvement of other nonphysicians as purveyors of mental health treatment. Starting with funding to World War II veterans from the GI bill, clinically oriented psychologists, social workers, and various counselors swarmed to the growing enterprise, far outnumbering psychiatrists (Goleman, 1990). The threat was not so much that other professions competed for scarce patients, but that these competitors brought with them various nonmedical interventions that they systematized as therapies, such as family therapy, gestalt therapy, milieu therapy, reality therapy, cognitive-behavioral therapy, and many, many others. These new forms of interpersonal helping, often used by psychiatrists as well, further de-medicalized therapy, showing that mental disorders and their treatment need not be the unique province of medicine or psychiatry. Could not a social worker as well as a psychiatrist help a family with an unruly child or a substance-abusing spouse? What, if any, unique role did psychiatrists play with regard to troubled clients who were not seen to need modification by drugs or electroshock? How were medical credentials and training relevant to the new, popular interventions?

By the 1960s psychiatry had succeeded in expanding its domain and acquiring new federal recognition. With the increased political salience, however, came increased scrutiny of its scientific grounding, effectiveness, and social purposes. At the historic moment of psychiatry's broader influence and institutional expansion, the essential core of the psychiatric enterprise came under attack, producing a broad crisis for the profession. The center of this crisis revolved around the seemingly simple, internal matter of the definition and diagnosis of mental disorder.

The Perfect Psychiatric Storm

Despite its greater prominence by 1960, psychiatry was still less prestigious than other fields of medicine, in which there were scientific discoveries of the causes of common diseases and breakthroughs in the prevention and effective treatment of many of them, such as the development of antibiotics and the near eradication of polio with a vaccine. In psychiatry, there were few solid examples of scientific "progress" or breakthrough discoveries, and, despite its political success, psychiatry remained a low-status branch of medicine. Furthermore, with the movement away from institutional care in state hospitals and toward community treatment (see chapter 3), psychiatry's identity was blending into the amorphous, somewhat undifferentiated mental health professions.

In part, these shortcomings of psychiatry stemmed from the fact that American psychiatry never needed to have a strong scientific infrastructure. Most psychiatric residents were trained to be therapists rather than scholars and researchers. Because Freud and his many adherents relied on case studies of individual patients, there was no well-established public health tradition of either epidemiological studies of the incidence and prevalence of mental disorders in the broad populations or of comparative clinical trials—carefully controlled experiments of the outcomes of different treatments.

At the same time, the massive discharge of residents of state asylums and the broad promises and claims about the wonders of community treatment (see chapter 3 for details) produced visibility that wasn't sought. For example, by the early 1970s there were constant news stories about the emergence of the visible homeless, many of whom might have resided in asylums in prior decades. In addition, doubts were raised about the clinical effectiveness or practicality of psychoanalytic therapy (Eysenck, 1952). But profound new challenges were brewing. The challenges came from many quarters and shook the foundations of psychiatry, particularly its scientific credibility, and created the perfect psychiatric storm. The questions had been around the halls of academia for decades but had generally been ignored. What exactly was mental illness? Why was it considered to lie within the jurisdiction of medicine? What evidence existed that psychiatrists could distinguish the mentally ill from the sane in ways that ordinary people could not? Paradoxically, Freud's legacy had so broadened the meaning of madness that psychiatry's primary construct had become even more ambiguous. (Although in America psychoanalysis had initially coupled with psychiatry, requiring psychoanalysts to possess a medical degree and usually a psychiatric specialty, in most of the rest of the world, professionals of all stripes and even laypersons could call themselves psychoanalysts after a course of study and personal analysis.) Within psychiatry itself, some mainstream figures recognized that the profession, on the verge of becoming more nationally prominent, was vulnerable in terms of its ability to define, identify, and diagnose mental illness (Kendell, 1975; Zigler & Phillips, 1961). Psychiatry's vulnerability was revealed sharply by a number of frontal assaults within a decade.

Assaults from the Academy

The physician and psychoanalyst Thomas Szasz, who became the most persistent and prolific critic of institutional psychiatry, argued vigorously that what psychiatrists were calling mental illnesses had no underlying physiological dysfunctions but were personally or socially unwanted, unpleasant, devalued behaviors (Szasz, 1961). Mental illnesses, Szasz argued, were just the latest nineteenth- and twentieth-century bogus claims by psychiatrists for defining as "medical" problems what were in reality, social, economic, ethical, and moral problems that all individuals face in the course of fashioning their existence and attempting to assert their autonomy. He asserted that mental illness is a "myth," in the sense that it is only a metaphor, an inappropriate analogy for describing human problems in living as if they constituted medical diseases, but he was not denying that these problems existed. This was a frontal attack on the Kraepelinian ambition. Szasz's publications quickly became some of the most widely read and cited critiques of psychiatry. His attack hit a nerve among psychiatrists, because no consensus existed on a definition of *mental illness,* and no physical evidence existed for classifying problems in living as bodily diseases requiring the attention of physicians. Although Szasz was quickly marginalized by the psychiatric establishment, his arguments were not easily rebutted and, partly because of his prodigious output and his longevity (1920–2012), still persist in the vigorous contemporary debates about psychiatric diagnosis, as they do in this book.

Social and behavioral scientists of many stripes joined the assault. Sociologists who had an interest in social responses to deviant behavior pushed the criticism of psychiatry further. Erving Goffman, with his collection of illuminating essays, *Asylums: Essays on the Social Situation of Mental Patients and Other Inmates*, was one of the first to cast a skeptical eye on psychiatric practices (Goffman, 1961). State hospitals were categorized, not with other medical institutions, but with "total institutions," such as prisons, monasteries, and battleships, in which near total control over every aspect of the lives of inmates transforms their identities. Within these institutions, patients had "moral careers" and had to devise ways of coping as they contended with the "daily round of petty contingencies to which they were subject" (p. x). Psychiatrists were part of the "tinkering trades," tinkering with hospitalized patients and their problems. As his language makes clear, Goffman debunked psychiatric practice, placing it not in the realm of science and medicine but squarely among agencies of coercive social control in charge of managing unsightly, unpleasant, and unwanted behavior.

This was a consistent theme among many other sociologists at the time, who discussed psychiatric treatment squarely as another form of social control, albeit under the guise of treatment, and theorized about its possible harms to people who might get labeled as mentally ill, including stigma and social rejection. One particularly provocative and widely read sociologist, Thomas Scheff (1966), proposed that mental illness was a form of "residual deviance," a mere collection of unusual behaviors that fit into no other social categories. Further, he suggested that being labeled as mentally ill could set in place a chain of social dynamics that could produce the very problems that psychiatrists were trying to treat. Scheff took the heart of psychiatrists' domain—the construct of mental illness—and insisted that it really served as a mask for society's ignorance about the nature of these unusual behaviors. Psychiatric diagnoses were only fancy labels for describing behaviors that baffled the public and mental health professionals.

Such disconcerting critiques of psychiatry came from other academic quarters as well. Foucault's *Madness and Civilization* (1965), Ivan Illich's *Medical Nemesis* (1975), and other popular works offered powerful critiques of psychiatry and medicine applied to the social world. R. D. Laing in *The Politics of Experience* (1967) turned madness on its head by suggesting that schizophrenia was an adaptive response to a disordered society. One young psychiatrist argued that psychiatry and the medical model it had adopted were dying and deserved a good Irish wake (Torrey, 1974).[3] These cultural critiques of psychiatry coincided with criticism that came from behavioral psychologists (Eysenck, 1952; Ullmann & Krasner, 1969), who argued that some of the "truths" of psychoanalytic theory (still at that time the main adopted paradigm of academic psychiatry) were bogus and that psychiatric practice appeared to be therapeutically ineffective.

Overall, these critiques targeted the heart of psychiatry. They suggested that psychiatry's core concepts were myths, that psychiatry's relationship to medical science had only historical connections, that psychiatry was more aptly characterized as a vast system of coercive social management, and that its paradigmatic practice methods (the talking cure and psychiatric confinement) were ineffective or worse.

For a decade or so, these criticisms stayed confined to academic debates among scholars critically sifting through evidence and arguments in the struggle to assert their views or find the truth. As serious as the conflicts were and as important to the psychiatric enterprise, they were generally ignored or treated as nihilistic. Unfortunately for the American Psychiatric Association, these debates broke into public view in ways that were entirely unexpected and anxiety-provoking to the psychiatric establishment. Two seemingly unrelated challenges to psychiatry erupted within a few years of each other, which opened a Pandora's box of vulnerability.

Public Embarrassment

The first challenge began in June 1969 with a police raid on the Stonewall Bar in New York City's Greenwich Village, a gathering spot for homosexuals. The raid incited a riot in which the gay community fought back, which symbolically marked the beginning of a new, more assertive phase in the struggle for gay rights. Psychiatry was not the target of gay community's wrath, although for some years gay activists had been raising questions with the medical and psychiatry associations about the psychoanalytic interpretations of homosexuality as a form of psychopathology (Bayer, 1981; Bayer & Spitzer, 1982). But within a year of the Stonewall Riot, the gay activists began confronting the American Psychiatric Association openly at its annual meetings, demanding that the APA remove homosexuality as a mental disorder in *DSM*. Most embarrassingly, their challenges were staged to attract media attention, which they did with smashing success. The novelty of the challenge was not lost on the media or the public. At a time when most gays were still in the closet, here was an activist gay group not simply revealing their homosexual identities publicly but challenging the psychiatric profession on scientific grounds. An entire group of people labeled as mentally ill by the American Psychiatric Association was disputing its psychiatric diagnosis. At the core of their challenge was a simple, easy-to-understand question: why was homosexuality a mental illness?

The question revived a serious and complex problem for the APA. What *is* a mental disorder? What are the criteria used to diagnose it? Are these criteria social and moral or medical in nature? What is the rationale for including some deviant behaviors and excluding others as illnesses in the official manual, the *DSM*? The gay community asked publicly and forcefully whether American psychiatry knew the difference between a mental illness and normality or social deviance. It was a question directed at the scientific integrity of psychiatry.

The unwanted media coverage demonstrated that the APA wasn't able to manage public relations nearly as well as the gay activists (Kutchins & Kirk, 1997). The APA and the *DSM* provided no immediate or persuasive answers. The second edition of the *DSM* (*DSM-II*), which was the ostensible target of the dispute, provided no guidance about why homosexuality was listed as a disorder. What was presumably a question that psychiatry had answered on the basis of psychiatric science was unmasked as a question of social values and political negotiations. After several years of embarrassing turmoil and fumbling by the APA, the resolution of the issue came not from science or new research, but from a vote of the members of the APA to drop homosexuality as a mental disorder in *DSM*. While this succeeded in ending the immediate controversy with the gay activists, dropping the diagnosis appeared to confirm that the constructions and the definitions of mental disorders were arbitrary matters—of personal opinions, group politics, and special interests in the APA—rather than matters of medicine, science, and evidence.

As with all political disputes among contending groups, there was behind-the-scenes scheming, negotiation, and compromise. In this case, a little-known psychiatrist from New York, Robert Spitzer, who initially believed that homosexuality was a mental illness, stepped forward as a mediator to manage the conflict about whether the diagnosis should be retained in *DSM*. Over a period of several years beginning in 1972, Spitzer inserted himself into the swirling controversy, meeting with gay activists, APA leaders, and psychiatrists on both sides of the battle on removing homosexuality from the *DSM*. He organized discussion sessions at psychiatric meetings and drafted compromise statements in an attempt to find a presentable rationale for removing the diagnosis from the *DSM*. In the end, he and others politically engineered the settlement to exclude homosexuality as a mental illness (Bayer, 1981; Kutchins & Kirk, 1997). Although the conflict did not disappear altogether for many years, it did bring an end to embarrassing publicity over this dispute. More importantly for Spitzer, he debuted in a role as master of diagnostic disputes, a role that he would reenact many times in the future.

The second eruption came on the heels of the dispute about homosexuality. It was initiated by a cleverly titled article, "Being Sane in Insane Places," that appeared in the world's most prestigious scientific journal, *Science* (Rosenhan, 1973). The article reported a study by Stanford University psychologist David Rosenhan in which he conspired with colleagues and graduate students to get them admitted to several psychiatric hospitals, without the hospitals knowing about the study. The pseudo-patients posed as having a minor symptom (hearing a "thud" sound or the word *empty*) at the emergency room. All were diagnosed as schizophrenic (one as manic-depressive) and hospitalized. All were prescribed medications. During their hospitalizations, the staff did not recognize them as sane or as inappropriately hospitalized, and pathologized many of their ordinary behaviors, such as asking staff when they would be released or writing their field notes. When discharged, the pseudo-patients were diagnosed with "schizophrenia in remission." Because it was an intriguing, easy-to-understand study and the findings were so striking, it was widely cited. The study reinforced the view that psychiatric judgments were not merely inadequate but almost laughable. Once again, the target of the joke was the scientific pretence of psychiatric diagnosis: psychiatrists could not distinguish the sane from the insane (or the study demonstrated that it was easy to fake mental illness, at least). Published in *Science*, the study's challenge could not be ignored. And it wasn't.

Two years after the Rosenhan study, a forceful rebuttal and defense of diagnosis appeared in a prominent psychology journal, the *Journal of Abnormal Psychology*, written by Robert Spitzer (1975), who himself had become concerned about the scientific basis of psychiatric diagnosis. By 1975, however, Spitzer was assuming a leadership role to revise the *DSM* for the American Psychiatric Association. He used the controversy created by Rosenhan's article to not only defend psychiatry, but to advance his own, as yet still private, agenda in reforming the diagnostic manual.

Rise of an Entrepreneur of Controversy

Robert Spitzer was a most unlikely rescuer of American psychiatry. His contribution to psychiatric history in the late twentieth century was not for developing some innovative theory of mental disorder, a new therapeutic approach, influential teaching, or significant scientific research. Nor was it established by his personal pedigree. His place in psychiatric history came about partially by chance and very much because of his bureaucratic persistence, single-mindedness, intelligence, and robust skills as a political actor. His major achievement, as first glimpsed in the homosexuality and Rosenhan disputes, was as an entrepreneur of diagnostic controversies. The achievement reaches its height as he created and managed a daunting series of political compromises between 1975 and 1980 that resulted in the landmark third edition of the diagnostic manual, the modern *DSM* (APA, 1980), which established the character of *DSM* for over thirty years into our day. He achieved this feat by working tirelessly on the technical classification of mental disorders, a task peripheral to psychiatric practitioners and largely ignored in academic psychiatry.

In 1966, Spitzer, who had trained as a psychoanalyst, became associated with this obscure codebook almost by accident in the Columbia University cafeteria while chatting with a colleague, Ernest Gruenberg, who was chairing the small group appointed to update the first 1952 edition of *DSM* (APA, 1952). Gruenberg invited Spitzer, who had no particular expertise regarding diagnosis, to be notetaker on the *DSM-II* committee. He did well in that role, and, when *DSM-II* was published in 1968, he was listed as a consultant. He also was called on to author an article describing the new edition to colleagues (Spitzer & Wilson, 1968, 1969). The second edition was infused with psycho-analytic terms and assumptions, reflecting the theoretical orientation of the leaders of the APA. This updating for the second edition of the diagnostic manual received very little notice in psychiatry and almost no publicity. As we have mentioned, classification of mental illness was not viewed as a vital or interesting topic.

But within a few years of the publication of *DSM-II* (1968), with the growing criticism of psychiatry in academic circles, the successful challenge to drop the homosexuality diagnosis, and the Rosenhan article in *Science*, psychiatric diagnosis would unexpectedly become ground zero for a major struggle within psychiatry. Spitzer, who had defended the APA and the *DSM* against the challenges by the gay community and Rosenhan, had made himself the APA's house expert on diagnosis. When in the 1970s, the APA decided it was time to revise the diagnostic manual, it asked Spitzer to serve as chair of the task force to produce the third edition.

At the time, psychoanalysis remained the reigning paradigm, although a re-emerging academic wing within psychiatry was emphasizing biological aspects of behavior and the growing use of psychotropic drugs. Spitzer, however, had become keenly interested in diagnosis and had been prepping for this assignment to revise *DSM*. He took on the task with gusto, taking strategic advantage of the fact that no one expected much from the work of this internal APA committee. As we will explain, the result of his work during the next five years made diagnosis singularly significant in psychiatry; reshaped training, research, and practice; and elevated the status of American psychiatry in ways that were completely unexpected. It also made the APA an unprecedented bundle of money. To many of his research colleagues, Spitzer became a psychiatric hero, "the most important psychiatrist of our time," according to one of his colleagues (Frances, 2010a).

The Rhetoric of Reliability and the Modern *DSM*

Because past revisions of the diagnostic manual were considered of little significance, Spitzer was given a free hand in appointing members to the *DSM-III* task force and to the many committees that were used in revising the manual. Selecting members of the task force was critical to his efforts. He drew heavily on a relatively small group of like-minded research psychiatrists (and a few psychologists) who also had concerns about the weaknesses of the manual (Kirk & Kutchins, 1992; Millon, 1983, 1986; Spiegel, 2005). Under Spitzer's firm leadership, within a year the task force had outlined a radically different architecture for the third edition of the *DSM*. In the following four years, they furnished this new edifice with thousands of new diagnostic details and procedures that would in time require political support for the transformation and the approval by various APA committees. Having recently emerged victorious from controversies surrounding homosexuality, Spitzer was undoubtedly aware of the struggles ahead as opponents of the revisions got wind of the radical changes that were being undertaken.

The Reliability Rationale

Since he had absolutely no mandate from the APA to engage in a major transformation of the *DSM*, Spitzer had to develop a compelling rationale. What was so wrong with *DSM-II* that required a total makeover? His answer, carefully developed over several years, was that the current classification system lacked "reliability" (Spitzer & Fleiss, 1974). This reliability problem had been a concern to only a few research-oriented psychiatrists and psychologists, such as the ones Spitzer had appointed to the task force. As mentioned previously, *reliability* refers to diagnostic consistency among clinicians: can psychiatrists using the *DSM* independently reach the same diagnoses for the same patients? If they can agree on the diagnoses of patients, there is diagnostic reliability. If there is substantial disagreement about the diagnoses for the same patients, the diagnostic system is said to be unreliable. Reliability is a minimal expectation for a science-based profession and is often easily achieved. Unreliability in diagnoses would impede research on the causes of disorders, on effective treatment for particular disorders, and on studies of the prevalence of disorders. Further, communication among clinicians about patients and their problems would be stymied, and the veracity of medical records and reimbursements for services for mental disorders would all be called into question. Psychiatry, which was expected to have responsibility for diagnosing and categorizing mental disorders, had the most to lose if its diagnostic system was considered unreliable.

It is important to realize, however, that reliability of diagnoses (consistency) was a simple problem compared to the specter of demonstrating the empirical existence of a putative category labeled *mental illness*, particularly since psychiatry's weak and inadequate definitions of *mental illness* were the target of critics. In the 1970s, as currently, the meaning or validity of mental illness was in dispute.

All members of Spitzer's task force understood the problem of having an unreliable *DSM*. Spitzer seized on this vulnerability and used it to gain crucial leverage in transforming the *DSM*. Nancy Andreasen, a prominent schizophrenia researcher and one of the initial members of Spitzer's task force, reports that at the very first meeting of the task force, as participants were introducing themselves and indicating what changes they thought needed to be made, the problem of reliability was raised, and, by the end of the very first meeting, there was unanimous agreement to create a different kind of manual (Andreasen, 1984, p.155).

Kappa: Measuring Unreliability

Spitzer had been issuing warnings about unreliability even before the task force convened and continued to do so until *DSM-III* was approved and published. One of his earliest warnings came in 1974 in the influential *British Journal of Psychiatry* (Spitzer & Fleiss, 1974). Along with his coauthor, the respected statistician Joseph Fleiss, Spitzer cautioned that any classification system, including *DSM*, had to be reliable. They emphasized that any unreliability in *DSM* would undermine its validity. Members of the task force, whom Spitzer had selected, needed little instruction about this problem; they were researchers and understood that to the extent that a classification system is unreliable, its *validity* is weakened. If people with the same troubles cannot be sorted into the same diagnostic categories, the validity of those categories is completely undermined. And validity is precisely the ingredient required for the scientific integrity of the concept of "mental illness." It was the validity of mental illness that had been questioned by Szasz, by critics of psychiatry, by the gay activists, and by Rosenhan, among many others. Improving reliability, the task force knew, would prop up the pivotal professional construct of madness until its validity could be more securely established.

Surely, the task force knew that not all problems confronting psychiatry could be addressed even by a major revision of *DSM*. But any major renovation, like the one contemplated by Spitzer and his inner circle, had to have a persuasive scientific rationale that would counter the substantial psychoanalytic faction of the profession who would oppose the changes they would make in *DSM*. Improving diagnostic reliability became that scientific rationale and defense of their plans.

Selecting diagnostic reliability for leverage had several advantages. First, no one could argue with the basic scientific principle of improving reliability. Second, an emerging series of studies were suggesting that diagnostic reliability was problematic, which provided some independent support for defining unreliability as a crucial problem. Third, focusing on the consistent use of diagnoses appeared to be a far easier problem to resolve than the conceptual challenges from Szasz, the cultural critics, or the various social scientists questioning the validity of the construct of mental illness. Fourth, unreliability appeared to many researchers to be largely a technical problem—getting agreement on diagnoses among clinicians—that seemed to be within the expertise of those who composed the *DSM* task force.

Spitzer began a campaign to elevate awareness of the importance of reliability so that he could use it effectively as the primary justification for the renovation of *DSM*. Having gained respect within the APA by being both an insider and a defender of psychiatric diagnosis, his opinion about the perils of unreliability had credibility. In his earlier article in the *British Journal of*

Psychiatry (Spitzer & Fleiss, 1974), he had reviewed seven available studies on diagnostic reliability and concluded that diagnostic reliability was troublingly low. The authors stressed that, without solving the unreliability problem, psychiatry was playing into the hands of the profession's severest critics. Using the data in the reviewed studies, they claimed that actual psychiatric diagnosis was in terrible shape and threatened the validity of diagnosis. If this conclusion was not alarming enough, they suggested that in routine clinical settings, unlike the research settings of the reviewed studies, reliability was probably worse.

Spitzer and Fleiss used a statistic, called kappa, as a tool to summarize the seven reliability studies, which had been published from the 1950 to the early 1970s. Researchers determine a kappa score by having pairs of clinicians independently assess a series of people coming into a mental health facility. They then tally up to what extent the two clinicians make the same or different diagnosis for each client. Of course, as in many games, there will be some level of agreement just by chance. Kappa is a statistical computation that discounts mere agreement by chance (it is called a chance-corrected measure) and provides a resulting measure of how close these pairs of clinicians achieve perfect (i.e., 100 percent) diagnostic agreement. Perfect agreement—perfect reliability—would result in a kappa score near or at 1.0. Levels of agreement that are no better than chance would have kappas of 0.0. Kappa then provides a method of comparing how much agreement is reached by clinicians and comparing the results of different diagnostic studies with each other.

Spitzer and Fleiss used this new tool to examine the level of reliability for different broad diagnostic (not the more specific) categories. This is similar to asking people to identify makes of automobiles using broad categories of automobile makers such as Ford, General Motors, or Toyota, rather than specific categories of cars, such as Mustang, Buick, or Camry. Using general categories will always produce higher agreement/reliability scores. For example, if two people looked at the same car and one said it was a Corvette and the other said it was an Impala, their responses would nonetheless be considered to indicate perfect agreement, since both cars are made by General Motors.

In the Spitzer and Fleiss review and in most subsequent reliability studies, reliability scores are usually reported for general diagnostic categories. In this case, they reported that no general categories had kappa levels that were "good," which appeared to mean scores somewhat above 0.75. Six kappa scores, averaging 0.74, were considered "only satisfactory," 12 with an average of 0.56 were "no better than fair," and the remaining 31, averaging 0.37, were described as "poor." The overall average mean for the nine general diagnostic categories was 0.53. Figure 4.1 presents a summary of the Spitzer and Fleiss data.

Figure 4.1
Interpretation of Kappa Reliability Levels: Early Studies (1950–1974)

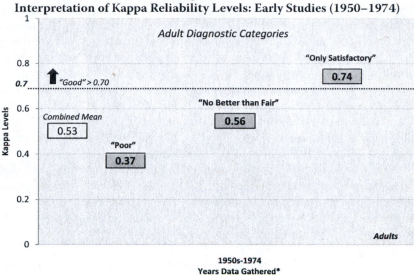

*Data reported in Spitzer & Fleiss (1974), *British Journal of Psychiatry.*

These damning conclusions were published just as Spitzer was being asked to chair the *DSM-III* task force. His attack on the reliability of *DSM-II* gave him the leverage he needed in the anticipated struggle to develop a new approach to diagnosis. It was a risky tactic, unless Spitzer and others had reasons to think that they could remedy the reliability problem. In fact, several small groups of research psychiatrists at Washington University and Columbia University had been working for years on just that problem and were about ready to announce in a series of important journal articles that their new approach to diagnosis remedied the problem of unreliability (Kirk & Kutchins, 1992). This group of like-minded experts formed an "invisible college" that eventually became referred to as neo-Kraepelinians (Andreasen, 1984; Blashfield, 1982; Klerman, 1986; Millon, 1986). They worked on codifying psychiatric diagnosis by creating a system of describing symptomatic behaviors, as a means of grouping patients into homogeneous categories that would facilitate the conduct of research to identify how patients differed biologically from normal people. This was the fulfillment of Kraepelin's agenda. The emphasis on improving the reliability of diagnosis, rather than on directly attempting to understand the causes and dynamics of disturbed behaviors (which Kraepelin assumed were at root distinct biological diseases), radically distinguished the neo-Kraepelinians from the professionally dominant psychoanalysts.

The neo-Kraepelinians had an explanation for why psychiatrists couldn't often agree on diagnoses: the diagnostic process was unregulated, unsystematic, and messy. For example, there was no standard method of conducting a psychiatric interview to reach a diagnosis. Clinicians gathered information about a patient's condition in disparate ways: they asked different questions, in different sequences, and with varying levels of probing. This resulted in different amounts and types of information from a patient. Clinicians also varied in how carefully they may have reviewed the patient's existing psychiatric records, whether they gathered information from other sources, like family members, teachers, employers, or other physicians. Consequently, independent clinicians were likely to each have information about a patient that differed in quality, extensiveness, and amount of detail. To Spitzer and these research psychiatrists, such different interviewing practices explained why diagnoses might be so inconsistent, so unreliable.

But there was a more profound reason for unreliability. Even if clinicians obtained exactly the same information, there were no established criteria for determining whether the person's behaviors constituted a mental illness, and if so, which type of illness. In short, there were no guiding criteria for making a diagnosis.

While these ambiguities were of great concern to Spitzer and the neo-Kraepelinians, they were not particularly troubling to psychotherapists, who viewed differences in clinical style as part of each therapist's methods of establishing rapport with different clients in order to provide effective help. Therapists had their own individual ways of interviewing, of understanding the meaning of what they learned from clients, and their own sense of what the diagnosis might be. The challenge for the *DSM-III* task force was to figure out how they could change the diagnostic thinking and behavior of all mental health practitioners, a debate that continues still (Jaffe, 2010).

Creating Descriptive Diagnosis

The solution that Spitzer and the task force created would become known as descriptive diagnosis. For the first time, they developed specific behavioral criteria to use for each diagnosis. These diagnostic criteria would represent specific rules for determining if a mental disorder was present and, if so, which one. They expected, with justification, that this standardization would improve reliability. By establishing new criteria for each mental disorder, they expected that these criteria would provide a framework to structure the assessment and diagnostic interviewing process. Structured interview guides were nothing new to social scientists, who for decades had used structured questionnaires in surveys to obtain more complete information in a standard format from each respondent. With these two diagnostic innovations—diagnostic criteria and structured interviews—Spitzer fully expected to greatly improve the reliability of *DSM*, and with it, the scientific reputation of psychiatry, and to pave the way for the rise of biopsychiatry.[4]

Task Force Struggles

The process of constructing the radically new manual and building sufficient support for it was a five-year, full-time struggle for Spitzer. Few research psychiatrists would have had the creativity, energy, fortitude, and political skill to accomplish such a revision, and fewer still would have been willing to devote their entire professional life to such a complicated challenge.

Although prior revisions of the manual had been simple administrative updates of a minor pamphlet, this third revision by comparison was a monumental struggle. As Spitzer and the task force created additional working groups and began circulating drafts of the work-in-progress, controversies erupted in print and behind the scenes, within psychiatry and elsewhere, demanding Spitzer's attention. For example, Spitzer offered a new definition of *mental disorder*, defined as a "subset of medical disorders," which caused an eruption by clinical psychologists who perceived this as an unfounded jurisdictional expansion, sweeping all manner of behavioral problems into medicine. Psychoanalysts were frequently critics of Spitzer's efforts, and they vigorously challenged the removal of the cherished term *neurosis* from the manual. Compromises had to be fashioned. Similarly, many groups with an interest in particular "disorders" lobbied the task force: gay activists monitored efforts to reinsert homosexuality as a disorder; black psychiatrists proposed that racism be included as a mental disorder; veterans pushed successfully for adding posttraumatic stress disorder; and so on. None of this whirl of interest groups and politicking had characterized prior revisions of *DSM*. All the while, Spitzer steadfastly held to his position that revising psychiatric diagnosis and *DSM* was a scientific enterprise and no longer an arbitrary exercise in stigma-producing labels.

The Unveiling of DSM-III

After five years and epic struggles, the third edition of the manual, *DSM-III*, was finally published. *DSM-III* (APA, 1980) contained features never seen in any previous edition. First among these was its sheer size, a whopping five hundred pages—over three times longer than the 1968 second edition (*DSM-II*) and sold for more than ten times the prior edition's price. The second notable feature was the listing of hundreds of names of individual psychiatrists, not only of the task force members, but of the APA officers, and every member of seventeen advisory committees, many formed after most of the major structural decisions about the manual had been made. This filled the first five pages of the new manual, deliberately conveying the impression that the manual was the product of a broad array of psychiatrists, not the handiwork of a few. The listings were also a bid for legitimacy, as the renovation that was being published had been very controversial. The third novel feature was a notable twelve-page introduction to *DSM-III*, written by Spitzer, which covered the history of the manual, the background for the third edition, the process of its development, and its new features, which were many, including a new multi-axial system, expanded text for each disorder, and scores of new mental disorders.

For the first time in any edition of *DSM*, in his introduction Spitzer emphasized that this edition was based on data gathered in field trials:

> " . . . interest in the development of this manual is due to awareness that DSM-III reflects an increased commitment in our field to reliance on data as the basis for understanding mental disorders" (APA, 1980, p. 1).

This important claim is echoed several times in his introduction. In justifying the character of the new manual, he notes that other contemporary classifications (like the ICD-9) were not "sufficiently detailed for clinical and research use" and did " . . . not make use of such recent major methodological developments as specified diagnostic criteria" (p. 2). He describes ten goals that the task force sought to achieve. The first was clinical usefulness, and the second was the reliability of diagnostic categories (p. 2). He acknowledges that even though the task force tried to rely on research evidence, task force members often differed in their interpretations of the findings (p. 3). No earlier edition of the manual had even invoked research or data. The great bulk of the new manual described the nearly three hundred specific mental disorders. Some were making their debut:

- Post-traumatic Stress Disorder, which was described as "symptoms following a psychologically traumatic event that is generally outside the range of usual human experience. The characteristic symptoms involve reexperiencing the traumatic events; numbing of responsiveness to, or reduced involvement with, the external world; and a variety of autonomic, dysphoric, or cognitive symptoms" (p. 236).
- Borderline Personality Disorder, which was described as a disorder "in which there is instability in a variety of areas, including interpersonal behavior, mood, and self-image. No single feature is invariably present" (p. 321).

And some old favorites (e.g., Inadequate Personality Disorder) were retired. Its full description in the previous edition of *DSM-II* stated that is was

- a behavior pattern "characterized by ineffectual responses to emotional, social, intellectual and physical demands. While the patient seems neither physically nor mentally deficient, he does manifest inadaptability, ineptness, poor judgment, social instability, and lack of physical and emotional stamina" (p. 44).

All of these above examples are similarly vague and ambiguous. But the most significant differences between the old and new edition was that for each disorder in the new *DSM-III* the manual provided detailed lists of diagnostic criteria, borrowing heavily from the work of the St. Louis and New York groups. These criteria constituted the necessary and sufficient behaviors/signs/symptoms that must be observed or reported in order to use the diagnoses appropriately. These criteria constituted the technical strategy designed to bolster the impaired status of psychiatric diagnosis. Figure 4.2 uses a type of depression to illustrate some of the dramatic changes between *DSM-II* to *DSM-III*.

Figure 4.2
Contrast of DSM-II and DSM-III

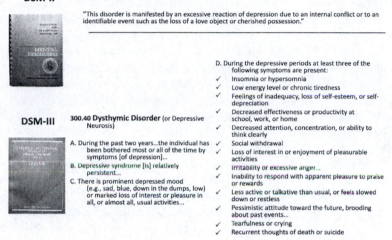

DSM-II 300.4 Depressive Neurosis

"This disorder is manifested by an excessive reaction of depression due to an internal conflict or to an identifiable event such as the loss of a love object or cherished possession."

D. During the depressive periods at least three of the following symptoms are present:
✓ Insomnia or hypersomnia
✓ Low energy level or chronic tiredness
✓ Feelings of inadequacy, loss of self-esteem, or self-depreciation
✓ Decreased effectiveness or productivity at school, work, or home

DSM-III 300.40 **Dysthymic Disorder** (or Depressive Neurosis)

✓ Decreased attention, concentration, or ability to think clearly
✓ Social withdrawal

A. During the past two years...the individual has been bothered most or all of the time by symptoms [of depression]...
B. Depressive syndrome [is] relatively persistent...
C. There is prominent depressed mood (e.g., sad, blue, down in the dumps, low) or marked loss of interest or pleasure in all, or almost all, usual activities...

✓ Loss of interest in or enjoyment of pleasurable activities
✓ Irritability or excessive anger...
✓ Inability to respond with apparent pleasure to praise or rewards
✓ Less active or talkative than usual, or feels slowed down or restless
✓ Pessimistic attitude toward the future, brooding about past events...
✓ Tearfulness or crying
✓ Recurrent thoughts of death or suicide

There are several noteworthy features in this comparison. The description in *DSM-II* was only one sentence, contained no specific criteria, included concepts based on psychoanalytic notions (e.g., neurosis internal conflict, love object), and revealed that depression was a *reaction* to something. None of this appears in *DSM-III*, which provides instead time frames and a list of supposedly more precise behaviors or feelings, with a minimum number required to make the diagnosis (at least three). This specificity was designed to aid clinicians in making diagnoses and to greatly improve consistency (i.e., reliability).

A Stunning Success?

The publication of the new manual was accompanied by the rhetoric of scientific victory. In the introduction to *DSM-III* and in other articles, Spitzer is explicit that the diagnostic criteria were to serve " . . . as guides for making each diagnosis since such criteria enhance interjudge diagnostic reliability" (APA, 1980, p. 8). He announces that for the first time, drafts of *DSM* had been tested in reliability field trials, involving over 12,000 patients who were evaluated by approximately 550 clinicians in 212 different facilities (p. 5). He claims that the data from these field trials indicate "far greater reliability" than had previously been obtained with *DSM-II* (p. 5). One publication about the field trials stressed that reliability was encouraging, was much better than had

Mad Science

been expected, and much higher than before (Spitzer, Forman, & Nee, 1979). In other articles, interviews, and presentations around the time of *DSM-III*'s publication, Spitzer and others repeated the claims of improved reliability (Spitzer, Williams, & Skodal, 1980; Talbot, 1980). By 1982 the reliability of *DSM-III* was said to be "extremely good" (Hyler, Williams, & Spitzer, 1982, p. 1276). At every turn, Spitzer and others used the prior reliability problems with diagnosis to promote the new manual as a great scientific advance. A few years later Spitzer boasted that the adoption of *DSM-III* had marked a signal achievement for psychiatry and represented an advance toward the fulfillment of the scientific aspirations of the profession and would eliminate the disarray surrounding psychiatric diagnosis (Bayer & Spitzer, 1985, p. 187).

Spitzer's rise to a position of control over psychiatric diagnosis had been solidified by his use of the problem of unreliability. Improving reliability had been his quest; it served as the scientific linchpin for the thorough renovation of the manual. The unique inclusion in the manual of the reliability appendix was of singular symbolic value. The data tables in the appendix were used as evidence that the task force and Spitzer had delivered on their promise. It was this claim of greater reliability that appeared to justify the diagnostic revolution.

This was a momentous scientific and political claim. The euphoria was not Spitzer's alone. It was infectious among those celebrating the *DSM-III*. Gerald Klerman, the highest-ranking psychiatrist in the federal government when *DSM-III* was published, gushed:

> In my opinion, the development of DSM-III represents a fateful point in the history of the American psychiatric profession . . . [the adoption of the new manual] represents a significant reaffirmation on the part of American psychiatry to its medical identity and its commitment to scientific medicine. (Klerman, 1984, p. 539)

Similarly, psychiatrist Gerald Maxmen claimed in *The New Psychiatrists* that *DSM-III* marked "the ascendance of scientific psychiatry" and that more than any other single event it demonstrated that psychiatry "had indeed undergone a revolution" (Maxmen, 1985, p. 35). With regard to the core problem of unreliability, Klerman made it clear: "In principle, the problem of reliability has been solved" (Klerman, 1984, 1986, pp. 25, 541).

Even critics of *DSM-III* readily accepted the claims that reliability was no longer problematic (Andreasen, 1984; Carson, 1991; Michels, 1984; Vaillant, 1984). For thirty years, there has been no diminishing of the belief that reliability had been greatly improved if not solved (Buckley, Michels, & MacKinnon, 2006). In 2002 those who would become the architects of *DSM-5* continued to praise *DSM-III*, saying that "the major advantage of adopting [*DSM-III*] was its improved reliability over prior classification systems" (Kupfer, First, & Regier, 2002, p. xviii). In the same book, others reaffirm that "when DSM-III was published in 1980, one of its most important advantages was a radical

148

improvement in the reliability of psychiatric diagnosis" (Rounsaville et al., 2002, p.13). And in March 2011, Carol Bernstein, president of the American Psychiatric Association, praised *DSM-III* for addressing "the pressing problem of interrater reliability in psychiatric diagnosis" and claimed that *DSM-III* "contributed significantly to improved diagnostic agreement" (Bernstein, 2011).

The Mad Science of Diagnostic Reliability

All of these recent claims about *DSM-III*'s radical improvement in reliability were made without citing a single study or source of evidence. There was another problem with all these claims: *reliability had not improved with DSM-III.*

How could such misinformation be so widely believed and disseminated? Apparently, no one actually examined critically the field trial data, nor tried to compare them with the earlier reliability levels of *DSM-II*. If they had, the justification for the diagnostic revolution would have collapsed. What the data actually show undermines what has been claimed about reliability for over thirty years. We will briefly present these data in summary fashion (for an earlier detailed analysis, see Kirk and Kutchins, 1992). Four original published sources report the results of different aspects of the *DSM-III* field trials (APA, 1980; Hyler et al., 1982; Spitzer & Forman, 1979; Spitzer et al., 1979). In addition, there is one unpublished summary (Williams, 1982) regarding personality disorders, which was found in a letter in the APA's *DSM* archives in Washington, DC. From the data reported in these sources, all of them developed by the *DSM* task force leaders, we compare the earlier, pre-*DSM-III* studies of reliability with the reliability of *DSM-III*.

The field trial data were collected in 1978–1979 and originally reported in two phases, first in an earlier report and then in an appendix to *DSM-III*. Within each phase, the results were organized separately for adults and children and for the major diagnostic categories of mental disorder (axis I) and the personality disorders (axis II). In summarizing these data, we retain the distinctions between adults and children, and between the major disorder categories and the personality disorders, but for simplicity we will combine the data from the two phases. Figure 4.3 consists of a bar graph of the average (mean) kappas (recall the earlier description of this statistic in which higher kappa scores represent better agreement, i.e., higher reliability) from the field trials for the diagnoses for adults. On the far left are the interpretative standards developed by Spitzer and Fleiss for the earlier reliability studies that we described previously (from figure 4.1). On the right are the *DSM-III* field trial data and a subsequent reliability study of *DSM* conducted several years later.

Several cautions should be raised about these data. First, these reliability studies were undertaken while the manual was being developed. The reports of the design, implementation, and findings were at times inconsistent and ambiguous. Second, aggregating data from many different clinical sites around the country, with little oversight or monitoring, creates various methodological problems (e.g., differences in base rates of disorders at different sites) that complicate the interpretation of the reliability statistics (kappa). Third, as mentioned before, the kappa measures of reliability in the field trials are based on the more forgiving general diagnostic categories, not on the specific diagnoses made by clinicians. For example, there are twelve types of personality disorder (e.g., antisocial, narcissistic, compulsive, and so forth). Even if two clinicians disagreed on which type of personality disorder a patient had, they still would have been scored as having perfect (kappa 1.0) agreement if they agreed that the patient had some type of personality disorder. Kappas based on the general class of disorder are liberal interpretations of reliability and are always much higher than the level of agreement with specific diagnoses. For all these reasons, it is prudent to view all the reliability measures as crude overestimates using crude data. Accordingly, we will use some ranges of average kappas calculated in different reasonable ways to describe reliability levels.

With that in mind, we now turn to figure 4.3, which contains the summaries of the reliability of adult diagnoses. For the major mental disorder categories, in both phases of the field trials, depending on how you calculate, the overall average kappa ranged from 0.55 to 0.72. This range of average scores comes from three different methods of calculating overall means. First, there are the field trial data (0.68 and 0.72 in each phase) in which actual calculation of the overall kappas is not provided, although it appears to be a kappa weighted by the number of patients in each category.[5]

Figure 4.3
Comparison of Reliability Levels (Kappa) for Early Studies and DSM-III

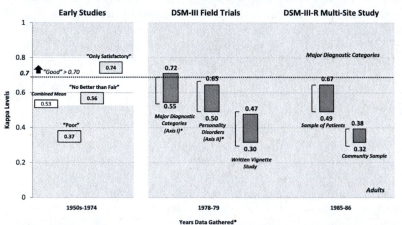

DSM-III field trial data for the major diagnostic categories and personality disorders are taken from appendix F in *DSM-III* (APA, 1980) and from a letter in the APA archives (Williams, 1982). Data for the Written Vignette Study comes from the *Archives of General Psychiatry* (Hyler, Williams & Spitzer, 1982). Data from the *DSM-III-R* Multi-Site Study is from the *Archives of General Psychiatry* (Williams et al., 1992).

A second method is to calculate kappa for all the major categories without weighting by simply adding their kappas and dividing by the number of total categories (0.63 and 0.55 for each phase). In addition, since many of the major categories had very few patients, the kappas are quite unstable estimates. So a third method was to recalculate the average kappas for categories that had at least six patients in each phase (0.59 and 0.66). These various kappas are in the range of kappas presented in figure 4.3 for major diagnostic categories for the field trials (from a low of 0.55 to a high of 0.72). The dark vertical blocks in figure 4.3 provide the general range of kappas from all the available sources, calculated in these different ways.

For the adult personality disorders, the kappa range represents the overall kappas from the appendix of *DSM-III* (0.56 and 0.65 for both phases) and from a mean calculated (0.50) from the list of individual kappas (n = 12) provided in the archival material, which covered both phases of the field trials.

The case summary study, which used written vignettes instead of live interviews and was conducted as part of the field trials, provided an additional source of information about diagnostic agreement among clinicians. It found lower levels of agreement (weighted kappa 0.47; unweighted mean kappa 0.30).

In other words, the *DSM-III* field trial data for adults do not support the claims that were made about far greater reliability. If they had, the three dark vertical bars in the center of figure 4.3 would have all been above the dotted horizontal line which Spitzer and Fleiss (1974) had earlier claimed represented "good reliability." In fact, by visual inspection one can clearly see that reliability remained at the same low level that existed before *DSM-III*. Let us recall that all these data were collected by the originators of *DSM-III*, who had a professional and personal stake in demonstrating superior reliability levels.

Perhaps because of these equivocal and disappointing results, another major reliability study was conduct several years after the publication of *DSM-III* by Spitzer and his associates. The later study, which its authors describe as the most rigorous and comprehensive reliability assessment ever conducted of *DSM*, gathered data in 1985–1986, using multiple clinical sites in Germany and the United States. It was published in 1992 (Williams et al., 1992), twelve years after the release of *DSM-III*. The findings were presented for two samples, one of 390 "patients" already in treatment (average weighted kappa of 0.61 and a range of overall kappas from the five sites of 0.49 to 0.67) and one of 202 people from a "community sample" (weighted kappa 0.37 and a range of overall kappas from the two sites of 0.32 to 0.38). These results are shown in the far right section of figure 4.3, under the heading Multi-Site Study. As the two dark vertical bars show, this later study again documents that no general improvement in reliability occurred in comparison to *DSM-II*.

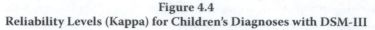

Figure 4.4
Reliability Levels (Kappa) for Children's Diagnoses with DSM-III

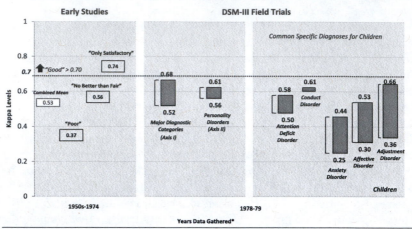

*Data for children's diagnoses come from appendix F in *DSM-III* (APA, 1980, p. 471). For the specific diagnoses the range of kappas comes from the means of the first and second phases of the field trial.

The results do not get any better when we examine the reliability reports for children; in fact, they are worse. Unfortunately, the field trials included few children: only seventy-one in phase I and fifty-five in phase II. Most of the diagnostic categories had fewer than five children, and many had only one or two, too few to allow for any meaningful recalculations. Here again, we combine both phases and provide the summary kappas that were offered in the *DSM* appendix on the field trials. For the major categories of disorder (0.72 and 0.43) and personality disorders (0.66 and 0.55), lower kappas were obtained in the second phase. Figure 4.4 provides these estimates. In addition, using only the categories with a larger number of children, we present the range of phase I and phase II kappas for five of the most common children's disorders. For example, Attention Deficit Disorder in the two phases had kappas of 0.58 and 0.50. The five vertical dark bars clearly show that none of the results reach kappa levels in the "good" range, and they are no better and perhaps worse than the disappointing adult results.

Achieving Success with Failure

As we have seen, the actual reliability data for the new *DSM* looks remarkably similar to the old *DSM*, clustering in the range of "no better than fair" and "poor." Almost none of the kappas fall above 0.70, a range earlier described by Spitzer as "good reliability." In sum, the often praised "far higher" or "extremely good" reliability of the modern *DSM* has become an institutionalized myth—unsupported by any convincing data—although those exaggerations conveniently served the ambitious purposes of the architects of *DSM*. The reliability myth, in fact, serves as a prototype of how science is used and misused in revising the manual: the scientific data really don't matter that much. The APA and others announced to the world that *DSM-III* was a scientific slam dunk, when, in fact, the ball didn't even come close to the basket.

After claiming success in solving the reliability problem, the topic was largely abandoned, perhaps conveniently because no one knew how to fix it. There was a plan funded by the MacArthur Foundation to conduct new reliability studies for *DSM-IV*, but the leaders quietly abandoned the effort without an explanation; no published results ever appeared (Kirk & Kutchins, 1992; Spiegel, 2005).

In subsequent decades, little evidence has appeared that mental health professionals in typical clinical settings can achieve high reliability with psychiatric diagnoses using any of the newer editions of the *DSM*. Nevertheless, a few subsequent studies that bear some semblance to earlier studies of the whole classification system continued to report diagnostic unreliability at levels similar to the pre-*DSM-III* studies (Regier, Kaelber, Roper, Rae, & Sartorius, 1994; Sartorius et al., 1993, p.116; Shear et al., 2000). The reliability of children's diagnoses are equally dismal (Spitzer, Davies, & Barkley, 1990; Kirk, 2004; Lahey, Applegate, Barkley, et al., 1994; Boyle et al., 1993; Ezpeleta, de la Osa, Domenech, Navarro, & Losilla, 1997; Kirk & Hsieh, 2004).

Other studies of diagnostic reliability appear occasionally in the journal literature, but these generally have limited relevance to the reliability of the *DSM* classification system as a whole as used by general mental health practitioners. Typically, these studies test the reliability of special measuring scales developed to identify a particular disorder or measure the consistency of diagnoses made under highly specialized circumstances or at special clinics focused only on a particular narrow group of disorders. For example, Mary Zanarini and her colleagues (Zanarini & Frankenburg, 2001; Zanarini et al., 2000) in several articles report generally high reliability scores (kappa) for personality disorders and other nonpsychotic disorders with *DSM-IV*. The underlying motive for the studies appeared to be to demonstrate that personality disorders could be diagnosed as reliably as other *DSM* disorders.

A careful reading of the studies reveals how high reliabilities were accomplished and why they cannot be generalized to general diagnostic practice. The results were obtained by maintaining rigorous control over the making of diagnoses. The study took place in university-related clinics and hospitals at Brown, Columbia, Harvard, and Yale, under the close supervision of the project coordinators. The study was, by design, a study of the reliability of two highly structured and well-developed interview protocols, Structured Clinical Interview for Axis I Disorders (SCID-I) and the Diagnostic Interview for Personality Disorders (DIPD-R), one of them—for personality disorders—developed by the lead author. Interviewers were graduate students (presumably in relevant disciplines) who were selected by the coordinators and underwent a week of intensive training in the use of the instruments, which contained over three hundred questions. This training was followed by additional training, supervised practice interviews, and close supervision throughout the study. Each interviewer had to be "certified" before they participated in the study. The instruments not only structure the questioning of clients but provide a specific scoring system that produces the "diagnosis." To test for inter-rater reliability, those trained to use the instrument participated on conjoint interviews (in which one person conducted the interview and the other observed), and each completed the instruments. At other times, those trained watched videotapes of prior interviews and their scores were compared. The patients for these interviews were selected by the project coordinator at each site.

Many structural and procedural aspects of these studies may account for the generally high reliability scores, among them the use of structured protocols that deliberately focus each interview, the careful selection of patients and interviewers, the use of conjoint interviews (which, technically, are not independent observations), the highly specialized nature of the research settings with highly motivated participants, and the leadership of the person who developed one of the instruments and had an obvious stake in its success. Under these special conditions and full technical control over the interviews and the scoring of answers, it is expected that interviewers would often reach agreement. Indeed, it would be surprising if they did not.

Does this mean that *DSM* itself is used reliably? None of these special research conditions apply to the real world of psychiatric diagnosis, in which individual clinicians with varying levels of training and perspectives are mandated to use *DSM* to screen a diverse array of clients walking into medical clinics, mental health centers, family service agencies, and so forth. Clinicians generally have different styles of interviewing, ask different questions, pursue different avenues for obtaining client information, and are supervised loosely, if at all. We will have more to say about this in the next chapter when we discuss *DSM-5*.

The Zanarini et al. (2000) diagnostic studies used the most highly trained and supervised interviewers working under the most controlled and protected circumstances. The relationship of the Zanarini et al. studies to actual clinical practice is about the same as comparing professional racecar drivers circling a race track at 150 miles per hour to granny moving her Volvo through city traffic. All are driving automobiles, just as all clinicians are making diagnoses, but no one ought to claim that there is much in common in their skills or in the setting.

Such studies of diagnostic instruments, whatever their usefulness for research purposes, have little bearing on the reliability of *DSM* as it is used by practitioners who are not mandated to use structured interview protocols and who see diverse patients walking into a clinic. As far as we know, there have been no new *DSM* reliability studies of the magnitude that Spitzer and his colleagues conducted over thirty years ago.[6]

The summary point is that there is little evidence that the signature objective of *DSM-III* to improve the reliability of psychiatric diagnosis was achieved. What was stated over a decade ago (Kutchins & Kirk, 1997) remains true:

> Mental health clinicians independently interviewing the same person in the community are as likely to agree as disagree that the person has a mental disorder and are as likely to agree as disagree on which of the over 300 disorders is present. . . . If the unreliability of diagnosis were widely recognized and if there were no scientific patina to DSM, the use of everyday behaviors as indicators of mental disorders would be more rigorously questioned by the public. The illusion that psychiatrists are in agreement when making diagnoses creates the appearance of a united professional consensus. In fact, there is considerable professional confusion. (p. 53)

The claims of achieving diagnostic reliability with the new editions of *DSM* are a prime example of mad science—a triumph of hope, marketing, and political rhetoric over the scientific evidence. After five years of bitter struggle to build support for the new *DSM-III*, its developers were certainly not about to reveal that the old bogeyman of unreliability was still around, big as life. Too much investment had already been made in the new manual, too many opponents defeated, too many reputations in jeopardy—and the business of diagnosis had to move forward. In addition, so few in the mental health professions understood the then-arcane language of reliability statistics or were in any position to assess the veracity of the developers' claims. In the process of promoting *DSM-III*, the claims were more the advertisements of entrepreneurs preparing to launch a new product, on which all their capital had been invested. Exaggeration, distortion, and bias should have been expected. In fact, it is a pattern that is replicated in the exaggerated claims of the effectiveness of community treatment (chapter 3) and drugs (chapters 6 and 7).

Twenty-five years after the launch of *DSM-III*, Spitzer admitted that he failed to solve the problem. "To say that we've solved the reliability problem is just not true," he said plainly (Spiegel, 2005, p. 63). "It's been improved . . . it's certainly not very good. There's still a real problem, and it's not clear how to solve the problem." Allen Frances, who worked on *DSM-III* and later chaired the task force that developed *DSM-IV*, pointed out in a 2005 interview that "without reliability the system is completely random, and the diagnoses mean almost nothing, because they're falsely labeling. You're better off not having a diagnostic system" (Spiegel, 2005). Nevertheless, he still claimed inaccurately that reliability had been improved, but acknowledged the ploy:

> To my way of thinking, the reliability of the DSM—although improved—has been oversold by some people. . . . From a cultural standpoint, reliability was a way of authenticating the DSM as a radical innovation. In a vacuum, to create criteria that were based on accepted wisdom as a first stab was fine, as long as you didn't take it too seriously. (p. 63)

Unfortunately, the vast majority took it very seriously. In the early twenty-first century, with the modern *DSM* completely institutionalized, its architects and entrepreneurs Spitzer and Frances could admit that diagnostic unreliability remains just as it was in the 1950s, a perplexing and unsolved problem that continues to undermine the validity of *DSM*.

The flawed new manual, however, became an undisputed marketing success, a runaway psychiatric bestseller. The APA sold 830,000 copies of *DSM-III* (Carey, 2008) and, given the price, grossed tens of millions of dollars. The APA commissioned a sequel from Spitzer, published in 1987 as *DSM-III-R* and in 1994 released *DSM-IV* and then a text revision in 2000 (*DSM-IV-TR*). *DSM* can now be found on the bookshelf of every mental health professional in America. It is reported that each year, sales of *DSM*s exceed $6.5 million (Greenberg, 2011).

The once obscure codebook is now an important instrument in shaping public mental health policy, guiding psychiatric—and much of psychology and social work—research and training, and determining the prevalence of mental disorders in the population. Moreover, because of insurance reimbursement requirements, *DSM* is used as the criteria for the financing of psychiatric treatment, hospitalization, and the use of medications. Furthermore, its categories have completely seeped into public discourse and shaped how behavioral problems of many kinds are described, understood, and anticipated to manifest themselves. Absolutely none of these indicators of acceptance and popularity pertained to its predecessor, *DSM-II*.

Troubling Consequences of Success

The success of *DSM-III* has spawned a cluster of unanticipated and very troubling consequences for people in need in help, for clinicians, and for our society. These will be explored in the next chapter. First, we will examine whether the descriptive approach to diagnosis introduced by *DSM-III* improved the validity of diagnosis as anticipated. Second, we will describe the alliance of American institutions that exploited *DSM* for their own purposes, while ensuring its success in the marketplace. For example, the APA embraced the new manual for restoring scientific respectability to psychiatry. Mental health clinicians and universities found that *DSM* provided a scientific-looking book for labeling human troubles and rapidly adopted it to authenticate their training and practices. The National Institute of Mental Health made the use of *DSM*'s criteria a requirement for funding research. The politically powerful drug industry rapidly exploited *DSM*'s expansive list of mental disorders and behaviors that could be labeled as symptoms and treated with expensive psychotropic drugs. The health insurance industry relied on the *DSM* to guide decisions about which disorders they would cover. The media, in news articles, magazines, and on television, provided a steady diet of stories about the "discovery" of new disorders and purported scientific advances in psychiatry and the wonders of new medications targeting the newly discovered disorders. We will then address the latest edition of the manual, *DSM-5*, and its controversies as it makes its way to publication in 2013. Is the new edition likely to be a diagnostic breakthrough or the inevitable collapse of descriptive psychiatry after a thirty-year reign? Finally, the social harms of *DSM* will be addressed.

Notes

1. The primary professionals working in mental health include psychiatrists, psychologists, social workers, and nurses. The number of professionals in each profession is elusive, depending on what levels of education are considered and which mental health service settings are included. One generally accepted estimate reports that in 2000 there were approximately 40,000 psychiatrists, 70,000 nurses, 70,000 social workers, and 88,000 licensed psychologists working in mental health services (Mechanic, 2008, pp. 12–17). Regardless of how these estimates are made, psychiatrists are always a small minority of mental health service providers in American.

2. In this regard, his model for mental illness was based on his work with Alois Alzheimer, who in his work on cadavers, identified the neurological disorder later known as Alzheimer's, as well as general paresis.

3. E. Fuller Torrey later became one of the most outspoken promoters of coercive and involuntary treatment in psychiatry, and an adherent of the view that schizophrenia had a viral origin. The private nonprofit Stanley Medical Research Institute, which he directs, has amassed one of the largest banks of brains in the world, and has spent over $300 million since 1989 on research on the "brain diseases" of schizophrenia, bipolar disorders, and depression, according to the Institute's website (http://www.stanleyresearch.org), but with no diagnostic brain lesions discovered so far through this effort.

4. Indeed, within a decade biopsychiatry had taken hold, as President George H.W. Bush and the NIMH proclaimed that the 1990s would be the "Decade of the Brain," and by 2005, the director of NIMH argued that psychiatrists needed to be trained as neuroscientists, not psychotherapists (Insel & Quirion, 2005).

5. Weighted kappa has technical advantages and disadvantages. The advantage is giving greater weight to those diagnostic categories in which more patients were placed. The disadvantage is that if many patients received their diagnoses in clinical sites with higher base rates for particular disorders (e.g., patients who were referred to an anxiety disorder clinic and were

therefore more likely to be diagnosed with anxiety disorders), the overall kappas from many different sites would be artificially inflated. Unweighted kappa gives equal status to each general diagnostic category.

6.   At least we were unable to locate any, and our queries to key *DSM-IV* participants revealed none.

References

American Psychiatric Association. (1952). *Diagnostic and statistical manual: Mental disorders.* Washington, DC: APA.

American Psychiatric Association. (1980). *Diagnostic and statistical manual of mental disorders, Third edition (DSM-III).* Washington, DC: American Psychiatric Association.

American Psychiatric Association. (2000). *Diagnostic and statistical manual of mental disorders, Fourth Edition (DSM-IV-TR).* Washington, DC: American Psychiatric Association.

Andreasen, N. C. (1984). *The broken brain: The biological revolution in psychiatry.* New York: Harper & Row.

Bayer, R. (1981). *Homosexuality and American psychiatry: The politics of diagnosis.* Princeton, NJ: Princeton University Press.

Bayer, R., & Spitzer, R. (1982). Edited correspondence on the status of homosexuality in *DSM-III. Journal of the History of the Behavioral Sciences, 18,* 32–52.

Bayer, R., & Spitzer, R. (1985). Neurosis, psychodynamics, and *DSM-III*: A history of the controversy. *Archives of General Psychiatry, 42,* 187–195.

Bernstein, C. A. (2011, March 4). Meta-structure in *DSM-5* process. *Psychiatric Times, 7.*

Blashfield, R. K. (1982). Feighner et al., invisible colleges, and the Matthew effect. *Schizophrenia Bulletin, 81*(1), 1–6.

Boyle, M. (2002). *Schizophrenia: A scientific delusion?* (2nd ed.). East Sussex, UK: Routledge.

Boyle, M., Offord, D., Racine, Y., Sanford, M., Szatmari, P., Fleming, J., et al. (1993). Evaluation of the diagnostic interview for children and adolescents for use in general population samples. *Journal of Abnormal Child Psychiatry, 21*(6), 663–681.

Buckley, P. J., Michels, R., & MacKinnon, R. A. (2006). Changes in the psychiatric landscape. *American Journal of Psychiatry, 163,* 757–760.

Carey, B. (2005, June 7). Most will be mentally ill at some point, study says. *New York Times, 1.*

Carey, B. (2008, December 18). Psychiatrists revise the book of human troubles. *New York Times.* Retrieved from http://www.nytimes.com/2008/12/18/health/18psych.html?pagewanted=all

Carlat, D. (2010). *Unhinged: The trouble with psychiatry—A doctor's revelations about a profession in crisis.* New York: Free Press.

Carson, R. (1991). Dilemmas in the pathway of the *DSM-IV. Journal of Abnormal Psychology, 100,* 302–307.

Eysenck, H. J. (1952). The effects of psychotherapy: An evaluation. *Journal of Consulting Psychology, 16,* 319–323.

Eysenck, H. J. (1986). A critique of contemporary classification and diagnosis. In T. Millon & G. Klerman (Eds.), *Contemporary directions in psychopathology* (pp. 73–98). New York: Guilford Press.

Ezpeleta, N., de la Osa, N., Domenech, J., Navarro, J., & Losilla, J. (1997). Diagnostic agreement between clinicians and the Diagnostic Interview for Children and Adolescents—DICA-R—in an outpatient sample. *Journal of Child Psychology and Psychiatry, 38*(4), 431–440.

Foucault, M. (1965). *Madness and civilization: A history of insanity in the age of reason.* New York: Random House.

Frances, A. (2010a, December 22). The most important psychiatrist of our time. *Psychiatric Times.* Retrieved from http://www.psychiatrictimes.com/blog/couchincrisis/content/article/10168/1766926?_EXT_4_comsort=of

Frances, A. (2010b, July 6). Normality is an endangered species: Psychiatric fads and overdiagnosis. *Psychiatric Times.* Retrieved from http://www.psychiatrictimes.com/display/article/10168/1598676

Freud, S. (1969). *The question of lay analysis.* New York: W. W. Norton.

Goffman, E. (1961). *Asylums: Essays on the social situation of mental patients and other inmates.* Garden City, NY: Anchor Books.

Goleman, D. (1990, May 17). New paths to mental health put strains on some healers. *New York Times,* A1, B12.

Greenberg, G. (2010). *Manufacturing depression: The secret history of a modern disease.* New York: Simon & Schuster.

Greenberg, G. (2011, January). Inside the battle to define mental illness. *Wired.* Retrieved from http://www.wired.com/magazine/2010/12/ff_dsmv/

Horwitz, A. V. (2002). *Creating mental illness.* Chicago: University of Chicago.

Horwitz, A. V. (2010). How an age of anxiety became an age of depression. *Milbank Quarterly, 88*(1), 112–138.

Horwitz, A. V., & Wakefield, J. C. (2012). *All we have to fear: Psychiatry's transformation of natural anxieties into mental disorders.* New York: Oxford University Press.

Hyler, S., Williams, J., & Spitzer, R. (1982). Reliability in the *DSM-III* field trials. *Archives of General Psychiatry, 39,* 1275–1278.

Illich, I. (1975). *Medical nemesis: The expropriation of health.* New York: Pantheon.

Insel, T. R., & Quirion, R. (2005). Psychiatry as a clinical neuroscience discipline. *JAMA, 294*(17), 2221–2224.

Jaffe, E. (2010, January 11). Of two minds. *Los Angeles Times,* E1, E6–E7.

Joint Commission on Mental Illness and Health. (1961). *Action for mental health.* New York: Basic Books.

Kendell, R. E. (1975). *The role of diagnosis in psychiatry.* Oxford: Blackwell Scientific Publications.

Kessler, R., McGonagle, K., Zhao, S., Nelson, C., Hughes, M., Eshleman, S., et al. (1994). Lifetime and 12-month prevalence of *DSM-III-R* psychiatric disorders in the United States: Results from the National Comorbidity Survey. *Archives of General Psychiatry, 51,* 153–164.

Kirk, S. A. (2004). Are children's *DSM* diagnoses accurate? *Brief Treatment and Crisis Intervention, 4,* 255–270.

Kirk, S. A., & Hsieh, D. K. (2004). Diagnostic consistency in assessing conduct disorder: An experiment on the effect of social context. *American Journal of Orthopsychiatry, 74*(1), 43–55.

Kirk, S. A., & Kutchins, H. (1992). *The selling of DSM: The rhetoric of science in psychiatry.* Hawthorne, NY: Aldine de Gruyter.

Klerman, G. (1984). The advantages of *DSM-III*. *American Journal of Psychiatry*, *141*, 539–542.

Klerman, G. (1986). Historical perspectives on contemporary schools of psychopathology. In T. Millon & G. Klerman (Eds.), *Contemporary directions in psychopathology*. New York: Guiford Press.

Kupfer, D. J., First, M. B., & Regier, D. A. (2002). Introduction. In D. J. Kupfer, M. B. First, & D. A. Regier (Eds.), *A research agenda for* DSM-V (pp. xv–xxiii). Washington, DC: American Psychiatric Association.

Kutchins, H., & Kirk, S. A. (1997). *Making us crazy:* DSM: *The psychiatric bible and the creation of mental disorders*. New York: Free Press.

Lahey, B., Applegate, B., Barkley, R., Garfinkel, B., McBurnett, K., Kerdyk, L., et al. (1994). *DSM-IV* field trials for oppositional defiant disorder and conduct disorder in children and adolescents. *American Journal of Psychiatry*, *151*, 1163–1171.

Lahey, B., Applegate, B., McBurnett, K., Biederman, J., Greenhill, L., Hynd, G., et al. (1994). *DSM-IV* field trials for attention-deficit/hyperactivity disorder in children and adolescents. *American Journal of Psychiatry*, *151*, 1673–1685.

Laing, R. D. (1967). *The politics of experience*. Baltimore: Penguin Books.

Luhrmann, T. M. (2000). *Of two minds: The growing disorder in American psychiatry*. New York: Knopf.

Maxmen, G. (1985). *The new psychiatrists*. New York: New American Library.

Mechanic, D. (2008). *Mental health and social policy: Beyond managed care* (5th ed.). Boston: Pearson.

Michels, R. (1984). First rebuttal. *American Journal of Psychiatry*, *141*, 548–551.

Millon, T. (1983). *DSM-III*: An insider's account. *American Psychologist*, *38*, 804–815.

Millon, T. (1986). On the past and future of the *DSM-III*: Personal recollections and projections. In T. Millon & G. Klerman (Eds.), *Contemporary directions in psychopathology: Toward the* DSM-IV (pp. 29–70). New York: Guilford Press.

Regier, D., Kaelber, C., Roper, M. T., Rae, D., & Sartorius, N. (1994). The ICD-10 clinical field trial for mental and behavioral disorders: Results in Canada and the United States. *American Journal of Psychiatry*, *151*, 1340–1350.

Rosenhan, D. L. (1973). On being sane in insane places. *Science*, *179*, 250–258.

Rounsaville, B., Alcarcon, R., Andrews, G., Jackson, J. S., Kendell, R. E., & Kendler, K. (2002). Basic nomenclature issues for *DSM-V*. In D. J. Kupfer, M. B. First, & D. A. Regier (Eds.), *A research agenda for* DSM-V (pp. 1–29). Washington, DC: American Psychiatric Association.

Sartorius, N., Kaelber, C. T., Cooper, J. E., Roper, M. T., Rae, D. S., Gulbinat, W., et al. (1993). Progress toward achieving a common language in psychiatry: Results from the field trial of the clinical guidelines accompanying the WHO classification of mental and behavioral disorders in ICD-10. *Archives of General Psychiatry*, *50*, 115–125.

Scheff, T. J. (1966). *Being mentally ill: A sociological theory*. Chicago: Aldine.

Shear, M., Greeno, C., Kang, J., Ludewig, D., Frank, E., Swartz, H., et al. (2000). Diagnosis of nonpsychotic patients in community clinics. *American Journal of Psychiatry*, *157*(4), 581–587.

Spiegel, A. (2005, January 3). The dictionary of disorder. *New Yorker*, 56–63.

Spitzer, R. (1975). On pseudoscience in science, logic in remission, and psychiatric diagnosis: A critique of Rosenhan's "On being sane in insane places." *Journal of Abnormal Psychology*, *84*, 442–452.

Spitzer, R., Davies, M., & Barkley, R. (1990). The *DSM-III-R* field trial of disruptive behavior disorders. *Journal of the American Academy of Child and Adolescent Psychiatry, 29*, 690–697.

Spitzer, R., & Forman, J. (1979). *DSM-III* field trials: II. Initial experiences with the multiaxial system. *American Journal of Psychiatry, 136*, 818–820.

Spitzer, R., Forman, J., & Nee, J. (1979). *DSM-III* field trials: I. Initial interrater diagnostic reliablity. *American Journal of Psychiatry, 136*, 815–817.

Spitzer, R., & Wilson, P. T. (1968). A guide to the American Psychiatric Association's new diagnostic nomenclature. *American Journal of Psychiatry, 124*, 1616–1629.

Spitzer, R., & Wilson, P. T. (1969). *DSM-II* revisited: A reply. *International Journal of Psychiatry, 7*, 421–426.

Spitzer, R. L., & Fleiss, J. L. (1974). A re-analysis of the reliability of psychiatry diagnosis. *British Journal of Psychiatry, 125*, 341–347.

Spitzer, R. L., Williams, J., & Skodal, A. (1980). *DSM-III*: The major achievements and an overview. *American Journal of Psychiatry, 137*, 151–164.

Szasz, T. (1961). *The myth of mental illness: Foundations of a theory of personal conduct*. New York: Hoeber-Harper.

Talbot, J. (1980). An in-depth look at *DSM-III*: An interview with Robert Spitzer. *Hospital and Community Psychiatry, 31*, 25–32.

Torrey, E. F. (1974). *The death of psychiatry*. New York: Penguin.

Ullmann, L. P., & Krasner, L. (1969). *A psychological approach to abnormal behavior*. Englewood Cliffs, NJ: Prentice-Hall.

Vaillant, G. (1984). The disadvantages of *DSM-III* outweigh its advantages. *American Journal of Psychiatry, 141*, 542–545.

Whitaker, R. (2010). *Anatomy of an epidemic: Magic bullets, psychiatric drugs, and the astonishing rise of mental illness in America*. New York: Crown.

Williams, J., Gibbon, M., First, M., Spitzer, R. L., Davies, L., Borus, J., et al. (1992). The structured clinical interview for *DSM-III-R* (SCID): II. Multi-site test-retest reliability. *Archives of General Psychiatry, 49*, 630–636.

Zanarini, M. C., & Frankenburg, F. R. (2001). Attainment and maintenance of reliability of Axis I and II disorders over the course of a longitudinal study. *Comprehensive Psychiatry, 42*(5), 369–374.

Zanarini, M. C., Skodal, A., Bender, D., Dolan, R., Sanislow, C., Schaefer, E., et al. (2000). The collaborative longitudinal personality disorders study: Reliability of Axis I and II diagnoses. *Journal of Personality Disorders, 14*(4), 291–299.

Zigler, E., & Phillips, L. (1961). Psychiatric diagnosis: A critique. *Journal of Abnormal and Social Psychology, 63*, 607–618.

Zilboorg, G. (1941). *A history of medical psychology*. New York: Norton.

5

The Failure of Descriptive Diagnosis

Introduction

The last chapter demonstrated how a particularly narrow scientific concern—diagnostic reliability—was used creatively by a few researchers to justify an entirely new approach to diagnosis. Descriptive diagnosis, as this approach was called, was developed by capitalizing on the vulnerabilities of psychiatry to scientific criticism. The new approach then benefited, not from improving reliability, but by merely claiming to have done so, using data that was difficult for outsiders to assess accurately. The details of the data, moreover, were quickly forgotten in the wave of celebration over the "scientific" nature of the new *DSM-III*. In this chapter we continue to follow the story of *DSM*'s evolution.

For the most part, we, too, will leave reliability behind and move, first, to a much larger and significant problem that emerges at every turn in the story, the problem of the meaning (i.e., the validity) of the modern *DSM* classification of mental disorders. Did the descriptive approach to diagnosis deliver on its promise to more accurately identify and describe valid markers of mental illness—and of different mental illnesses? Did the new manual improve clinical practice, lead to more effective treatment, and allow researchers to make scientific breakthroughs in understanding the claimed biological and medical causes of mental disorders? In short, has all the effort and subsequent celebration been matched by major scientific or clinical advances?

We answer these questions by first examining the "diagnostic criteria" that are the signature characteristic of all *DSM* editions since 1980. Then, after understanding how and why the diagnostic criteria have failed to ensure diagnostic validity, we turn to the institutional investors and supporters of *DSM*, who collectively ignored these scientific failures, thus ensuring that the flawed manual became viewed as indispensible to mental health thinking and practice. With this as background, we finally examine the current efforts to produce the *DSM-5*, due in 2013. The controversies surrounding the *DSM-5* illuminate many of the inherent and inevitable problems of descriptive diagnosis and the profound mistakes that are made when the anguishes, fears, worries, and sufferings of human beings are—on the basis of no more than the beliefs of psychiatric observers in late-twentieth-century America—classified as disorders of the brain.

Are Psychiatric Diagnoses Valid?

Unreliability is an important diagnostic problem because it undermines the validity of the construct of mental disorder. The diagnostic criteria were attempts to improve reliability, but, more importantly, to buttress validity. The gay activists who asked the APA why homosexuality was defined as a mental disorder were questioning the *validity* of a psychiatric diagnosis. They wanted to know exactly how *DSM* distinguished between mental disorder and non-disorder, that is, how *DSM* established diagnostic validity, or the *truth* of diagnosis. As discussed, *DSM-III* first addressed this problem by dodging it, then by removing homosexuality from the diagnostic manual, and later by providing criteria for each disorder. *DSM-III*, as we noted in chapter 1, also for the first time offered a definition of the concept of mental disorder. Unfortunately, this definition invoked other undefined notions. For example, in addition to meeting specific criteria, all disorders had to be "clinically significant," associated with "distress" yet not be an "expectable . . . response to an event," and also had to be the result of biological, behavioral, or psychological "dysfunction." The problem was that *none of these additional requirements was defined at all*. So rather than clarifying or anchoring the concept of mental disorder in a solid foundation, the *DSM* definition further obscured matters (Bolton, 2008; McNally, 2011). In order to know what the APA/*DSM* considers a valid mental disorder, one must therefore examine the diagnostic criteria for each disorder, which themselves do not represent any coherent framework.

Scientific tradition requires that assertion about the validity of concepts, such as "mental illness," cannot rest on mere personal opinion or even group consensus but must be supported by an independent body of theory and evidence. This is an extremely important point to note, as misunderstandings about how validity is established may blind many to a fundamental problem with the *DSM*. To state that mental illness is a valid concept (that it truly identifies a phenomenon of nature), means that some body of *evidence* has been amassed according to the guidelines of a specific biomedical *theory*, and then has survived rigorous tests devised upon the notion that the specific theory might be false. Then and only then might we entertain with some confidence that behaviors now defined as symptoms of mental disorders might "truly" be the manifestations of diseases or brain disorders. This has not occurred. But history, of course, is littered with people's assumptions and even certainties about things that later are shown to be untrue, to be invalid.

The classification of mental illnesses, such as *DSM*, must be *tested* if it is to be considered valid. Unlike a pontifical statement, it cannot be accepted on faith. The modern *DSM*, beginning in 1980, could identify no neuropsychological or medical or remotely physiological criteria for any of its categories of mental illness—which would buttress the idea that these categories pointed to real phenomena of nature rather than being mere ideas arising out of speech, faith, belief, or expediency. It offered no explicit theory of cause, nor pointed to any body of evidence to justify its claim that its description of mental disorders was scientifically valid. Instead, it offered (false) claims of greatly improved reliability, which was really only a preliminary issue to the central issue of whether the hundreds of specific diagnostic criteria had any bearing on the validity of presumed illnesses. The claims of improved reliability were false, but even if true, they were not adequate pillars on which to rest claims that psychiatric diagnosis was now "scientific."

To be sure, the diagnostic practices of its predecessor *DSM-II* were a hodgepodge; that 1968 version of the manual offered little specific guidance in making diagnoses, giving at most a few sentences, although these sentences did suggest prototypes of the disorders. But to the research psychiatrists who dominated the deliberations that produced *DSM-III*, such brevity in describing diagnostic categories undermined claims that diagnosis was scientific and that "real mental disorders" actually existed *out there*, independently of the ideas American psychiatrists might have about such matters. The new descriptive formats that they developed were expected to add more precision to diagnosis, improve reliability, and buttress claims about validity.

Although *DSM* avoids making any definitive statements about the actual meaning of the lists of diagnostic criteria, their primary function surely was to identify presumably valid cases of mental illness, or, conversely, screen out cases in which mental disorder was not present. *The criteria are the essence of descriptive diagnosis.* That is why NIMH and psychiatric leaders routinely use these criteria in research that determines how many people in the population are mentally ill and why clinicians use the criteria to claim reimbursement from insurance companies for the treatment of mental disorders. In short, *DSM*'s diagnostic criteria *are* the established definitions of mental disorders in the United States.

Do these criteria ensure diagnostic validity? The answer is, no. *DSM*'s diagnostic criteria do not establish the validity of any disorders. If they did do so, the controversy over homosexuality could have been quickly resolved by a simple diagnostic list of homosexual feelings and behaviors. But a simple listing of behaviors would not have convinced the scientific community or gay activists *why* the behavior represented a mental illness. *Describing a set of behaviors and labeling them as pathological symptoms never establishes the validity of an illness.* At a minimum, one would need to identify a cluster of medical signs and symptoms consistently occurring together (a syndrome)—the minimal requirement for a medical disorder—and linking them empirically to an underlying, demonstrable physiological dysfunction.

DSM offers behavioral diagnostic criteria as if they confirm the existence of a valid disorder, when the criteria merely describe what is claimed a priori to be an illness. Descriptive diagnosis is a tautology that distracts observers from recognizing that *DSM* offers no indicators that establish the validity of any psychiatric illness, although they may typically point to distresses, worries, or misbehaviors.

Many other reasons help explain why lists of criteria for *DSM* disorders have not established the validity of the illness categories. Over the following pages we will discuss some of the major ones.

Ambiguity of Criteria

Throughout the *DSM* the diagnostic criteria are ambiguous, which can be problematic. For example, if the Internal Revenue Service stipulated that taxpayers were expected to pay their "fair share" of taxes without providing guidance about what that meant, individuals and tax professionals would have vastly different interpretations of the meaning of *fair share* and how to determine it. The diagnostic criteria in *DSM* generally fail to specify the conditions under which the criteria would be met, meaning that clinicians ultimately provide their own interpretation. For example, the first two criteria for Generalized Anxiety Disorder include "excessive anxiety" that the person finds "difficult to control." How exactly does a clinician determine what is excessive or how difficult it is to control? How much control? Similarly, with Histrionic Personality Disorder, which can be identified by criteria such as when a person "is uncomfortable in situations in which he or she is not the center of attention," "displays rapidly shifting and shallow expressions of emotions," or "shows self-dramatization." How uncomfortable? What is a shallow expression? What exactly constitutes self-dramatization? Clinicians and others would find it very difficult to know exactly when such criteria are sufficiently manifested, thus producing unreliability in diagnosis and undercutting the validity of the presumed personality disorder.

Redundancy of Criteria

DSM requires that disorders meet multiple criteria. The ostensible purpose is that multiple criteria are supposed to raise the threshold for the use of each diagnosis, making it appear that the *DSM* standards will ensure validity (i.e., those diagnosed with a disorder would be clearly different from those without a diagnosis). For example, using only one behavioral criterion would be viewed as unjustifiable because it would produce many false negatives (cases diagnosed with the disorder but not "really" having the disorder). By using multiple criteria, *DSM* conveys that it is enhancing the validity of diagnosis. Any careful reading of these lists of criteria, however, finds that many supposedly different criteria are merely the same stated differently.

For example, the first of five criteria for the diagnosis "Social Phobia (Social Anxiety Disorder)" is:

- a marked and persistent fear of one or more social or performance situations in which the person is exposed to unfamiliar people or to possible scrutiny by others. The individual fears that he or she will act in a way (or show anxiety symptoms) that will be humiliating or embarrassing. (APA, 2000, p. 456)

So the first criterion is whether the person if fearful and anxious about some social situation. We will ignore that the *DSM* provides no specification about the nature of "fear" or its many different contexts and types.

The additional four criteria just reiterate elements of the first criteria:

- "a feared social situation provoking anxiety;
- the person recognizes that there is unreasonable fear;
- the feared situation is avoided or endured with anxiety; and
- the feared social situation interferes with the person's normal routine or he is distressed about the phobia (APA, 2000, p. 456)."

In other words, there are not five criteria to be met but only one—and that one criterion is actually contained in the title of the disorder. This redundancy is so blatant that one thinks this must be a rare mistake in the manual. But it is not.

One of the most common diagnoses for children is Attention-Deficit/Hyperactivity Disorder (ADHD). There are three subtypes: Inattention, Hyperactivity, and Impulsivity. For each type there are supposedly different criteria. For Inattention six criteria must be met to use the diagnosis. The first criterion for Inattention is:

- "often fails to give close attention to details or makes careless mistakes in schoolwork, work, or other activities."

But this is restated in other criteria:

- "difficulty sustaining attention,"
- "does not seem to listen,"
- "fails to finish school work,"
- "avoids . . . tasks that require sustained mental effort,"
- is "easily distracted," and
- is "forgetful in daily activities (APA, 2000, p. 92)."

Six of the nine criteria are explicit or clearly implied by the first criteria. What at first appears to be a stringent threshold for use of the diagnosis, supposedly enhancing validity, is in reality one criterion restated in different ways. Little wonder that 10 percent of schoolchildren in the United States are labeled with the diagnosis (Pastor & Reuben, 2008).

The redundancy also occurs in the criteria for Hyperactivity, where six of nine criteria must be met. The first criterion is "often fidgets with hands or feet or squirms in seat." Other criteria are implicit in the first:

- "often leaves seat,"
- "often runs about,"
- "has difficulty playing . . . quietly,"
- "often on the go," and
- "often talks excessively (APA, 2000, p. 92)."

Apparently, the developers of this list then ran out of synonyms for fidgeting, which *The Random House Unabridged Dictionary* (Author, 1987) defines as: "to move about restlessly, nervously, or impatiently."

Similarly, there are three criteria for Impulsivity, which also reflect, upon a cursory inspection, the same criterion:

- "often blurts out answers before questions have been completed,"
- "often has difficulty awaiting turn," and
- "often interrupts or intrudes on others (APA, 2000, p. 92)."

In the case of ADHD, therefore, there is really only one or maybe two criteria, and they are both implied in the title of the disorder. The title of the disorder says all the architects of *DSM* intended to say about this category. The point is that lists containing multiple criteria provide a false sense of validity by appearing to use substantively different criteria. Using synonyms as criteria does not enhance validity any more than using a checklist of synonyms for *ghost—spirit, ghoul,* or *poltergeist*—would enhance the validity of the category *ghost.*

Ignoring Social Context of Behaviors

Descriptive psychiatry requires the implausible belief that the meaning and causes of observable behaviors can be understood and used as symptoms of *mental disorder* without paying attention to the social context of the behaviors themselves, and of course the meaning of the behaviors to the person and those who observe the person. For example, is it a sign of mental illness if a devout Christian converses intimately with God, a young woman becomes extremely morose after learning that she is afflicted with a terminal illness, or a child severely misbehaves in an abusive, alcohol-drenched, chaotic household? *DSM's* almost total neglect of the interpersonal, social, cultural, and physical environment ensures that the diagnostic criteria are susceptible to what psychologists have called the fundamental attribution error. That common error is interpreting the behaviors of others as due to their own personality and personal tendencies, rather than as responses to their social circumstances (Levy, 2010; Ryan, 1971; Weiner, 1995). That error, of course, is compounded when those making the attribution lack the time, the skills, or the genuine interest to listen to people's own uncertain, groping explanations of why they behave as they do.

DSM has placed the fundamental attribution error as the cornerstone of descriptive diagnosis. For example, all the major epidemiological surveys that purport to establish the prevalence of mental illness in the population rest on simple counts of whether the diagnostic criteria are met or not. *DSM* assumes that individuals' social class, past life experiences, current social context, ethnic and cultural identity, religious beliefs, loves and losses, aspirations and frustrations, intentions and excuses, competence and failure, joys and heartaches—as these individuals see them and understand them and have acted on these perceptions *and* as others have responded—are irrelevant to the issue of knowing precisely what ails them. None of these dimensions of experience is explored in determining whether people's behavior meets the established criteria for some presumed mental disorder. The diagnostic criteria, for the most part, are *devoid of context* (Jacobs & Cohen, 2010). Certainly some clinicians rightfully explore these personal and contextual dimensions in their assessment interviews, but when they need to make a diagnosis, they are required to assume that some mental illness exists and then to conform only to the checklists of criteria. Descriptive psychiatry, in fact, was designed to minimize clinical intuition and inferences and to push clinicians into assuming that human troubles inevitably constitute signs of disorder. Neglecting to value the importance of social context in understanding human behavior is absurd and only undermines the validity of *DSM* (Bolton, 2008; Greenberg, 2010; Horwitz & Wakefield, 2007; Horwitz & Wakefield, 2012; Hsieh & Kirk, 2003; Jacobs & Cohen, 2012; Kirk, Wakefield, Hsieh, & Pottick, 1999; Kirmayer & Young, 1999; Lane, 2007; Wakefield, Pottick, & Kirk, 2002).

Arbitrary Cutting Points and False Positives

Apart from their ambiguity, redundancy, and neglect of social context, using multiple diagnostic criteria supposedly helps to identify valid cases of mental illness. Some *DSM* disorders require that only a few criteria are met, whereas other disorders require many. The number of required criteria is arbitrary: just as disorders are created and deleted with each revision of the manual, so too are the type and number of criteria. There is no established method or standards that *DSM* uses in deciding how many criteria should be required for any disorder. This is because no scientific links or any other indicators exist that psychiatric researchers themselves consider important between the diagnostic criteria and any specific biological pathology (or anything biological). Without that scientific foundation, the decision about the number of criteria is essentially a practical and public relations problem.

It is self evident that when more criteria are required, fewer people will qualify as having the disorder (if, as we have shown earlier, the criteria are not merely synonyms); with fewer criteria, more people will be labeled as mentally ill. For example, *DSM-IV* requires that any three of fifteen criteria be met to diagnose a child with Conduct Disorder. Why three and not two, five, or seven? Probably, if only one was required many children would qualify for the mental illness, but if seven were required fewer would be defined as ill. The makers of *DSM* recognize this, and use cutoff numbers so that not too many children are defined as disordered—causing public skepticism and scientific rebuke—and not so few children that funding for research and services might be decreased because the problem seems rare. Again, this is not a decision driven by scientific findings but rather a public relations, economic, and political judgment.

In general, the developers of *DSM* select cutoff points that boost the number of people that can be labeled as mentally ill using the *DSM*. Even by their own estimates, which assume that *DSM* is describing valid "disorders" (an assumption that we do not make), they acknowledge that the diagnostic system makes two types of misdiagnosis. The first, mentioned previously, is what is called a false negative, which is to falsely identify a child as not having a presumed "disorder" when they actually do have such a disorder. The second, called a false positive, is falsely identifying some child as having a presumed "disorder" when they do not have that disorder. Using several standard computations, the rate of both types of errors can be calculated. For example, looking at the list of criteria for disorders for children and adolescents in *DSM-IV* (Kirk, 2004), the misdiagnosis or error rate for the diagnosis of ADHD is about 38 percent, for Conduct Disorder about 11 percent, and for Oppositional Defiant Disorder about 21 percent. (Of course, these computations *assume* that the diagnostic categories are valid.) The overwhelmingly more frequent error is identifying children as mentally ill who are not. For example, with ADHD, for every 1,000 children screened using the *DSM* criteria, about 4.5 with ADHD would be incorrectly diagnosed as not having it (false negatives), but 370 kids who don't have ADHD would be misdiagnosed with it (false positives). These errors rates were known before the criteria for *DSM-IV* were selected. In other words, the makers of *DSM-IV* chose cutoff points for *DSM* children's disorders that routinely exaggerate the prevalence of presumed mental disorder in the population. The ambiguity and redundancy of criteria, the neglect of social context in identifying the meaning of behaviors, and the arbitrary method of establishing cutoff points contribute to additional, more profound problems with validity of *DSM* categories.

Heterogeneity within Categories

The fundamental objective of *DSM*'s categorical approach was to capture people who all had the same presumed mental illness. Studying them as a group, it was hoped, would lead to the validation of the disease category by discovering some underlying biological marker that would validate the categories as existing in nature by distinguishing those who have the illness from others without the illness (Rounsaville et al., 2002). This was the Kraepelinian goal: to discover biological markers (hopefully *causal*) to confirm the existence of the diseases in those in whom diseases were hypothesized to exist and the inexistence of such markers in others.

This hasn't happened. There are no known biological markers for any category. This observation is not only a Szaszian attack on the myth of the validity of mental disease; it is today the oft-repeated conclusion of current leaders of psychiatry. After thirty years of research using the modern *DSM* categories, there is agreement among the researchers who have looked at the problem that the *DSM* categories *do not* group together people with distinguishing characteristics (Regier, Narrow, Kuhl, & Kupfer, 2009; Jablensky, 2012; Rounsaville et al., 2002).

It is easy to understand why this lack of homogeneity within categories arose. First, there may be no distinguishing characteristic underlying the *DSM* madness categories to be found. If the categories themselves are invalid, precisely sorting types of behavior into them won't make them meaningful. Recall that many women were identified and sorted into an earlier category of "witches," but that sorting did nothing to establish the validity of the idea of witches. Second, as we have said, the criteria used for the sorting are ambiguous, redundant, and arbitrary. Third, the use of multiple criteria, that is, multiple behaviors, provides many entrances into the same category. For example, for Conduct Disorder for children, any three of fifteen different behaviors must be observed. But three of fifteen allows for many different combinations. In fact, it allows for precisely 455 different combinations of children's behaviors in diagnosing a child with Conduct Disorder. Heterogeneity of children should be expected. The only consistency to be observed with Conduct Disorder is that clinicians use the same diagnosis for many different types of children and behaviors. Common problems such as this undermine the validity of *DSM* categories.

Comorbidity among Categories

In addition to heterogeneity within categories, there is comorbidity across *DSM* categories. Comorbidity refers to people having more than one "disease," more than one morbid condition. Since some *DSM* categories share diagnostic criteria (behaviors asserted to be representative "symptoms"), some people either meet the required criteria for more than one category or have some but not enough symptoms to "qualify" for any one *DSM* disease category. In short, many people don't fit neatly into the *DSM* categories. This is not merely the case of the occasional person having more than one "independent" illness at the same time. This is a much more extensive and common problem, undermining the *DSM* assumption of discrete categories of illness. In fact, studies (Kessler, Chiu, Kemler, & Walters, 2005) have found comorbidity in about half of people diagnosed, suggesting, as one researcher said, that "there is no empirical evidence" for "natural boundaries between major syndromes," and that "the categorical approach is fundamentally flawed" (Cloninger, 1999, as cited in Rounsaville et al., 2002, p. 12).

DSM provides various tactics for categorizing messy cases. One is a catchall option within most categories: NOS "Not Otherwise Specified." If a person doesn't meet the required specific criteria demanded by *DSM*, clinicians can use NOS. Another tactic, added in *DSM-IV* (p. xxiii) allows clinicians to use a category even if the problem "falls just short" of the full criteria. In these ways, the entire effort of the modern *DSM* to specify required diagnostic criteria can be ignored at any time by any clinician by using NOS or the "just falls short" options.

Underlying Dimensionality

The categorical system has not carved nature at its joints, as is expected of any scientific classification system. The evidence is accumulating that there may not be joints to be found for presumed mental illnesses. There is growing recognition among researchers, including those crafting the *DSM-5*, that almost all of the phenomena of concern to psychiatry—behaviors, moods, perceptions, emotions, cognition—are better conceptualized as continua, ranging from the less intense (more frequently noticed) to the more intense (less frequently noticed), without any clear discontinuities along the way. If sharp discontinuities of feelings and behaviors were found, it might suggest some natural cutoff points at the boundaries of normal and unusual, lend some empirical validation to the disease categorical approach. We find this in most categories of serious physical illness, where there are independent tests to determine whether one has a cancerous tumor or not, pneumonia or not, tuberculosis or not. The exceptions tend to be around "illnesses" for which drug companies with a profitable product to sell until the patent on the product expires have lobbied powerfully to establish lower cutoff scores from physical tests for such things as bone density, high blood pressure, and cholesterol levels (Healy, 2012). In doing so, these drug companies greatly reshape the understanding of disease while extending their markets and profits (Greene, 2007).

In psychiatry, by contrast, we do not find natural discontinuities or bimodal distributions of anxiety, insomnia, irritability, or sadness or most other relevant experiences. Even hearing voices or thinking that others mean to harm us is a widely distributed phenomenon (Luhrmann, 2010). The dimensionality of the "symptoms" used in *DSM* suggests that the categorical system is problematic and that the attempt to distinguish disorder from nondisorder is arbitrary (Bolton, 2008). As we will see, most of the struggles over *DSM-5* are, in fact, disputes over where the arbitrary boundaries should be drawn between phenomena that have not been validated as disease categories.

Description Is Not Explanation

The modern *DSM* purports to provide guidance in identifying valid instances of mental illness. The manual explicitly claims that it is "atheoretical," terminology that was used to imply that the categories did not contain any inferences about the "causes" of the disease, no theory about what it is or why it occurred. That's why it is known as "descriptive diagnosis." This is about all the manual could officially claim, because there is no convincing scientific evidence concerning what causes people to feel or act in ways that are uncomfortable to themselves or bothersome to others. But in practice, clinicians use *DSM*, because it does offer "medical" explanations for behavior, although it does so in a tautological manner.[1]

Imagine that you go to your physician complaining of a sore throat. The physician listens to your complaint and explains that you have Sore Throat Disorder. You inquire how he reached the conclusion about your illness, and he responds, "Because you have a sore throat." This diagnostic reasoning would strike you as a joke, because, in medicine, when possible symptoms are noted, the physician uses independent procedures to gather information about the presence of some underlying disorder that might explain your symptom. For example, he might give you a physical exam or order blood tests, X-rays, throat cultures, or various invasive physical probes. If the physical tests and probes confirm that there is some underlying pathology, the physician can then conclude reasonably that your symptoms were caused by the pathology, perhaps in this case an infection triggered by some virus or bacteria. Even if the ultimate cause of the pathology is unknown, we can explain the symptoms as a result of the observable, tested pathology. The point here is that a symptom (a complaint, a behavior) explains nothing by itself. The symptom might have several underlying causes. And in the absence of a physical sign—which itself may also have several different underlying causes—the symptom is an extremely poor guide to determine what, if anything, is the matter.

Contrast this with diagnosis in psychiatry. You take your young son to a psychiatrist and complain that he doesn't pay attention, doesn't listen, and is fidgety most of the time. The psychiatrist listens to your story and shares that disturbing news that your child's behaviors are due to a mental disorder: Not Paying Attention Disorder. You may be comforted to learn of the diagnosis that explains your child's behavior, but you ask the psychiatrist how he reached this conclusion. He explains that he reached the diagnosis because the boy doesn't pay attention.

This is precisely how children are diagnosed with Attention-Deficit/ Hyperactivity Disorder (ADHD). To use the diagnosis of ADHD, a child must exhibit at least six behaviors from a longer list in *DSM*, such as he often fidgets or "often fails to give close attention to details" or "often does not seem to listen"—redundant criteria—as we have pointed out in detail. If the child meets the criteria, the child is said to "have" the underlying disease of ADHD. But no independent tests can verify any underlying mental disorder; the very symptoms used to construct the alleged mental disorder confirm the presence of the disease. Why does the child fidget and not listen? Because he has ADHD, the construct that uses these descriptions as its defining criteria. How do we know he has ADHD? Because parents and teachers state that he fidgets and doesn't listen. The acceptance of this patently circular reasoning by countless experts, authorities, and parents in America and increasingly around the world is a sad measure of the scientific "progress" that has been achieved in mental health.

This tautological ruse with ADHD is not confined to children's disorders. Psychiatric diagnosis in general is the equivalent of Sore Throat Disorder. It is description masquerading as explanation. In psychology, this is called the nominal fallacy, in which naming is presented as explaining (Levy, 2010). *DSM* has made the nominal fallacy another foundation stone. Naming and describing a phenomenon as a mental disorder does not in any way confirm the validity of diagnosis or of the existence of a presumed disorder.

The Successful Marketing of Failure

One would reasonably expect that these glaring weaknesses of descriptive psychiatry—unreliability and invalidity due to ambiguous and redundant criteria that ignore social context; the lack of homogeneity within categories and comorbidity across categories; arbitrary decisions about cutoff points biased in favor of false positives; and where merely naming is passed off as explaining—would have completely undermined the credibility of the modern *DSM* and that the APA's ownership and monopoly over the terrain of madness would be called into question.

When such serious flaws are found with other consumer products, such as were allegedly seen with Toyota's automobiles, this would justify a recall, a suspension of sales, an independent scientific review, and a search for a different manufacturing approach. Instead, *DSM* has been a huge success and created an epidemic of labeling people as mentally ill (Whitaker, 2010). In thirty years, *DSM* went from a meaningless codebook to a veritable bible on madness and misbehavior. Ironically, the serious flaws of *DSM* have been exploited to extend its use. If there are no solid conceptual or empirical standards for what should be considered a psychiatric "brain" disorder, if the diagnostic criteria are ambiguous, if any troublesome behavior can be designated as a "symptom," and if clinicians have wide latitude and financial incentives to find disorder, the *DSM* becomes a handy dictionary of disorders with a scientific patina only provided by the APA. It is then understandable that with each edition, the list of disorders and the criteria expand, the thresholds for diagnosis become less stringent, and proposals for new "recently discovered" brain disorders pour in—binge eating, shopping disorder, psychosis risk syndrome, road rage, temper dysregulation disorder, and more. Many people, professions, and programs are stakeholders, and they relentlessly push for more psychiatric brain disorders—that is, for more *names* of entities to be accepted as brain disorders.

Nothing in the turgid text or detail of the modern *DSM* can possibly account for its huge success. Nor was there ever any solid scientific evidence of its vast superiority. Its success was that it found an eager market among powerful groups, institutions, and organizations, and perhaps fed on an insatiable urge to medicalize that which is difficult to understand. Let's look briefly at these groups and institutions and some of their actions.

American Psychiatric Association

The boosters of *DSM* in 1980 skillfully used the professional journals of the American Psychiatric Association as part of the promotion of the manual. Instead of a scientific journal functioning as an arbiter of truth and tests for truth, the APA-sponsored *American Journal of Psychiatry* promoted a commercial product in which it had a financial stake (for details, see Kirk & Kutchins, 1992: 185–187). Rarely would you see in a scientific article, as one did in 1980, a footnote directing readers to the sales department of the APA and instructing them in precisely how much money they needed to send to the APA for a copy (Spitzer, Williams, & Skodal, 1980). The APA's leadership, however, had not given Spitzer a mandate to radically change the diagnostic system, not sanctioned the methods he used to accomplish it, or welcomed the controversies he created behind the scenes and publicly. Nevertheless, by the time the new manual was approved, the APA rallied behind Spitzer's efforts.

Spitzer had proved himself an able advocate and a tireless crusader. The task force he chaired and the committees he created and coordinated were composed of many of the rising scientific elite of psychiatry. Although psychoanalytic factions of the profession and many psychologists were skeptical about the nature of the new manual, the APA could hardly turn its back on a diagnostic effort that was being billed as a great scientific achievement and as a way for psychiatry to take the upper hand in a battle with critics. Spitzer offered irresistible products: scientific respectability and the illusion of supportive data. After 1987, however, Spitzer's personal stamp on the manual and strong control over the processes of revision began to grow uncomfortable for the APA and the APA replaced Spitzer as the chief *DSM* guru with another *DSM* insider, Allen Frances, an expert on personality disorders, who was chosen to guide the development of *DSM-IV* (Spiegel, 2005).

The APA's rapid embrace of the *DSM* was only part of what propelled its success. Mental health professionals were easy converts or draftees, and it was their purchasing of the manual that created a multimillion-dollar commercial windfall for the APA. Psychiatrists were only a small proportion of the professionals in the burgeoning mental health professions during these decades (Goleman, 1990). Although most clinicians weren't embroiled in the academic debates over the meaning of *mental illness* or the reliability of diagnoses, they were aware of the growing attention of the public to mental health and the growing popularity of psychotherapy in its many forms. The reestablishment of the credibility of psychiatric diagnosis, under the medical imprimatur of the APA, provided a plausible defense for all these clinicians, not only for psychiatrists. The new *DSM* gave them all a handy scientific-looking codebook that provided a rationale for labeling human troubles as true "mental disorders" and a medical justification for their helping services, along with a renewed sense of respectability and status. Whatever the concerns of psychologists about the increased medicalization of behavioral problems or of social workers about the emphasis on internal pathology to the neglect of the social environment, clinicians eventually lined up to buy the new tome and to use it, in part because they had little choice. The more *DSM* was used, the more it had to be used. The use of *DSM* was rapidly adopted and required by clinics and agencies, and those in private practice needed it as well, since filing a specific, recognizable, and codified diagnosis quickly became a requirement for insurance reimbursement for services rendered. For clinicians, *DSM* migrated from codebook to bankbook.

National Institute of Mental Health

In addition to the APA, a chorus of institutional voices sang praises to the biomedical revolution in psychiatry and helped establish *DSM*'s dominance (see, for example, Whitaker, 2010, pp. 276–280). The first was the NIMH. As the federal government's major advocate for mental health research and services, NIMH played a marginal role in the development of *DSM-III*, although indirectly it funded many of the psychiatric studies that brought attention to the problems of psychiatric diagnoses. NIMH, after all, had a stake in finding a better scientific grounding for diagnoses as a way of organizing knowledge about mental illness. The claims made about *DSM-III* were music to the bureaucratic ears of officials at NIMH, and NIMH signed on as a booster. Shortly thereafter, NIMH made the use of *DSM*'s criteria a virtual requirement for those seeking funding for research on treatment, diagnoses, and epidemiology.

Big Pharma

The second institutional investor was comprised of multinational drug companies. Although the role of pharmaceutical companies in psychiatric research is now pervasive (Carey, 2006; L. Cosgrove, Krimsky, Vijayaraghavan, & Schneider, 2006; Healy, 2012), as it is in most areas of medical research, the role of the drug industry in the original development of *DSM-III* is obscure (though some studies, as in the case of panic disorder, do exist, see Jacobs, 1995, pp. 441–442). Nevertheless, the creation of *DSM-III* and the expanding number of disorders with lists of vague diagnostic criteria was an incredible gift to the pharmaceutical industry, offering not only scientific respectability to diagnosis, but also an opportunity for the expansion of the range of behaviors that might be legitimately labeled as symptoms of disorders and thereby treated with patented and prescribed psychoactive medications (see chapter 6 and 7). *DSM* gained prominence as these companies, part of one of the largest and richest industries in the world, exploited the expansion of mental disorders (Angell, 2011a, 2011b).

Health Insurance Industry

The third institutional investor in *DSM* was the health insurance industry, both public (e.g., Medicaid) and private. As more insurance policies began to include coverage for psychiatric treatment of some mental disorders, the insurance industry relied on the *DSM* to guide decisions about what distinguishes a mental disorder from other human problems. Also, the industry appreciated the lists of diagnostic criteria, which put constraints on mental health professionals using diagnostic labels indiscriminately. Thus, the appearance of a new "reliable" diagnostic system with lists of diagnostic criteria provided guidance to insurance companies sorting out whether reimbursement claims from mental health clients represented help with "genuine" psychiatric illness or merely with ordinary problems in living for which insurance would not pay. For example, parents seeking help for managing an unruly child might consult friends, teachers, or members of the clergy but would normally not seek, nor would companies pay for, professional services unless that child was officially labeled as having a mental disorder, such as Attention-Deficit Disorder. The new revised *DSM* gave insurance companies two tools. One was a list of specific behavioral criteria that had to be met before a diagnosis was used, providing the appearance that objective criteria, rather than clinicians' vague judgments, were employed to distinguish illness from other problems in living. Second, the expanded list of disorders forced insurance companies to select which specific disorders they would pay for and which they would not cover. Few insurance plans will cover all of the disorders in *DSM;* most cover only the more "serious" ones or the more popular ones; and most impose sharp limits on the number of treatment visits in a given time period. Thus, despite the potential expansion of disorders that the drug companies encouraged, the insurance companies could use *DSM* selectively to regulate their exposure to financial risk and costs.

Two federal laws, the Mental Health Parity and Addiction Equity Act of 2008 and the Patient Protection and Affordable Care Act of 2010 are likely to alter the insurance terrain in unpredictable ways. The first legislation insists that insurance coverage for mental disorders have "parity" with the coverage for physical diseases, and the second is the massive health reform legislation introduced by President Barack Obama. Although too early to know as of this writing, it is likely that *DSM*'s uses will increase through these initiatives and that the demand for and cost of treatment for mental disorders will increase. Conversely, to limit their costs, insurance companies might begin to insist that, in addition to diagnoses, measures of actual disability or impairment and their reversal determine eligibility for insurance coverage of mental disorders. Similarly, measures of efficacy as determined by clients, rather than only asserted in the professional literature, might be used by insurance companies to determine whether a given treatment for a mental health problem receives coverage. We will return to some of these issues in the concluding chapter of this book.

News Media

The fourth institutional investor was the news media, which has provided the public with a steady diet of stories about purported scientific advances in psychiatry since the 1960s. If one had asked ordinary people on the street in 1960 whether they had ever heard of the *Diagnostic and Statistical Manual of Mental Disorders*, only a few would have expressed any recognition. Today, many would not only say that they had heard of it, but most likely they would also be able to say which *DSM* disorders they qualify for. The *DSM* criteria sets for psychiatric diagnosis frequently appear in magazine and newspaper articles and are featured in stories on television. Pharmaceutical companies advertise these criteria in ubiquitous TV ads to increase their markets of people seeking and taking psychiatric drugs.

The APA, mental health professions, NIMH, drug and insurance companies, and the news media were all using *DSM* for their own disparate and often inconsistent institutional purposes: as a declaration of professional jurisdiction; medical dictionary of disorders; compendium of human troubles; administrative codebook; textbook and training manual; protocol for research funding; justification for prescription medications; insurance reimbursement claim form; and as a legal tool in forensic settings. Together this alignment of powerful professional, governmental, and commercial institutions—perhaps accurately termed the biomedical or biopsychiatric industrial complex—ensured the expansion of *DSM* because, even though each member may have had a different agenda, all were united to promote the idea that deviant or strange behavior should be understood as a medical illness subject to government-supported medical authority and intervention. Remarkably, little public opposition arose. Although *DSM-III* and *DSM-IV* completely failed to deliver on their scientific promises and claims, their marketing was effective, pervasive, and unstoppable.

DSM-5 and the "Best and Latest Scientific Research"

Science is always the ostensible rationale for revising *DSM*. Ever since Robert Spitzer first claimed science as the rationale to reform the *DSM* in the 1970s, each subsequent revision (*DSM-III-R*, *DSM-IV*) was justified by claiming that the manual needed to incorporate new scientific knowledge. As implausible as that rationale has been, it is nearly impossible to assess before the revision is published. Even afterward, the manual contains no footnotes directing the curious to the scientific data on which hundreds of decisions were made. Despite criticisms of each edition, the promoters of *DSM* hope that among the vast armies of users the manual, like religious dogma, will be accepted gratefully and uncritically.

Something different emerged for the next edition, *DSM-5*. Work on *DSM-5* began five years after the publication of *DSM-IV* in 1994. Discussion about the next revision began among the director of NIMH, the medical director of the APA, and the chair of the APA's committee on psychiatric diagnosis who jointly organized a *DSM-5* Research Planning Conference in 1999 to "set research priorities" (APA, 2008). Over the next years, they set up planning work groups, commissioned a series of white papers, and sponsored over a dozen conferences to discuss and develop a research agenda for *DSM-5*. The APA stressed the global nature of the efforts, which involved consultations with the World Health Organization (WHO), the World Psychiatric Association (WPA), and others. NIMH was asked to fund a series of "research planning conferences that would focus on the research evidence for revisions of specific diagnostic areas" (APA, 2008). NIMH, the National Institute on Drug Abuse (NIDA), and the National Institute on Alcoholism and Alcohol Abuse (NIAAA) provided over $1 million. Originally expected by 2010, the publication of *DSM-5* has been pushed back several times as political and scientific problems have mounted. The latest date posted by the APA as of this writing is May 2013, making the gestation period for the next edition nearly three times longer than it took Robert Spitzer to give birth to *DSM-III*.

Selected experts were invited to participate in the important initial planning conference, but, curiously for a purportedly scientific effort, those closely involved in the development of *DSM-IV* were not included, "to encourage thinking beyond the current DSM-IV framework" (APA, 2008). We will return to this matter shortly.

In 2006 the APA president appointed Drs. David J. Kupfer and Darrel A. Regier, prominent insiders at the APA and NIMH who had key roles in prior *DSM* editions, as the chair and vice chair of the *DSM-5* task force. Kupfer and Regier then nominated other APA members as chairs of the various work groups and as members of the central task force. The rhetoric of the APA was similar to that used in prior revisions. There were assurances that the diagnostic categories "will evolve to better reflect new scientific understanding," that there were "no pre-set limitation on the nature and degree of change that work groups could recommend," that their work would encourage "research questions and hypotheses . . . that can be "investigated through literature reviews and analyses of existing data," and that "they will also develop research plans, which can be further tested in DSM-V field trials involving direct data collection." Based on this "comprehensive review of scientific advancements, targeted research analyses, and clinical expertise, the work groups will develop draft DSM-V diagnostic criteria" (APA, 2008).

In May 2008 the APA announced the appointment of most members to all the major committees, "more than 120 world-renowned scientific researchers and clinicians" to "examine the extent to which this new research warrants modifying the current organization of disorders, descriptions of disorders and the criteria for diagnosis" (from APA press release: "APA names DSM-V work group members: Experts to revise manual for diagnosis of mental disorders" May 1, 2008).

Conflicts of Interest

One element of these APA announcements, however, had never appeared in prior *DSM* revisions, namely, that in order to avoid any "conflicts of inter-est" all task force and work group members had to "disclose all significant relationships with entities that have an interest in psychiatric diagnoses and treatments." Further, no participant was allowed to be paid more than $10,000 per year from "industry sources" while working on the revision. The APA press release provided reassurance that "we have made every effort to ensure that DSM-V will be based on the *best and latest scientific research*, and to eliminate conflicts of interest in its development" (May 1, 2008; emphasis added). Investigative journalists had already documented that the pockets of the APA, psychiatric leaders and organizations, and leading officials at NIMH and elsewhere were bulging with drug money (Willman, 2004a, 2004b; see chapters 6 and 7). The APA's announcement about avoid-ing conflicts of interest and voluntary disclosures had the appearance of a requirement forced onto the APA after a series of disturbing public revela-tions (see also Cosgrove et al., 2006).

For years drug industry ties to psychiatry had been hidden, although there was increasing evidence of financial conflicts of interest in medical research (Bekelman, Li, & Goss, 2003; Campbell et al., 2007; Campbell et al., 2006; Rothman, 2008). Drugs firms make billions of dollars marketing psychoactive drugs to primary care physicians and psychiatrists. For example, prescriptions for powerful antipsychotic drugs rose to 54 million in 2011, with total US sales of $18.2 billion (Friedman, 2012). As the *DSM-5* revision got underway, however, there was a cascade of negative revelations about psychiatry and the drug industry. For example, in 2007, it was revealed that psychiatrists top the list of medical specialists in accepting gifts from drug companies (Harris, 2007), and in 2010 a study in the *Archives of Internal Medicine* found that nearly 80 percent of psychiatrists had some kind of a relationship with drug companies (Graham, 2010). A congressional investigation, led by Senator Grassley, uncovered a series of conflicts of interest in psychiatry, which were reported by most major newspapers. These articles documented hidden financial payments by drug companies to influential psychiatrists at Harvard, Stanford, and Emory universities, and elsewhere.

Take the case of Charles B. Nemeroff, who resigned from his position as chair of the psychiatry department at Emory University after it was disclosed (Harris, 2008b) that he had received funds from drug companies without revealing them as required by the university and by NIMH, which also funded his research. In this and other cases, the universities and the NIMH began internal investigations. To the authors of this book, the reactions of the universities and of NIMH appear as disingenuous as that of the APA. For example, Emory University claimed to have been misled about Nemeroff's extensive involvement with drug companies though he was hardly secretive about his conflicts of interest (which were probably taken to constitute business-as-usual in that academic field). For example, in his 2004 book, *The Peace of Mind Prescription: An Authoritative Guide to Finding the Most Effective Treatment for Anxiety and Depression* (Charney, Nemeroff, & with Braun, 2004), Nemeroff provides a footnote in the introduction that lists the drug companies (and one research group primarily funded by the drug industry) from whom he received support. They include the following:

- Abbott Laboratories
- AFSP
- AstraZeneca
- Bristol-Myers Squibb
- Corcept
- Cypress Biosciences
- Eli Lilly
- Forest Laboratories
- GaxoSmithKline
- Janssen Pharmaceutica
- Merck
- NARSAD
- Pfizer
- Wyeth-Ayerst
- Acadia Pharmaceuticals
- Neurocrine Biosciences
- Novartis
- Organon
- Otsuka
- Sanofi
- Scirex
- Somerset

As an indicator of how little Nemeroff's history of undisclosed payoffs bothered the psychiatric community, shortly after he was forced to resign from Emory University as department chair and his NIMH funding was suspended, Nemeroff was recruited by the University of Miami as chair of its psychiatry department. Thomas Insel, the director of NIMH, even recommended him for that position (Basken, 2010).

Another scandal involved P. Trey Sunderland, the head of the NIH's geriatric psychiatry branch, who was charged by federal prosecutors for taking $285,000 in fees from a drug company, Pfizer, without the permission or knowledge of NIH (Wilson, 2006). Another public embarrassment was caused by Frederick Goodwin, the former director of NIMH, who was a radio celebrity on National Public Radio (NPR). In 2008, NPR fired him when it learned that he promoted the off-label use of mood stabilizers for children on the radio without disclosing that he had received more than $1 million from drug manufacturers since 2000 (Harris, 2008a).

Still another public relations disaster involved Harvard psychiatrist Joseph Biederman, the leading promoter of labeling children with bipolar disorder, a diagnosis which had rarely been applied to children (Harris & Carey, 2008). His promotion was credited with the dramatic increase of the use of that unusual diagnosis, which directly encouraged the off-label use of antipsychotic and anticonvulsant drugs for children—drugs with commonly dangerous effects. It was revealed by the congressional investigation that Biederman and his drug industry-funded research center had received millions of dollars from companies that profited handsomely from his advocacy (Harris, 2008c).

Although the APA is not directly responsible for these unethical practices by individual members, universities, or federal research institutes that regularly choose to look the other way or do not enforce their own rules, it also benefits from drug industry money. The US congressional investigation requested that leading medical associations reveal details about the amount of money that they and their directors receive from drug makers (Harris, 2009b). The APA receives 30 percent of its $62 million budget from pharmaceutical companies in ad revenues, convention support, and other income. Its own president in 2010, Alan Schatzberg of Stanford University, had $4.8 million in stock holdings in a drug company that he had cofounded. A huge proportion of the costs for the required continued education of psychiatrists and other physicians are paid by drug companies (Carlat, 2007). In addition, the APA and other publishers of medical journals have been faulted for failing to reveal conflicts of interest among authors of research articles funded by or conducted by drug companies; failing to prevent the publishing of articles ghostwritten by drug company employees (Wilson, 2009), and failing to reveal that drug companies' studies that don't support their products have been suppressed or manipulated (*The Economist*, 2008). Even when an APA committee made fourteen recommendations designed to regulate and significantly curtail conflicts of interest between psychiatrists and the pharmaceutical industry, the APA Assembly, its governing body, quashed the report before it could even be discussed and debated (Cassels, 2010). Universities, too, are not blameless; they have also failed to control conflicts of interest (Basken, 2009b; Harris, 2009; Monastersky, 2008), because they too are not immune to the attractions of money.

The actions of many drug companies have been described as criminal and have resulted in about $7 billion in fines or penalties for illegal off-label marketing and overcharging government health programs between 2004 and 2009 alone (Bloomberg.com, 2009; *New York Times*, 2010). There is rising concern that drug companies have corrupted medical research (Angell, 2004; Barber, 2008; Whitaker, 2010). A coalition of concerned scientists and ethicists petitioned NIH to investigate the many conflicts of interest that pervade medicine, including ghostwritten articles, physician payoffs, and the use of hired academic opinion leaders, such as Goodwin, Biederman, and Nemeroff, to increase markets for drugs (Basken, 2009a).

It was then—as a defensive reaction to these unfolding investigations of corruption and conflict of interest and to a study that uncovered that a majority of the psychiatrists who had served on the *DSM-IV* task force had financial ties to drug companies (Cosgrove et al., 2006)—that the APA responded with a conflict-of-interest policy for those working on *DSM-5*. (Note: in 2010, the APA officially changed *DSM-V* to *DSM-5*.). A response from the APA was needed, since another study had shown that psychiatrists were more likely than other medical specialists to receive payoffs from drug companies. To defend the profession, the APA requested that all of the participants in the *DSM-5* work groups sign a pledge (APA, 2012) to limit the income they receive from pharmaceutical companies. But the agreements are hardly reassuring. Each task force member pledged to take no more than *$10,000 a year* from drug manufacturers during the at least five-year process. Few observers would doubt that $50,000 or more might influence judgment. Among some public figures or public servants, such conflicts could lead to criminal conviction and prison sentences. There are other loopholes: there is no limit to the amount of money that participants can receive in "unrestricted" research funds from the same companies, nor is there a limit to how much they had received in prior years or will be paid in years immediately following the release of *DSM-5*.

Many principal members of the *DSM-5* task force have had lucrative relationships with many drug companies. The Center for Science in the Public Interest reported that twenty-eight members of the *DSM-5* task force are reported to have drug industry ties (Kaplan, 2009). The APA disclosure forms were incomplete and misleading, according to a report in *U.S. News and World Report* (Garber, 2007). For instance, they didn't reveal the drug industry funds that were funneled through other companies to the task force chair, David Kupfer. Also, the forms do not reveal how much money changed hands—as if the difference between $500 and $500,000 is irrelevant. Finally, disclosures were voluntary. In short, the APA's feeble attempt to control conflicts of interest in the revision of *DSM* only called attention to the wave of influence from the drug industry that permeates the psychiatric establishment. In fact, the most recent study (Cosgrove & Krimsky, 2012) of conflicts of interest among those working on *DSM-5* reports that 69 percent of the participants have ties with pharmaceutical companies, a one-fifth *increase* over the previous edition.

Secrecy and Attacks from Insiders

Although Robert Spitzer was removed from *DSM* oversight by the APA in the late 1980s, he resurrected himself with *DSM-5*. This time, instead of effectively managing political controversies created by outsiders, he created one himself. In September 2008 Spitzer sent an open letter (via e-mail) to a wide swath of mental health professionals, accusing the APA and the *DSM-5* task force of revising the next edition of *DSM* in secret (Spitzer, 2008). His letter was the purported outgrowth of his frustration in attempting to have the task force leaders, David Kupfer and Darrel Regier, make public the minutes of *DSM* meetings. Apparently they had refused his requests by invoking the need "to maintain DSM-V confidentiality." In his letter, Spitzer revealed that all those involved in the *DSM* revision process had been required to sign a confidentiality agreement that prohibited them from disclosing anything about the *DSM-5* to anyone, including the spiritual godfather of the modern *DSM*, Spitzer himself. Spitzer found this unprecedented, puzzling, and "ludicrous." He argued that an open and transparent process would allow for wide critical review—the very "foundation of science." He stated:

> It is ironic that one of the most widespread (and in my view unfair) criticisms of DSM-III and progeny has been the process of decision-making by committee. This silly new "confidentiality" policy plays right into the hands of these critics and fuels cynicism about the decision-making process—except that in this case, in contrast to decision making for the revision of prior DSMs, the cynicism may be well justified. (Spitzer, 2008)

It was clearly Spitzer's intention to create a political controversy for the APA and the *DSM-5* participants. And he did. Newspapers picked up the story (Carey, 2008; Grossman, 2008; Lane, 2008). But so did the other *DSM* guru, Allen Frances, who had guided the development of *DSM-IV*. Both Spitzer and Frances, the two psychiatrists in charge of *DSM* for thirty years, opened a public attack on those working on *DSM-5*. Their attack is worth describing in some detail, because it borrows heavily from those who have been psychiatry's severest critics, portending yet another impending crisis in American psychiatry.

For years, outside critics and some marginalized psychiatrists have been accusing psychiatry of engaging in the systematic medicalization of normality (Boyle, 2002; Breggin & Breggin, 1994; Caplan, 1995; Caplan & Cosgrove, 2004; Chodoff, 2002; Cohen, 1990, 1994; Conrad, 2007; Kutchins & Kirk, 1997; Szasz, 2007). Now those accusations were coming from insiders who had promoted and worked for the American Psychiatric Association. On June 19, 2009, Spitzer circulated a new long essay by Allen Frances that struck at the very heart of *DSM*'s weaknesses. Frances forecast "grave problems in the DSM-V goals, methods and products" that if not corrected would "lead to many damaging unintended consequences," and he described a psychiatric debacle that he feared was in the making (Frances, 2009c). Someone who spent decades developing and strengthening the *DSM* enterprise had transformed himself into a critic of that enterprise. As Greenberg (2011) quipped, Frances was "hurling grenades into the bunker where he spent his entire career."

First, Frances accused the leaders of *DSM-5* of soaring ambition and remarkably weak methodology. He thought the task force leaders' claim that the next revision would be a "paradigm shift" was absurd. The simple truth, he said, is that "there can be no dramatic improvements in psychiatric diagnosis until we make a fundamental leap in our understanding of what causes mental disorders." The advances in neuroscience, he said, "are still not relevant to the clinical practicalities of everyday psychiatric diagnosis." He reminded them of the "disappointing fact that not even one biological test is ready for inclusion in the criteria sets of DSM-5." No paradigm shift can occur now, he argued, because "descriptive diagnosis is simply not equipped to carry us much further than it already has" (Frances, 2009c). He questioned the advantage of moving toward dimensional ratings, arguing that introducing more complexity into the manual would not be a paradigm shift and would probably be ignored by busy clinicians.

Most of his essay focused on the great risks to psychiatry if the rumors behind the secret revision process were true. First, if the revisions were not based on substantial evidence, any "innovations" would likely be trivial and arbitrary while requiring unnecessary efforts by clinicians, educators, and researchers to adopt new diagnostic procedures.

Frances went further: he cautioned in an astounding mea culpa that changes in the *DSM-IV* diagnostic criteria had created three false epidemics: those of autistic disorder, ADHD, and bipolar disorder. He warned that the drug industry was ready to pounce on every change in criteria that "could conceivably lead to a marketing advantage . . . to promote drug sales." He predicted "many new 'epidemics' based on changes in DSM-V" (Frances, 2009c).

Frances worried that little new research or field testing of *DSM-5* using any new criteria sets or studies of reliability or prevalence would occur (eventually there were field trials, as we will discuss in a moment). He discounted research in university settings as not generalizable to normal practice settings. He faulted the *DSM-5* work groups for using inconsistent standards to make changes and of ignoring many research papers prepared in the last revision. He fretted about *DSM-5*'s "shallow foundation" and "embarrassing post publication surprises." He pointed to some representative examples of *DSM-5*'s "most reckless suggestion," namely its inclusion of many new categories to capture "the milder subthreshold versions of the existing more severe official disorders." He argued that recognizing milder versions of disorders would "flood the world with new false positives" and prevalence rates would "skyrocket," resulting in "*a wholesale imperial medicalization of normality . . . a bonanza for the pharmaceutical industry.*" (emphasis added). "Psychiatry," he asserted, "should not be in the business of inadvertently manufacturing mental disorders." Frances also criticized the proposal to add a "prodromal" or so-called pre-psychotic category. "This is a drug company's dream come true," providing "ways of penetrating the huge new markets with medications having largely unproven benefit and very substantial side effects" (Frances, 2009c).

As if this weren't damning enough, Frances continued to press his concerns about what appeared to be a runaway train of diagnoses. He castigated the task force for even considering the expansion of the "behavioral addictions" (to shopping, sex, food, internet, etc.) and other proposals for new, questionable disorders or expansion of existing ones. He concluded by worrying about the "extremely puzzling" secrecy of the whole process and confided that he had "little confidence" in the current *DSM-5* leadership. He and Spitzer called on the APA to establish an external review committee to monitor the progress of *DSM-5* (Frances, 2009c).

This early and unexpectedly forceful public attack on *DSM-5* did not go unanswered by the APA and the task force leaders (Schatzberg, Scully, Kupfer, & Regier, 2009), who nonetheless avoided responding to the core of Frances's critique. The APA leaders claimed that the *DSM-5* process was "the most open and inclusive ever," implicitly comparing theirs to the prior ones of Spitzer and Frances, and that their new process was "scientific." They explained that the key difference was that their "focus is not on keeping things as they are" but on determining what was wrong with the current *DSM* and trying to correct it, implying that Spitzer and Frances were merely wedded to their own prior work. Instead, the APA leaders said without providing specific details, the *DSM-5* would optimize clinical utility and be guided by research evidence. They then counterpunched: "The DSM-III categorical diagnoses with operational criteria were a major advance for our field, but they are now holding us back because the system has not kept up with current thinking" (Schatzberg et al., 2009). The APA leaders ended their rebuttal by implying that Spitzer and Frances's critique was motivated by financial conflicts of interest, noting that the two were still getting royalties on earlier *DSM*-associated products that would end with the publication of *DSM-5*.

Warning the Research Community

Spitzer's reply to the APA focused on terrain that he knew well: field trials. After acknowledging that the APA's response had "taken an ugly turn" (Spitzer, 2009), Spitzer resumed his attack on the APA's secrecy. If the *DSM-5* process was the most open and inclusive ever, he asked, why were the leaders of the APA unwilling to reveal any details of the field trials that were scheduled to begin imminently? As Spitzer knew from personal experience, the field trials were complicated to conduct in the process of a manual revision, but they also were useful in providing a scientific patina to the hundreds of decisions that were being made. There was no conceivable reason that the plans for the field trials should not be made public. He asked pointedly: what proposals are being tested in trials; what is the empirical basis for the trials; what is the planned methodology of the trials; and what are the questions being asked of the trials—reliability, validity, rate of false positives? Spitzer offered two possible reasons why the APA remained silent concerning these simple scientific questions: (1) the APA leaders were shielding themselves from criticism or (2) they did not yet know the answers to those questions. In short, Spitzer was striking at the heart of the APA's scientific pretense.

The rancor continued in the *Psychiatric Times* between the prominent inside defenders and inside critics of the *DSM-5* process. (See the variety of responses at http://www.psychiatrictimes.com.) Allen Frances was compelled to defend his motivations for his criticisms, pointing out that his royalties on products from *DSM-IV* were no more than the conflict-of-interest policies for everyone working on *DSM-5*. He argued that there were profound risks to psychiatry of making ill-considered changes to the diagnostic manual. He also reiterated that "descriptive psychiatry had reached its limits of usefulness" and that at best the new task force should strive to "do no harm" (Frances, 2009b). Six months later, Frances issued an alert to the research community, based on his "several converging, anonymous . . . sources" (Frances, 2009a).

Using the gambit of an investigative reporter relying on insider informants, he relayed to the psychiatric community that the APA was about to release a draft of options for *DSM-5* on the web in January and February 2010 and that the research community would only have a month to respond, an exceedingly brief review period for such an important document. He also leaked the news that the field trials had been postponed, that the proposal for external funding for the trials had been rejected, that early drafts of diagnostic criteria sets displayed their drafters' inability to write clearly and consistently, and that the final publication of *DSM-5* had been set back to 2013. He repeated his warnings that there was much harm that an ill-considered *DSM* could bring to the practice and research communities in the form of the further "medicalizing normality and trivializing psychiatric diagnosis" and again noted the influence of the drug industry and the excessive use of medications that are potentially dangerous. He ended by encouraging the research community to be prepared to apply "pressure" on the *DSM-5* process by pointing out specific problems when the draft was released. And then Frances stated:

> The APA realizes that it holds the franchise to publish the DSMs only by historical accident, and that this is easily revocable if enough interested organizations lose confidence in its competence and its ability to control its inherent conflict of interest. (Frances, 2009a)

Frances's warnings proved correct. In February 2010 the APA released a draft of *DSM-5* on its website, which contained scores of pages and documents and solicited comments. It provided less than two months for comments on the exceedingly complex document. And, as forecast, it announced the postponement of both the field trials and the publication of *DSM-5*. The media immediately began covering issues raised by the draft (Carey, 2010b).

What even a cursory review of the draft of *DSM-5* revealed was that Spitzer and Frances's fears were well grounded. Everything that Frances fretted over was included in the draft and more. While the developers of *DSM-5* invited private comments about the draft directly on its own website—comments that would be available to them alone and not to the interested psychiatric community—Frances immediately began publishing scathing critiques of its contents (Frances, 2010a, 2010d). He said that the plans for field trials had at least six "seriously disabling limitations" and one fatal one (Frances, 2010b). Among the six disabling limitations, three focused on reliability: namely, that unclear diagnostic criteria would lower reliability, that field trials in average clinical settings were likely to show low reliability and "undercut the credibility" of diagnosis, and that reliability studies in special research settings would not be generalizable. Two other limitations were that the design of the field trials were unfocused and would not provide much useful information and that the complexity and logistics of the field trials would postpone the manual by at least a year. The most serious and fatal problem was that the new manual would lead to a tsunami of overdiagnosis.

In another article, Frances argued that normal grief would be diagnosed as a mental disorder in *DSM-5* and would invite harmful, unneeded medical intervention (2010c). Other critics jumped on the proposed changes to the personality disorders section of *DSM*, in which five of the ten existing disorders would be eliminated and the others would be given different names

(Carey, 2010a; Zanor, 2010). This proposal was a stunning admission of the invalidity of one of psychiatry's key set of disorders. In a commentary in the APA's flagship journal, seven prominent experts questioned the changes being proposed for the personality disorders (Shedler et al., 2010; Shedler et al., 2011; Skodal, 2011). Even members of the *DSM-5* task force worried about "monumental screwups that will turn the field into a laughingstock," but would not go on record for fear of retaliation, according to Gary Greenberg, who interviewed them (Greenberg, 2011).

On several critical fronts, the leaders of the *DSM-5* had to acknowledge limitations, some profoundly unsettling, while acting as if great progress was being made. For example, in a commentary in the APA's flagship journal, Kupfer and Regier acknowledge that when they began planning the revision they expected that scientific advances in genetics, neuroimaging, and pathophysiology during the last twenty-five years would "mitigate" the known limitations of *DSM* (Kupfer & Regier, 2011). They anticipated that this knowledge would help to provide a more valid classification of mental disorder, one at long last grounded on *some* neuroscience findings. They conceded that this was currently not possible. Rather than admit failure, they noted proudly that NIMH would be continuing to search for this elusive neurobiology and that "we believe this initiative will be very informative for subsequent versions" (p. 673) of the manual. They acknowledged that "it is difficult to assess how quickly progress will come about . . . but genetic data are clearly not yet ready for clinical applications" (p. 673). They continued: "Can we ask psychiatrists to use genetic markers to assist in diagnosing a patient with schizophrenia? At this point in time, the answer is no." But they reassured readers that the time is "soon coming," that like the Bible, *DSM* is a "living document," a "work in progress" that will incorporate "dramatic neuroscience discovery" (p. 674). This is *DSM*'s, and psychiatry's, perennial promise: valid psychiatric diagnosis is just around the next (neuro)science corner.

Even if neuroscience isn't ready for prime time, the *DSM-5* task force posted on its website the proposed changes to the *DSM* and invited feedback from any interested parties. This posting was itself claimed as some achievement, although it was, for the most part, a public relations process. In periodic reports, Kupfer offered positive and upbeat news of *DSM-5* developments, largely ignoring the storms that were brewing. For example, in the August 2011 commentary (Kupfer, 2011), he says that the "feedback was so successful" that they received "visits" from 125,000 individuals. He mentions, however, that only 2,120 (less than 2 percent) made comments or asked questions. Curiously, most frequent comments were about sexual and gender identity disorders. Some comments were concerned with insurance reimbursement, some with pathologization, some promoted particular diagnoses, and others were from consumers talking about their own experiences. Nonetheless, Kupfer conveys excitement about these comments and reassures everyone that they are "sorting through all submissions." He asserts, "The importance of public and professional input into DSM-5 cannot be understated" (Kupfer, 2011). The importance, of course, is in appearing to be responsive, while keeping the work and the decision processes of the committees essentially private.

But the appearance of openness and vacuous press releases didn't quell concerns about the revisions of the *DSM*; in fact, the concerns intensified as questions arose about the "science" of diagnosis and its social implications. One unlikely example was the emergence of controversy about Asperger's syndrome, a "disorder" that *DSM-IV* had defined as a mild form of autism.

Like childhood bipolar disorder, the likelihood that children were diagnosed with autism, defined as a pervasive developmental disorder, had been increasing rapidly for at least a decade, without convincing evidence about whether this was due to increasing incidence, better surveillance by clinicians, or the overuse of *DSM*'s broadened definition of autism (Carey, 2012d; *New York Times* Editorial, 2012; Steinberg, 2012; Zarembo, 2011). The *DSM-5* task force proposed that the definition of *autism* be narrowed (DSM Task Force, 2012) to avoid defining socially awkward children (i.e., shy, timid, or having trouble relating to peers) as autistic. This proposal provoked a public battle that played out in blogs and newspapers across the country (e.g., Nugent, 2012), pitting those questioning why social awkwardness, whatever its disadvantages, should be considered as a serious mental disorder against those concerned that more restricted boundaries of autism would disqualify some children for state-funded education and support. This controversy highlighted that defining any behaviors as symptoms of a mental disorder provides a medical rationale for providing services. Drawing the arbitrary boundaries for mental disorders controls the allocation of billions of dollars in health, educational, and social services (Carey, 2012b).

As mentioned above, another controversy emerged about the diagnosis of depression. In prior editions of *DSM*, the criteria for Major Depressive Episode (APA, 1994, p. 323) acknowledged that "symptoms" of depression could result from the loss of a loved one but that normal sadness should not be viewed as a mental disorder. Excluding normal bereavement from mental disorders was a rare acknowledgment by the developers of the manual that the social context of behaviors should be taken into account. The new *DSM-5* proposal, however, eliminated the bereavement exclusion and thus would allow normal grief to be considered a mental disorder.

The media and the experts immediately challenged this proposal (Carey, 2012a; Frances, 2010c), suggesting that the APA appeared to be pathologizing normal sadness following the death of a loved one. The controversy was furthered by a detailed analysis of the empirical evidence (Wakefield & First, 2012), which showed that the *DSM-5* proposal was based on faulty and misinterpreted data and rested on no convincing scientific evidence.

Such concerns about the *DSM-5* proposals came not just from a few newspaper columnists, concerned families, or psychiatric experts, nor did they include only a few controversial categories. Mental health professional organizations began questioning the entire medical orientation of the *DSM*. For example, the Society for Humanistic Psychology (2012) of the American Psychological Association circulated a ten-page detailed critique and petition online against the *DSM-5*. The American Counseling Association (2012) publicized its own concerns. The British Psychological Society distributed a detailed document questioning the "medicalization of . . . natural and normal responses" of people, "which do not reflect illnesses so much as normal individual variations." Their response continues:

> The putative diagnoses presented in DSM-V are clearly based largely on social norms, with "symptoms" that all rely on subjective judgments, with little confirmatory physical "signs" or evidence of biological causation. The criteria are not value-free, but rather reflect current normative social expectations. . . . diagnoses are plagued by problems of reliability, validity, prognostic value, and co-morbidity. (British Psychological Society, 2011, p. 2)

Even the prestigious medical journal *Lancet* joined the fray, publishing an (anonymous) editorial calling the medicalization of grief in the forthcoming *DSM-5* "not only dangerously simplistic, but also flawed" (*Lancet*, 2012).

Among the whirl of criticism, few voices were as persistent or public as that of Allen Frances, the former leader of the *DSM-IV*. Nor could other critics match his "insider" status. Frances first began writing regular blogs appearing in the online *Psychiatric Times* (available at www.psychiatrytimes.com) and another series entitled "DSM5 in Distress" for *Psychology Today* (available at www.psychologytoday.com). In dozens of blog posts, he relentlessly criticized the *DSM-5* task force, dozens of proposals for changes in the manual, and the APA for ignoring or mishandling the rising chorus of public and expert criticisms. In March 2012, he wrote:

> In fact, my criticisms of DSM-5 arise precisely from its obvious failure to be an impartial, meticulous, and consensus academic endeavor. DSM-5 has suffered from a fatal combination of excessive ambition, sloppy method, and closed process. It fully deserves the concerted opposition it has generated from 47 professional organizations, the world press, the Society of Biological Psychiatry, *The Lancet*, and the general public. (Frances, 2012a)

Even long-forgotten scientific issues stimulated new conflicts. After thirty years of neglect since the publication of *DSM-III*, the *DSM-5* task force created an unexpected controversy over the reliability of diagnoses. The *DSM-5* designers had decided to conduct field trials that would include tests of the reliability of the proposed diagnoses. As these trials were nearing completion, but before any results were reported publicly, the co-chairs and other members of the *DSM-5* task force published a commentary in the January 2012 issue of *American Journal of Psychiatry (AJP)*, lowering the expectations for "acceptable" levels of reliability (Kraemer, Kupfer, Clarke, Narrow, & Regier, 2012). As we described in chapter 4 (table 4-1), the standards previously promulgated for interpreting studies of reliability were that "good" reliability was achieved with kappa scores above 0.70; "no better than fair" for scores around 0.50; and "poor" for scores around 0.40 and less. For *DSM-5*, however, Kraemer et al (2012) now suggested that scores of 0.80 "would be almost miraculous"; between 0.60 and 0.80 "would be cause for celebration"; between 0.40 and 0.60 would be a "realistic goal"; while "between 0.20 and 0.40 would be acceptable" (p. 14). With this type of grade inflation, "poor" scores disappear. This effort to significantly lower expectations—presented as dispassionate technical analysis—did not go unnoticed. In a letter to the editor in *AJP*, Robert Spitzer and associates questioned depicting kappas around 0.4 as "the standards of what is acceptable reliability in medicine" (Spitzer, Williams, & Endicott, 2012). They concluded: "Calling for psychiatry to accept kappa values that are characterized as unreliable in other fields of medicine is taking a step backward" (p. 537).

Allen Frances reminded *Psychiatric Times* readers that the chair of the *DSM-5* task force, responding to those who worried that final decisions about diagnoses had already been made prior to the field trials, had reassured them that the early draft of the manual contained proposals that wouldn't necessarily "end up in the DSM-5. If they don't achieve a level of reliability, clinician acceptability, and utility, it's unlikely they'll go forward" (Frances, 2012c). Similarly, the head of the *DSM-5* oversight committee stated in an interview in 2010, "It's going to be based on the work of the field trials—based on the assessment and analysis of them. I don't think anyone is going to say we've got to go forward if we get crappy results" (as quoted by Frances, 2012b). Apparently, in the continuing mad science of diagnostic reliability, one approach to avoiding "crappy results" is simply to redefine them as acceptable results.

In May 2012 at the APA annual meeting in Philadelphia, the *DSM-5* task force unveiled some preliminary reliability findings from the field trials. With the announced lowering of standards as the prelude, it shouldn't have surprised observers that the findings, appearing to be "crappy," were now defined as "acceptable." *Medscape Medical News* called them "mixed," and Darrel Regier, the task force co-chair, offered various explanations for disappointing results (Brauser, 2012). For example, in the limited data released,[2] only a single category reached the standards applied to *DSM-II* and *DSM-III* ("good" kappas were at or above 0.70): Major Neurocognitive

Disorder (for organic mental disorder), with a kappa of 0.78. The other results were as follows:

Adults Diagnoses

Schizophrenia	0.46
Schizoaffective	0.50
Bipolar I Disorder	0.54
Major Depressive Disorder	0.32
General Anxiety Disorder	0.20
PTSD	0.67
Alcohol Use Disorder	0.40
Borderline Personality Disorder	0.55
Antisocial Personality Disorder	0.22
Obsessive-Compulsive Personality Disorder	0.31

Children and Adolescence Diagnoses

Autism Spectrum Disorder	0.69
ADHD	0.61
Oppositional Defiant Disorder	0.41
Conduct Disorder	0.48
Disruptive Mood Disorder	0.50
Major Depression Disorder	0.29

What is readily apparent from this partial peek at the initial data is that the *DSM-5* task force had nothing to cheer about. Conducting a few limited studies usually provides a scientific patina to the development of new editions of *DSM*, but in this case the results undercut the efforts. Forty years after the invention of descriptive diagnosis, with the major objective to greatly improve reliability, the *DSM-5* field trial results, no matter how they were spinned, showed that there was no general trend toward higher reliability over the 1980 *DSM-III*. In addition, with some high-profile diagnostic categories, there were worrisome findings. Schizophrenia, Schizoaffective, and Bipolar disorders for adults—the bedrock diagnoses of psychosis—were between 0.46 and 0.54, which would have placed them in the lower range of major diagnostic classes in the *DSM-III* field trials (see table 4-3). Major Depressive Disorder and General Anxiety Disorder presented enormous scientific and political problems, with kappas of 0.32 and 0.20, a range that by every past standard would easily be classified as unacceptable or poor, raising the problem of how to justify even including these diagnostic categories in *DSM*. The task force is hardly likely to abandon these diagnoses, regardless of their unstable scientific grounding. They constitute two of the most prevalent diagnoses made

(Kessler et al., 2005) and provide an enormous population target for the marketing of psychiatric drugs. Despite the earlier struggles to alter and improve the diagnosis of personality disorders, their reliability was dismal, lower than the *DSM-III* field trials (see table 4-3). Similarly, the children's disorders saw no improvement over the middling levels of *DSM-III* (see table 4-4).

The release of information about the field trials at the annual convention and the growing concerns and protests over the direction of *DSM-5* was reflected in generally negative media coverage (Jabr, 2012; Urbina, 2012). The prior week, the *Washington Post* ran an op-ed by Paula Caplan: "Psychiatry's bible, the *DSM*, is doing more harm than good" (Caplan, 2012), and Allen Frances's op-ed in the *New York Times* on May 12, 2012, blasted the *DSM-5* and proposed that the APA "should no longer be permitted to call all the shots" and that ownership of the *DSM* needs to be lodged in an independent, scientific organization, such as the Department of Health and Human Services or the World Health Organization (Frances, 2012b).

In the face of widespread criticism, the task force, "in a rare step," according to the *New York Times* (Carey, 2012c), backed away from several controversial proposals that they vigorously championed for several years. Frances blogged on *Psychology Today*, "Wonderful news: DSM 5 finally begins its belated and necessary retreat" (Frances, 2012d). Although Frances was encouraged, he listed a dozen other proposals that he thought had serious flaws. The APA had backed away from a new "psychosis risk" disorder, tweaked slightly major depression in response to concerns that it was pathologizing normal sadness, and nixed a new "mixed anxiety depressive disorder." But it held firm to the narrowing of its definition of autism and to much of the rest of its proposals. Whether there will be other proposals withdrawn or significantly modified by the task force is unclear as this is written. In May 2012 the task force gave the public only several more weeks to review the hundreds of changes to the manual, perhaps the last public exposure to *DSM-5* until it is publicly released at the APA annual meeting in May 2013. David Kupfer, the co-chair, invited "patients and their loved ones, professionals, and the general public . . . to review the proposed changes, and let us know their thoughts" (Kupfer, 2012). There is no reason to assume that the controversies will cease during the final year, nor that the APA will conduct new field trials on all or any of the recently altered diagnostic categories, because it would again delay publication.

What is most striking about all the controversies over *DSM-5* and all its prior editions is that the conflicts are not really about science or empirical evidence about the reliability of psychiatric diagnoses. The evidence suggests that reliability has worsened over time, undermining the validity of the classification system. In a truly scientific endeavor, this would send the *DSM-5* task force back to the drawing board. True science does not require publication deadlines, press releases, public relations specialists, reviews by the public nor by patients or their loved ones. Science stands or falls on the empirical outcome of rigorous tests of claims, regardless of popular opinion.

On the other hand, proposals in a democracy to fundamentally alter social and economic policy do require such public scrutiny, precisely because the decisions are rooted deeply in social values that may be informed by science but cannot be decided by scientific evidence. For example, revising the United States tax code can only be accomplished in a process that involves many strong institutional stakeholders concerned primarily with their own self-interests and their own social values. In such a process, controversy, conflict, distortions, and public relations campaigns are unavoidable.

DSM is like a tax code masquerading as a scientific classification system. Contending psychiatric factions and opinion leaders argue over specific criteria for substance, mood, anxiety, or personality disorders, as if through debate or field trials they can "get it right," can truly "discover" the true nature of medical disease categories of mental illness. The various criteria being debated are largely meaningless. This is because, as we have argued, the existence of a *disease* of mental illness has never been established or satisfactorily defined, so on what basis can anyone "scientifically" judge the validity of one classification of an illusion against a slightly revised one? The self interests of the psychiatric stakeholders—the APA, mental health professions, clients, insurance companies, pharmaceutical industries, and government—will inevitably determine the decisions that are made, as would be the case in any major tax code revision. Madness, whatever its nature and whatever its social uses, resides deeply in human distress and in our social norms and values. The current squabbles about *DSM* are largely scientifically meaningless, although they are certainly meaningful in terms of the threats to the dominance of American psychiatry in controlling the business of mental illness.

We have documented in detail the controversies over the revision of *DSM-5* because they are more visible than the diagnostic controversies of the past, although the dynamics are similar. The Internet, of course, has magnified that visibility, making it easier to see how the leaders of the latest *DSM* revision maneuver through a political minefield of contending parties while steadfastly claiming that they are being driven by "scientific evidence." And, similar to prior revisions, it remains unclear what exactly the evidence is or how it is connected to any of the task force's decisions. *DSM* is more than a classification system of purported disease; it is also an expression of professional power within American psychiatry and the pharmaceutical industry, as both seek relentlessly to expand the reach of the manual among the US population as a target of medical intervention.

Harms of *DSM*

DSM provides a method of identifying presumed afflictions, as the APA, pharmaceuticals, and NIMH expand surveillance of the population, screening children in schools and enlisting general medical practitioners to be on the lookout for mental troubles among children and adults. Psychiatric experts are expected to find hidden diseases in people harboring mental illnesses by noting signs that often consist of common expressions of emotions and behaviors. These experts claim to act in the best interests of the community and the person in need, although in some cases the remedies they offer may involve considerable harm.

Part of *DSM*'s success can be attributed to the willingness of the public, disordered and non-disordered alike, to accept this psychiatric reframing of what is the matter and when intervention is needed. It seems clear that the public has generally accepted the medicalization of many problems in living. Part of this undoubtedly started with the popularization of psychology in American society, which communicated an essentially hopeful message. The language of psychology encourages the public to view myriad personal troubles as normal events in the struggles of living, not—as in former times—as signs of immorality, failure, or personal weakness. Self-help and self-improvement books encourage people to be optimistic that life is malleable and that things can be improved. The public is told that they are not prisoners of fate, that although human travail and anguish have many sources—poverty, bad parenting, troubled childhoods, and the common stresses of life—people can overcome adversity and improve their circumstances. This view accepts human pain and struggle as inevitable but within the abilities of people, perhaps with assistance, to overcome. Human agency is emphasized.

Psychiatry's discourse of brain disorder is rapidly supplanting the psychological perspective, though the conquest is not yet complete. The discourse of disease removes normal troubles from an arena in which the individual can overcome personal problems with encouragement, support, education, and discipline. In its place, human troubles are sequestered in an arena of disease, pathology, and medical prescriptions. The NIMH, the APA, and the pharmaceutical companies, using the modern *DSM*, have forcefully promoted the view that even mild forms of discomfort, anxiety, sadness, and misbehavior should be redefined as illness or impending disease, and those with difficulties should ask their doctors for the medication that "is right for you," before their "condition" deteriorates and they become targets of coercive intervention. Human agency has shrunk to require only that the individual seek professional help, as directed by state and other agencies working in tandem with psychiatric organizations. The doctor will take responsibility from there. Capitalizing on the high prestige of medical science and on people's obvious and natural desire to lessen pain and disability, psychiatry encourages the fantasy that human anguish is a disease that can be effectively treated.

The *DSM* facilitates this ideological maneuver with a novel method of counting troublesome behaviors and converting them into treatable pathology. With the development, recycling, and marketing of psychoactive medications (see chapters 6 and 7), descriptive diagnosis has melded parallel systems of beliefs for physical and mental illnesses. Without definitively identifying the existence of its putative brain disorders or understanding their presumed causes, the *DSM* provides the illusion that the diagnostic criteria validly distinguish pathology from normality. And many people, including mental health professionals, unable or unwilling to exercise their critical faculties, mistake the illusion for reality. In addition to how psychiatry and *DSM* shaped popular views of life's struggles and the role of human agency, the *DSM* has distorted other realms of activity.

Distortion of Research

Ironically, one of the early criticisms of *DSM* was that it was designed as a research, not a clinical, tool. In fact, the *DSM* became a prominent clinical tool for financing care and marketing medications, but its scientific weaknesses, as we have seen, have distorted and undermined research.

The *DSM*'s diagnostic criteria have shaped psychiatric research for thirty years, but, because of its unreliability and thus its indeterminable validity, *DSM* has undermined the integrity of the studies it has spawned. Having valid categories of disorder matters fundamentally in epidemiological research, for example, which must sort people consistently into categories (i.e., the disordered versus the non-disordered) on which predictions and other scientific or practical efforts will rest. If the diagnostic criteria do not or, as we have argued, cannot validly identify who is disordered, epidemiological research based on them is largely meaningless, except as a sociopolitical tool for psychiatric expansionism (Horwitz & Wakefield, 2007; Whitaker, 2010).

Other forms of research are also impaired when they rely on *DSM*. For example, in research that compares the effectiveness of different forms of treatments, often using complex designs called randomized clinical trials, patients must be carefully selected with similar problems and then randomly assigned to different treatment or control groups. Following several weeks or months of treatment, patients are assessed to see how they are functioning and whether those receiving different treatments had different outcomes. If their diagnoses are unreliable or invalid, the patients selected for the study would be too heterogeneous in general and in their responses to the same treatment, undermining the conclusions that the researchers may reach. There is emerging evidence that this, in fact, has happened.

For example, several years before the official launch of the *DSM-5* task force, the APA and NIMH commissioned six white papers to stimulate research and planning for the upcoming edition to "fundamentally alter the limited classification paradigm [*DSM-IV*] now in use" and to ". . . search for new approaches to an understanding of the etiological and pathophysiological mechanism . . . to improve the validity of our diagnoses" (Kupfer, First, & Regier, 2002). These quotes are from the opening of the introductory paragraph of the volume containing the white papers and written by two of the psychiatrists who would eventually be selected to co-chair the *DSM-5* task force. Why would they suggest the need to fundamentally alter *DSM*, search for new approaches, or improve validity, unless, after thirty years of monumental commercial success and dominance, the current *DSM* is, after all, fundamentally flawed and based on a defective approach that has limited validity?

In fact, the opening chapters of their book, A *Research Agenda for* DSM-V, Kupfer and his associates (2002) admit that research has not been able to document the validity of the *DSM* classification system (Kupfer et al., 2002). They note the following: that research has not discovered common etiologies for the major *DSM* disorder categories; that not one laboratory marker has been discovered for any *DSM*-defined syndrome; that studies have found disorder categories overlap, undermining the belief that these disorders have distinct causes; that there are high degrees of short-term instability for many disorders; that there is lack of specific treatments: the same treatment, drugs, or psychotherapy are used for many supposedly different disorders; and that even studies of twins have contradicted the *DSM* assumption that different disorders have different underlying genetic bases.[3] All of these findings suggest that the *DSM* classification system is of questionable validity.

No modern (or older) edition of *DSM* has produced scientific break-throughs. Kupfer et al. (2002) conclude that "researchers' slavish adoption of DSM-IV definitions may have hindered research in the etiology of mental disorders," and that "research exclusively focused on refining the DSM-defined syndromes may never be successful in uncovering their underlying etiologies." They argue that the reification of *DSM* entities "is more likely to obscure than to elucidate research findings" (pages xviii–xix). More recently, in attempts to gain leverage to make dramatic changes, the developers of *DSM-5* continue to attack the validity of prior editions of *DSM* (Regier et al., 2009; Schatzberg et al., 2009). They argue that because of fundamental validity problems, *DSM* has hindered psychiatric research. With so much concern about the validity of *DSM*, even those at the center of the *DSM* enterprise appear to admit that they don't know what the *DSM*-defined disorders really are. Unfortunately, however, they want the public to believe that they can solve these problems by tinkering yet again with the diagnostic criteria. Can they *really* believe this? These scholars read and understand the same literature that the authors of this book read and understand. In our view, the most plausible reason for more tinkering with *DSM* categories is that psychiatry must go on.

Distortion of Records and Help

The psychiatric research enterprise is not the only institutional investor to be misled by a false sense of diagnostic accuracy. With the wholesale adoption of *DSM* by hospitals, clinics, and private and government insurance programs, inaccurate and invalid psychiatric diagnoses have been indelibly written into the medical records of millions of children and adults who seek help with all manner of human troubles, many of which neither the clinicians nor the clients themselves view as mental illnesses. Nonetheless, because medical insurance coverage requires that a diagnosed physical or mental disease is being treated, primary care physicians, psychiatrists, and other mental health professionals routinely scan the *DSM* looking for a diagnosis that can be used for reimbursement (Braun & Cox, 2005; Greenberg, 2010; Kirk & Kutchins, 1988; Rost et al., 1994). Regardless of the validity of the diagnosis, clinicians are paid to provide services to these clients. Clinicians, clinics, hospitals, and clients may accrue some benefits, but the residue of false and misleading psychiatric diagnoses distort the medical records of many whose only distinguishing feature was to have requested assistance from a service or professional who formally diagnosed them, which can easily cause future legal and employment problems. Moreover, the practice of deliberate misdiagnosis raises ethical issues for the mental health professionals who use questionable diagnoses to gain reimbursement for services.

The harms of surveillance and misleading diagnoses extend far beyond psychiatry. Much disagreement exists in the medical community about the costs and benefits of mammograms to detect breast cancer in women and the PSA blood test to detect prostate cancer for men. The diagnostic tests are not definitive; very few of those screened will enjoy any benefit, and many of those screened will be subjected to medical procedures that are worrisome, costly, and probably unwarranted (Aschwanden, 2011; Woolston, 2011).

In psychiatry the problems are probably more severe, because the diagnostic gamesmanship that is common to many clinicians and clinics is totally unnecessary to provide help for people who actually need it. Psychiatric diagnosis is, in fact, not needed in order to help the vast majority of those currently labeled as mentally disordered. A former president of the APA was asked in a recent interview how he used *DSM*. He said that his secretary had just asked him for the diagnosis of a patient he's been seeing in treatment for several months in order for her to send a bill to the insurance company. He "hadn't really formulated it," but scanned *DSM* and suggested that the patient had obsessive-compulsive disorder.

> Interviewer: "Did it change the way you treated her?"
> Psychiatrist: "No."
> Interviewer: "So what would you say was the value of the diagnosis?"
> Psychiatrist: "I got paid." (Greenberg, 2011)

A case for requiring a psychiatric diagnosis for the receipt of services would only be legitimate if an identifiable medical problem existed, the diagnosis pointed to a specific underlying "pathology" causing the "symptoms," and if without knowing the diagnosis, clinicians might provide harmful, less effective help for the person. None of these conditions is true for the vast majority of people who seek assistance for problems in living from clinical psychologists, social workers, marriage and family counselors, psychiatrists, or others. *DSM* diagnoses describe behaviors unconnected to any known biological causes or medical conditions; the treatments used on those diagnosed with mental disorders are nonspecific to the diagnosis (including the uses of psychoactive drugs, as discussed in the next chapters); and clinicians provide similar services and interventions across diagnostic categories, from bipolar disorder to mood, anxiety, and personality disorders. In fact, the placebo effect may rank as the most generally effective treatment in psychiatry and certainly the one with the fewest and least harmful side effects (Fournier et al., 2010; Greenberg, 2010).

Moreover, providing help to children, adults, and families who may be troubled generally consists of offering support, advice, clarifying emotions and thoughts, exploring options, and linking the person to other supports and helping resources. Clinicians have known for decades that the natural ingredients of helping come from providing a tolerant and safe environment, conveying a sense of respect and trust, and offering assistance in a manner that is warm, nonjudgmental, and empathic. A *DSM* diagnosis is largely irrelevant to the helping relationship.

Counseling and psychotherapy do not require a specific diagnosis, are not improved by a specific diagnosis, and are not made more effective by a specific diagnosis. The helping relationship is certainly enhanced when clinicians develop a broad understanding of the person's life space, family, friends and social ties, struggles, pain, and failures, and of sources of strength and resiliency. This was true prior to the transformation of *DSM* and remains true today. In a recent study by the World Health Organization and the World Psychiatric Association (Reed, Correia, Esparza, Saxena, & Maj, 2011), an overwhelming majority of the nearly 5,000 psychiatrists from forty-four countries preferred classifications that were designed for clinical use, not research purposes, which allowed for more flexible diagnostic criteria and fewer than a hundred categories, versus the current three hundred. Whether they favor one hundred or three hundred diagnoses, these clinicians may not be critiquing the dominant disease model. However, they seem to be suggesting that *DSM*-type classifications add little except administrative distraction to the generic helping process. We know of no evidence showing that people diagnosed by *DSM* are more likely to receive effective treatment than they would otherwise receive.

Conclusion

Thirty years after *DSM-III* revolutionized American psychiatry by claiming to have solved the fundamental problem of diagnostic reliability and thus to have taken a great leap toward establishing diagnostic validity, mental health professionals still can't reliably agree on diagnoses—or even on what constitutes a mental disorder, much less establish diagnostic validity. The rhetoric about diagnosis has *never* matched the actual science. The old promises of progress have remained unfulfilled, as yet more new promises are made by the architects of the forthcoming *DSM-5*.

The quest of biological psychiatry, adopted and aided by *DSM*, is to claim a brain disease for every human trouble. From Kraepelin to NIMH's *Decade of the Brain*, the perennial promise is that brain diseases will be discovered. Despite decades of failure to confirm that misbehaviors and emotional turmoil are caused by disordered brains—a search floated on the massive stream of funding from the federal government and the drug industry—the effort has never lost momentum and even enthusiasm, as if the key to human misery will be discovered. The failure for the enterprise to deliver on its promises has not discouraged efforts to support it, which suggests that it is at its core a moral crusade.

A corollary illusion is that every "symptom," every expression of anguish and anger, hurt and heartache, exuberance and despair is presumed to be linked to some unknown biochemical pathology. And while the causal links are elusive, those who are anxious, scared, sad, lonely, inept, or frustrated, can, in the meantime, occasionally find comfort in any one of a number of pharmaceutical remedies.

The APA and the pharmaceutical industry appear to be on a quest to find disease and disorder everywhere. Descriptive psychiatry has enticed the public to swallow the myth that all manner of human troubles are not the inevitable nature of the human comedy: they are expugnable illnesses. The implicit ideal of the healthy, normal, and truly happy camper is someone who, properly treated, will harbor no serious worry or animosities, no sadness over losses or failed ambitions, no disappointments with children or spouses, no doubts about themselves or conflicts with others, and certainly no strange ideas or behaviors. Children should be well-behaved, bright and attractive, and have flawless DNA. These "normal" people will only have orgasms that are perfectly controlled and properly timed and directed. Their moods will be mellow in all circumstances, and bad hair days will be a thing of the past.

Could anyone truly be swayed by these illusions, duped into believing that problems are solved when they are not? The history that we have reviewed previously and mankind's perennial follies suggest a resounding yes. *DSM* has become so encrusted into the American public's and professionals' views of madness, into how services are arranged and financed to help people, that it has become almost impossible to think about a world without a diagnostic manual of mental disorders. But perhaps it is time to consider a radical alternative by asking some questions. Are we really well-served by a *DSM* that provides a dictionary of fictitious brain disorders as a guide to describe, name, understand, or cope with human adversity? Is it really necessary to place people into illness categories to provide them with humane and effective help if they need and request it?

Notes

1. Even clinicians who do not have a medical orientation, or are uninterested in making a *DSM* diagnosis, or even those who believe *DSM* diagnoses are invalid frequently end up making such diagnoses, because these clinicians and their patients operate within a biomedical industrial complex (see Gomory, Wong, Cohen, and Lacasse, 2011). See also discussion in this chapter under "Distortion of Records and Help."
2. The initial presentation of these data took place at the annual meetings, with PowerPoint slides of the data. Neither the full data nor the methodological details have been published as this is written. Published news accounts have presented slightly different kappas, thus these initial partial results are tentative.
3. It is beyond the scope of this book to undertake a critique of genetic hypotheses of mental disorders, and especially the validity of twin studies upon which the inadequate notion of "heritability" rests and is used misleadingly and incoherently to claim that various human behaviors and actions have "genetic causes." For this purpose, see, for example, Jay Joseph, *The gene illusion*.

References

American Counseling Association (2012). retrieved 4-30-12 http://www.counseling.org/PressRoom/NewsReleases.aspx?AGuid=315a280b-4d0b-48af-9421-1f7d3f01b4b7

American Psychiatric Association. (1994). *Diagnostic and statistical manual of mental disorders, Fourth edition (DSM-IV)*. Washington, DC: American Psychiatric Association.

American Psychiatric Association. (2008). *DSM V: The Future Manual.* Retrieved September 30, 2008 from www.dsm5.org

American Psychiatric Association. (2000). *Diagnostic and statistical manual of mental disorders, Fourth edition, Text revision (DSM-IV-TR)*. Washington, DC: American Psychiatric Association.

American Psychiatric Association. (2012). Retrieved 5-19-12 at: http://www.DSM5.org/about/Pages/BoardofTrusteePrinciples.aspx)

Angell, M. (2004). *The truth about the drug companies: How they deceive us and what to do about it.* New York: Random House.

Angell, M. (2011a, June 23). The epidemic of mental illness: Why? *New York Review of Books.*

Angell, M. (2011b, July 14). The illusions of psychiatry. *New York Review of Books.*

Aschwanden, C. (2011, March 7). Mammograms: Debate rages on about the merits of screening women in their 40s. *Los Angeles Times.*

Author. (Ed.). (1987) *Random House unabridged dictionary (2nd ed.).* New York: Random House.

Barber, C. (2008). *Comfortably numb: How psychiatry is medicating a nation.* New York: Pantheon Books.

Basken, P. (2009a, November 17). Ethicists prod NIH to spend money investigating conflicts of interest. *Chronicle of Higher Education.*

Basken, P. (2009b, November 19). Federal audit faults universities over researchers' financial conflicts of interest. *Chronicle of Higher Education.*

Basken, P. (2010, June 6). As he worked to strengthen ethics rules, NIMH director aided a leading transgressor. *Chronicle of Higher Education.*

Bekelman, J. E., Li, Y., & Goss, C. P. (2003). Scope and impact of financial conflicts of interest in biomedical research. *JAMA 289*(4), 454–465.

Bloomberg.com. (2009). Big Pharma's crime spree. Retrieved at: www.bloomberg. com, December, 2009.

Bolton, D. (2008). *What is mental disorder? An essay in philosophy, science, and values.* New York: Oxford University Press.

Boyle, M. (2002). *Schizophrenia: A scientific delusion?* (2nd ed.). East Sussex, UK: Routledge.

Braun, S. A., & Cox, J. A. (2005). Managed mental health care: Intentional misdiagnosis of mental disorders. *Journal of Counseling & Development, 83*(4), 425–433.

Brauser, D. (2012). *DSM-5* field trials generate mixed results. *Medscape Medical News Psychiatry,* retrieved from www.medscape.com/viewarticle/763519?src=mpnews&spon=12

Breggin, P. R., & Breggin, G. R. (1994). *Talking back to Prozac: What doctors won't tell you about today's most controversial drug.* New York: St. Martin's Press.

British Psychological Society. (2011). *Response to the American Psychiatric Association:* DSM-5. Retrieved from http://www.bps.org.uk/news/psychologists-petition-against-dsm-5

Campbell, E. G., Weissman, J. S., Ehringhaus, S., Rao, S. R., Moy, B., Feibelmann, S. et al. (2007). Institutional academic-industry relationships. *JAMA, 298*(15), 1779–1786.

Campbell, E. G., Weissman, J. S., Vogeli, C., Clarridge, B. R., Abraham, M., Marder, J. E. et al. (2006). Financial relationships between institutional review board members and industry. *New England Journal of Medicine, 355*(22), 2321–2329.

Caplan, P. J. (1995). *They say you're crazy: How the world's most powerful psychiatrists decide who's normal.* Reading, MA: Addison-Wesley.

Caplan, P. J. (2012, April 27). Psychiatry's bible, the *DSM,* is doing more harm than good. *Washington Post.*

Caplan, P. J., & Cosgrove, L. (Eds.). (2004). *Bias in psychiatric diagnosis.* Lanham: Jason Aronson.

Carey, B. (2006, April 20). Study finds a link of drug makers to psychiatrists. *New York Times.*

Carey, B. (2008, December 18). Psychiatrists revise the book of human troubles. *New York Times.*

Carey, B. (2010a, December 4). Narcissism: The malady of me. *New York Times.*

Carey, B. (2010b, February 10). Revising book on disorders of the mind. *New York Times.*

Carey, B. (2012a, January 24). Grief could join list of disorders. *New York Times.*

Carey, B. (2012b, January 20). New definition of autism may exclude many, study suggests. *New York Times.*

Carey, B. (2012c, May 9). Psychiatric manual drafters back down on diagnoses. *New York Times.*

Carey, B. (2012d, March 29). Rate of autism diagnoses has climbed, study finds. *New York Times.*

Carlat, D. (2007, June 13). Diagnosis: Conflict of interest. *New York Times.* http://www.nytimes.com/2007/06/13/opinion/13carlat.html

Cassels, C. (2010, June 11). APA assembly rejects proposed conflict of interest recommendations. *Medscape Medical News,* retrieved from http://www.medscape.com

Charney, D. S., Nemeroff, C. B., & with Braun, S. (2004). *The peace of mind prescription: An authoritative guide to finding the most effective treatment for anxiety and depression.* Boston: Houghton Mifflin.

Chodoff, P. (2002). The medicalization of human condition. *Psychiatric Services, 53*(5), 627–628.

Cloninger, C.R. (1999). A new conceptual paradigm from genetics and psycho-biology for the science of mental health. *New Zealand Journal of Psychiatry, 33* (August): 174-186.

Cohen, D. (1990). *Challenging the therapeutic state: Critical perspectives on psychiatry and the mental health system. Journal of Mind and Behavior* (Special double issue), *11*(3–4).

Cohen, D. (1994). *Challenging the therapeutic state, part two: Further disquisitions on the mental health system. Journal of Mind and Behavior* (Special double issue), *15*(1–2).

Conflicts of interest in continuing medical education. (2008, December 16). *Inside Higher Ed.*

Conrad, P. (2007). *The medicalization of society: On the transformation of human conditions into treatable disorders.* Baltimore: Johns Hopkins University Press.

Cosgrove, L., & Krimsky, S. (2012). A comparison of *DSM-IV* and *DSM-5* panel members' financial association with industry: A pernicious problem persists. *PLoS Medicine, 9*(3), e1001190.

Cosgrove, L., Krimsky, S., Vijayaraghavan, M., & Schneider, L. (2006). Financial ties between *DSM-IV* panel members and the pharmaceutical industry. *Psychotherapy and Psychosomatics, 75,* 154–160.

DSM Task Force. (2012). Retrieved April 30, 2012 at http://www.*DSM5*.org/ProposedRevision/Pages/proposedrevision.aspx?rid=94

Fournier, J. C., DeRubeis, R. J., Hollon, S. D., Dimidjian, S., Amsterdam, J. D., Shelton, R. C., et al. (2010). Antidepressant drug effects and depression security: A patient-level meta-analysis. *JAMA, 303*(1), 47–53.

Frances, A. (2009a, December 3). Alert to the research community: Be prepared to weigh in on *DSM-V. Psychiatric Times.* http://www.psychiatrictimes.com/display/article/10168/1493263.

Frances, A. (2009b, July 9). Dr. Frances responds to Dr. Carpenter: A sharp difference of opinion. *Psychiatric Times.* http://www.psychiatrictimes.com/display/article/10168/1426935.

Frances, A. (2009c, June 26). A warning sign on the road to *DSM-V*: Beware of its unintended consequences. *Psychiatric Times.* http://www.psychiatrictimes.com/display/article/10168/1425378

Frances, A. (2010a, March 19). *DSM*-5 and "psychosis risk syndrome": Not ready for prime time. *Psychiatric Times*. http://www.psychiatrictimes.com/display/article/10168/1541615

Frances, A. (2010b, May 7). The *DSM-5* field trial proposal—An expensive waste of time. *Psychiatric Times*. http://www.psychiatrictimes.com/print/article/10168/1565512?GUID=461C7A1F-D4E4-4939-B081-C3B02B079BD8&remember me=1&printable=true

Frances, A. (2010c, August 14). Good grief. *New York Times*.

Frances, A. (2010d, February 11). Opening Pandora's box: The 19 worst suggestions for *DSM-5*. *Psychiatric Times*. http://www.psychiatrictimes.com/dsm/content/article/10168/1522341

Frances, A. (2010e, June 2). Psychiatric fads and overdiagnosis. *Psychology Today: DSM5 in Distress*. http://www.psychologytoday.com/blog/dsm5-in-distress/201006/psychiatric-fads-and-overdiagnosis

Frances, A. (2012a, March 16). Am I a dangerous man? *Psychology Today: DSM5 in Distress*. http://www.psychologytoday.com/blog/dsm5-in-distress/201203/am-i-dangerous-man.

Frances, A. (2012b, May 12). Diagnosing the DSM. *New York Times*.

Frances, A. (2012c, January 18). A response to "How reliable is reliable enough?" *Psychiatric Times*. http://www.psychiatrictimes.com/blog/frances/content/article/10168/2019475

Frances, A. (2012d). Wonderful news: *DSM-5* finally begins its belated and necessary retreat. *Psychology Today: DSM5 in Distress*. http://www.psychologytoday.com/blog/dsm5-in-distress/201205/wonderful-news-dsm-5-finally-begins-its-belated-and-necessary-retreat

Friedman, R.A. (2012). A call for caution on antipsychotic drugs. *New York Times*, September 24. http://www.nytimes.com/2012/09/25/health/a-call-for-caution-in-the-use-of-antipsychotic-drugs.html?_r=0

Garber, K. (2007, December 20). Who's behind the bible of mental illness: Critics say the touted efforts against conflicts fall short. *U.S. News*.http://health.usnews.com/health-news/articles/2007/12/20/whos-behind-the-bible-of-mental-illness

Goleman, D. (1990, May 17). New paths to mental health put strains on some healers. *New York Times*, pp. A1, B12.

Gomory, T., Wong, S. E., Cohen, D., & Lacasse, J. R. (2011). Clinical social work and the biomedical industrial complex. *Journal of Sociology and Social Welfare*, *38*(4), 135–165.

Graham, J. (2010, November 13). Doctors' ties to drug industry still strong. *Los Angeles Times*.

Greenberg, G. (2010). *Manufacturing depression: The secret history of a modern disease*. New York: Simon & Schuster.

Greenberg, G. (2011, January). Inside the battle to define mental illness. *Wired*. http://www.wired.com/magazine/2010/12/ff_dsmv/

Greene, J. A. (2007). *Prescribing by numbers: Drugs and the definition of disease*. Baltimore: Johns Hopkins University Press.

Grossman, R. (2008, December 29). Psychiatry manual's secrecy criticized. *Los Angeles Times*.

Harris, G. (2007, June 27). Psychiatrists top list in drug maker gifts. *New York Times*. http://www.nytimes.com/2007/06/27/health/psychology/27doctors.html

Harris, G. (2008a, November 21). Radio host has drug company ties. *New York Times.* http://www.nytimes.com/2008/11/22/health/22radio.html?em

Harris, G. (2008b, October 3). Top psychiatrist didn't report drug makers' pay. *New York Times.* http://www.nytimes.com/2008/10/04/health/policy/04drug.html?_r=1&oref=slogin

Harris, G. (2008c, November 24). Research center tied to drug company. *New York Times.* http://www.nytimes.com/2008/11/25/health/25psych.html?pagewanted=all

Harris, G. (2009, November 19). Academic researchers' conflicts of interest go unreported. *New York Times.* http://www.nytimes.com/2008/11/25/health/25psych.html?pagewanted=all

Harris, G. (2009b, December 7). Senator Grassley seeks financial details from medical groups. *New York Times.* http://www.nytimes.com/2009/12/07/health/policy/07grassley.html?scp=2&sq=Senator+Grassley%2C+12-7-09&st=nyt

Harris, G., & Carey, B. (2008, June 8). Child experts fail to reveal full drug pay. *New York Times.* http://www.nytimes.com/2008/06/08/us/08conflict.html?pagewanted=all

Healy, D. (2012). *Pharmageddon.* Berkeley: University of California Press.

Horwitz, A. V., & Wakefield, J. C. (2007). *The loss of sadness: How psychiatry transformed normal sorrow into depressive disorder.* New York: Oxford University Press.

Horwitz, A.V. & Wakefield, J.C. (2012). *All we have to fear: Psychiatry's transformation of natural anxieties into mental disorders.* New York: Oxford University Press.

Hsieh, D. K., & Kirk, S. A. (2003). The effect of social context on psychiatrists' judgments of adolescent antisocial behavior. *Journal of Child Psychology and Psychiatry, 44*(6), 877–887.

Jablensky, A. (2012). The disease entity in psychiatry: Fact or fiction? *Epidemiology and Psychiatric Sciences, 21*(3), 251–264. doi:10.1017/S2045796012000339

Jabr, F. (2012, May 6). Field tests for revised psychiatric guide reveal reliability problems for two major diagnoses. *Scientific American.* http://blogs.scientificamerican.com/observations/2012/05/06/field-tests-for-revised-psychiatric-guide-reveal-reliability-problems-for-two-major-diagnoses/

Jacobs, D. H. (1995). Psychiatric drugging: Forty years of pseudo-science, self-interest, and indifference to harm. *Journal of Mind and Behavior, 16*(4), 421–470.

Jacobs, D. H., & Cohen, D. (2012). The end of neo-Kraepelinism. *Ethical Human Psychology & Psychiatry, 14*(2), 87–90. doi: 10.1891/1559-4343.14.2.87

Jacobs, D. H., & Cohen, D. (2010). Does "psychological dysfunction" mean anything? A critical essay on pathology vs. agency. *Journal of Humanistic Psychology, 50*(3), 312–334.

Joseph, J. (2004). *The gene illusion.* Algora Publishing.

Kaplan, A. (2009, January 1). *DSM* controversies. *Psychiatric Times.* http://www.psychiatrictimes.com/display/article/10168/1364926

Kessler, R., Chiu, W., Kemler, O., & Walters, E. (2005). Prevalence, severity, and comorbidity of 12-month *DSM-IV* disorders in the National Comorbidity Survey replication. *Archives of General Psychiatry, 62*(6), 617–627.

Kirk, S. A. (2004). Are children's *DSM* diagnoses accurate? *Brief Treatment and Crisis Intervention, 4*(3), 255–270.

Kirk, S. A., & Kutchins, H. (1988). Deliberate misdiagnosis in mental health practice. *Social Service Review, 62*(2), 225–237.

Kirk, S. A., & Kutchins, H. (1992). *The selling of DSM: The rhetoric of science in psychiatry.* Hawthorne, NY: Aldine de Gruyter.

Kirk, S. A., Wakefield, J. C., Hsieh, D., & Pottick, K. (1999). Social context and social workers' judgment of mental disorder. *Social Service Review, 73*, 82–104.

Kirmayer, J. L., & Young, A. (1999). Culture and context in the evolutionary concept of mental disorder. *Journal of Abnormal Psychology, 108*, 446–452.

Kraemer, H. C., Kupfer, D. J., Clarke, D. E., Narrow, W. E., & Regier, D. A. (2012). *DSM-5:* How reliable is reliable enough? *American Journal of Psychiatry, 169*(1), 13–15.

Kupfer, D. J. (2011, August 19). Public feedback on *DSM-5* provides crucial piece of the puzzle. *Psychiatric Times.*

Kupfer, D. J. (2012, May 4). *DSM* field trials providing ample critical data. *Psychiatric News.* Retrieved from http://psychnews.psychiatryonline.org/newsarticle.aspx?articleid=1130382

Kupfer, D. J., First, M. B., & Regier, D. A. (2002). Introduction. In D. J. Kupfer, M. B. First, & D. A. Regier (Eds.), *A research agenda for DSM-V* (pp. xv–xxiii). Washington, DC: American Psychiatric Association.

Kupfer, D. J., & Regier, D. A. (2011). Neuroscience, clinical evidence, and the future of psychiatric classification in *DSM-5*. *American Journal of Psychiatry, 168*(7), 672–674.

Kutchins, H., & Kirk, S. A. (1997). *Making us crazy:* DSM: *The psychiatric bible and the creation of mental disorders.* New York: Free Press.

Lancet. (2012). Living with grief. Retrieved from http://www.thelancet.com/journals/lancet/article/PIIS0140-6736(12)60248-7/fulltext

Lane, C. (2007). *Shyness: How normal behavior became a sickness.* New Haven: Yale University Press.

Lane, C. (2008, November 16). Wrangling over psychiatry's bible. *Los Angeles Times.*

Levy, D. A. (2010). *Tools of critical thinking: Metathoughts for psychology.* Long Grove, IL: Waveland Press.

Luhrmann, T. (2010). *Ethnographic case study.* Paper presented at the Cultural and Biological Contexts of Psychiatric Disorders.

McNally, R. J. (2011). *What is mental illness?* Cambridge: Harvard.

Monastersky, R. (2008, October 31). Hidden payments to university researchers draw new fire. *Chronicle of Higher Education.*

New York Times (Associated Press). (2010, April 29). Drug makers to pay fine of $81 million. http://www.nytimes.com/2010/04/30/business/30fine.html.

New York Times (Editorial). (2012, April 1). The puzzle of more autism cases.

Nugent, B. (2012, January 31). I had Asperger Syndrome. Briefly. *New York Times.*

Pastor, R. N., & Reuben, C. A. (2008). *Attention deficit disorder and learning disability: United States, 1996–2006.* Retrieved from National Center for Health Statistics website: http://www.cdc.gov/nchs/data/series/sr_10/sr10_237.pdf

Reed, G., Correia, J., Esparza, P., Saxena, S., & Maj, M. (2011). The WPA-WHO global survey of psychiatrists' attitudes towards mental disorders classification. *World Psychiatry, 10*(2), 118–131.

Regier, D. A., Narrow, W. E., Kuhl, E. A., & Kupfer, D. J. (2009). The conceptual development of *DSM-V*. *American Journal of Psychiatry, 166*(6), 645–650.

Rost, K., Smith, R., Matthews, D. B., & Guise, B. (1994). The deliberate misdiagnosis of major depression in primary care. *Annals of Family Medicine, 3*(4), 333–337.

Rothman, D. J. (2008). Academic medical centers and financial conflicts of interest. *JAMA, 299*(6), 695–697.

Rounsaville, B., Alcarcon, R., Andrews, G., Jackson, J. S., Kendell, R. E., & Kendler, K. (2002). Basic nomenclature issues for *DSM-V*. In D. J. Kupfer, M. B. First, & D. A. Regier (Eds.), *A research agenda for* DSM-V (pp. 1–29). Washington, DC: American Psychiatric Association.

Ryan, W. (1971). *Blaming the victim.* New York: Vintage Books.

Schatzberg, A., Scully, J., Kupfer, D. J., & Regier, D. A. (2009, July 1). Setting the record straight: A response to Frances' commentary on DSM-V. *Psychiatric Times.* http://www.psychiatrictimes.com/display/article/10168/1425806.

Shedler, J., Beck, A., Fonagy, P., Gabbard, G. O., Gunderson, J., Kernberg, O., et al. (2010). Personality disorders in *DSM-5. American Journal of Psychiatry, 167*(September), 1026–1028.

Shedler, J., Beck, A., Fonagy, P., Gabbard, G. O., Kernberg, O., Michels, R., et al. (2011). Response to Skodol letter. *American Journal of Psychiatry, 168*(1), 97–98.

Skodal, A. (2011). Revision of the personality disorder model for *DSM-5. American Journal of Psychiatry, 168*(1), 97.

Society for Humanistic Psychology. (2012). Retrieved 4-30-12 http://www.ipetitions.com/petition/*DSM5*/].

Spiegel, A. (2005, January 3). The dictionary of disorder. *The New Yorker,* 56–63.

Spitzer, R., Williams, J., & Skodal, A. (1980). *DSM-III*: The major achievements and an overview. *American Journal of Psychiatry, 137,* 151–164.

Spitzer, R.L. (2008). Psychiatrists revise diagnostic manual—In secret, Retrieved on 9-25-08 and posted at http://taxa.epi.umn.edu/~mbmiller/sscpnet/20080909 Spitzer.

Spitzer, R. L. (2009). APA and *DSM-V*: Empty promises. *Psychiatric Times.*

Spitzer, R. L., Williams, J., & Endicott, J. (2012). Standards for *DSM-5* reliability. *American Journal of Psychiatry, 169*(5), 537.

Steinberg, P. (2012, January 31). Asperger's history of over-diagnosis. *New York Times.*

Szasz, T. (2007). *The medicalization of everyday life: Selected essays.* Syracuse, NY: Syracuse University Press.

The Economist. (2008, November 29). Absence of evidence, p. 82.

The puzzle of more autism cases. (2012, April 1). *New York Times.*

Urbina, I. (2012, May 12). New guidelines may sharply increase addiction diagnoses. *New York Times.*

Wakefield, J. C., & First, M. B. (2012). Validity of the bereavement exclusion to major depression: Does the empirical evidence support the proposal to eliminate the exclusion in *DSM-5? World Psychiatry, 11,* 3–10.

Wakefield, J. C., Pottick, K., & Kirk, S. A. (2002). Should the *DSM-IV* diagnostic criteria for conduct disorder consider social context? *American Journal of Psychiatry, 159,* 380–386.

Weiner, B. (1995). *Judgments of responsibility: A foundation for a theory of social conduct*. New York: Guilford Press.

Whitaker, R. (2010). *Anatomy of an epidemic: Magic bullets, psychiatric drugs, and the astonishing rise of mental illness in America*. New York: Crown.

Willman, D. (2004a, December 22). $508,050 from Pfizer, but no "Outside Positions to Note." *Los Angeles Times*.

Willman, D. (2004b, December 22). The National Institutes of Health: Public servant or private marketer? *Los Angeles Times*.

Wilson, D. (2006, December 5). NIH scientist charged with conflict. *Los Angeles Times*.

Wilson, D. (2009, November 18). Medical schools quizzed on ghostwriting. *New York Times*. http://query.nytimes.com/gst/fullpage.html?res=9404EFDA173A F93BA25752C1A96F9C8B63&scp=1&sq=medical+schools+quizzed+on+gh ostingwriting&st=nyt

Woolston, C. (2011, March 7). PSA: Do the blood tests actually save lives? The medical community is divided. *Los Angeles Times*.

Zanor, C. (2010, November 29). A fate that narcissists will hate: Being ignored. *New York Times*.

Zarembo, A. (2011, December 11–16). Discovering autism (4 part series). *Los Angeles Times*.

6

Dancing with Drugs

Introduction

Like other "advances" in community treatment and diagnosis that we deconstruct in this book, the promises of the scientific drug treatment of distress, madness, and misbehavior rest on uncritically accepted claims, not well-tested evidence. The popular success of prescribed psychoactive drugs does not rest on scientific demonstrations of efficacy in the treatment of medical disorders. The success results from the synergistic combination of ideological, cultural, and commercial forces. Bearing down from above came shoddy science, uncritical practitioners with a monopoly on drug pre-scriptions, the minting of new mental disorders, ubiquitous drug market-ing, co-opted regulatory agencies, and plain fraud. Surging up from below and augmented by a newly emerging health consumerism came people's indefatigable desires for psychoactive drugs, the powerful but dismissed power of placebo, and the reverberation of myriad personal narratives of drug-induced transformation, recovery, and cure.

The merging of these forces created the conviction among the educated and not-so-educated that such popular success could only rest on a solid scientific foundation. It was and remains inconceivable to many observers that consumers and insurers might spend billions of dollars on placebos with brand names—or worse, on drugs that produce waves of iatrogenic (that is, doctor- or treatment-induced) diseases. Indeed, over the past half century the psychoactive medicines enterprise was constantly justified by appeals to science, but its foundations did not rest on science as a search for truth, as an effort to test hypotheses rigorously, or as a means to understand biological or social facts. As for the specific field directly concerned with the investi-gation of psychiatric drug treatment, clinical psychopharmacology, many of its practitioners and researchers engaged in nothing less than the studious avoidance of evident facts about distress, psychoactive drugs, healing, and the power of suggestion.

In this chapter, we lay out the mental health system's current crisis with regard to psychiatric drugs: the emerging consensus that the latest prescribed

211

psychiatric drugs do not necessarily improve the targeted symptoms of people diagnosed with major mental disorders. We review recent studies conducted with United States federal government funding that attempted to assess what sort of improvement the major modern classes of psychiatric drugs were actually bringing about in such people. We then place their findings in the context of the long-standing promotion of drugs by the pharmaceutical industry, and psychiatry's enthusiastic role as the industry's junior partner. Yet as our initial comments in this chapter suggest, the story of the widespread adoption of apparently ineffective drugs as paradigmatic treatments is complex and involves many other interacting forces and players. *It is also not a new story in psychiatry.* We try to paint this more complex yet recurring story in chapter 7, which also looks at the dubious distinctions made between "dangerous drugs" and "approved medications" throughout the century and examines how some particular psychoactive substances become constructed and promoted as FDA-approved medications.

We present two complementary but different critiques of the current disease-centered approach to conceiving of the beneficial effects of prescribed psychiatric drugs. The first, in this chapter, focuses on the continuously documented but continuously avoided power of placebo. The second, focusing on the striking and subtle psychoactive effects of psychiatric drugs, suggests that placing these drugs squarely within the broader ecological niche of *all psychoactive drugs* could go far to increase our understanding of how drugs "work" to relieve distress while creating new opportunities for a truly patient-centered psychopharmacology (Moncrieff & Cohen, 2009; Moncrieff, 2008).

Yet Another "Seige Cycle"

That psychoactive drugs used as prescribed medicines often do not have the beneficial impact on mental disorders (however defined) claimed by proponents and promoters of drugs is relatively easy to demonstrate: the most touted studies show that the desired outcomes of modern drug treatment do not reveal improvement when compared with outcomes of treatments from the pre-drug era, or with outcomes from older or discarded drugs, and in some cases the recent outcomes appear worse. For example, when followed for one year, depressed persons who are drug-treated experience more depressive episodes, and longer ones, than depressed persons who remain drug-free (Patten, 2004). Very long-term follow-up studies of ten years' duration or more of depressed people show no worse outcomes for drug-free than drug-treated individuals (Hughes & Cohen, 2009). In the largest real-world study of the drug treatment of depression funded by the NIMH, it appears that not more than 3 percent of the more than four thousand subjects who underwent drug treatment managed to stay in the study, improve, and be considered to stay well for one year (Nierenberg et al., 2008). Improvement rates in drug treatment studies of schizophrenic patients during the late 1980s to the mid-1990s were identical to rates observed in studies conducted between sixty and one hundred years earlier (Hegarty et al., 1994). When British psychiatrist David Healy (2009) investigated changes over the past fifty years around his own hospital in North Wales, he observed the following: compulsory psychiatric detentions were up 300 percent, admissions for serious mental illness were up 700 percent, while admissions overall were up 1500 percent. Suicide rates among patients diagnosed with schizophrenia were up 2000 percent. General death rate among patients considered seriously mentally ill had "risen substantially." Healy added that all studies find that the death rate of schizophrenic patients increases with the number of drugs given. He concluded: "What we are seeing now is not what happens when treatments work" (2009, pp. 32–33).

Such assessments have not only come from mental health professionals known for their critical views. Thomas Insel, director of the NIMH, acknowledged in 2009 the failure of the pharmacological agents that have dominated mental health treatment since the 1960s. Insel asked: "Is there any evidence to support that progress in psychiatry leads to reductions in morbidity or disability in people with serious mental illness?" To answer, he reviewed recent US national studies involving interviews with participants in several thousand households. He made the dramatic assertion that "there is no evidence for reduced morbidity or mortality from any mental illness" (2009, p. 129). "The results demonstrate no change in the prevalence of mental illness between 1992 and 2002, but increased rates of treatment. . . . Curiously, despite increased treatment, there was no evidence for decreased disability" (pp. 128–129). Concerning mortality, Insel noted that persons diagnosed with serious mental illness die from thirteen to thirty-two years earlier than people in the general population, and that suicide rates have not decreased.

In this respect, the official realization of disappointing effects from widely promoted drugs fits what French historians Christian Bachman and Anne Coppel have called the "path of stigmatization" (1989, p. 109), which they believe characterizes how psychoactive drugs move over time in society. More pointedly, Dutch historians Toine Pieters and Stephen Snelders (2005) have named this a "Seige cycle," after German psychiatrist Max Seige, who suggested as early as 1912 the idea of a cyclical dynamic of the careers of such drugs. A Seige cycle is characterized by initial enthusiasm and therapeutic optimism leading to widespread use, subsequent negative appraisal, and finally, limited use or an outright ban. Seige's insight is notable, given the few drugs he must have considered as examples by this date. The opiates, morphine especially, exemplify this path: at the start, a "uniquely efficacious" drug; at the end, "addicted victims"[1] (Chast, 1995).

Thomas Szasz (1974) as well as drug scholar Richard DeGrandpre (2007) have also commented on the trajectories of drugs from panaceas to panapathogens (but sometimes also back to panaceas as is the case with the medical use of morphine today and the renewed psychiatric interest in hallucinogens, see Tierney, 2010), despite an identical scientific understanding of their pharmacology at the start as at the end of the trajectory. These authors argue that the social-ceremonial aims of psychoactive drugs may far outweigh—whether in personal lives, professional interest, or public policy spheres—their actual pharmacological effects. We find these insights intriguing and will be applying them throughout our analysis of psychiatry's portrayals of the prescription of its favorite psychoactive drugs as evidence-based treatment.

The preceding paragraphs suggest that there is nothing unusual about the inability to show, in scientific studies conducted after psychoactive drugs have been in widespread use for years and decades, that these drugs do not necessarily decrease disability—that in fact they may be responsible for excess disability. This pattern may have occurred with every class of drugs introduced in psychiatric practice since the turn of the twentieth century. Disappointing findings of effectiveness and findings of excess (iatrogenic) morbidity have also regularly been used to justify and promote the adoption of newer drugs or drug classes, on the promise of improved effectiveness and reduced toxicity. Being unfamiliar with history or being too closely wedded to a particular school of thought, or both, many people within and outside of the mental health system may therefore have confused the *popularity* of psychiatric drugs with the *validity of the claim* that psychiatric drugs constitute specific, effective treatments for specific disorders. In our view, this latter belief is a major impediment to understanding any genuine treatment functions and accomplishments of psychiatry today, and we deconstruct it in this and in the following chapter.

One Drug after Another

Starting roughly in the 1920s with the introduction of the sedative barbiturates into routine medical practice, crops of new-and-improved psychiatric drugs have been prescribed to an increasing number of people. The stimulating amphetamines were introduced in the 1940s. In the 1950s came the neuroleptics (or antipsychotics) and the tricyclic antidepressants (TCAs), launching a new confidence in biological psychiatry. In the 1960s the tranquilizing benzodiazepines were introduced, making large new inroads into general medical practice. In the 1980s, the serotonin-reuptake inhibitors (SSRIs), initially approved as antidepressants, extended biological psychiatry's conquest-by-medication and in the 1990s, the second-generation antipsychotics and anticonvulsant "mood stabilizers" mopped up virtually all remaining pockets of resistance. Insel's appraisal of progress, or the lack thereof, was published in 2009.

Prescriptions written for antidepressants in the United States numbered about 40 million in 1988, the year Prozac was launched, compared to

264 million in 2011 (IMS Health, 2012). Five years earlier, antidepressants had become the most prescribed class of drugs in the United States (Centers for Disease Control and Prevention, 2006)—more often prescribed than antibiotics or drugs to treat heart disease. Looking only at the short interval between 1998 and 2004, the number of noninstitutionalized Americans purchasing products from the psychiatric drug classes of antidepressants, antipsychotics, benzodiazepines, and stimulants increased from 22 million to 38 million (Stagnitti, 2007). The really notable changes occurred among children. In the mid-1980s, less than 1 percent of children were taking any psychiatric drugs, usually stimulants and benzodiazepines. Twenty years later, depending on the specific age group considered, 8–12 percent of youths were being medicated with psychiatric drugs. Indeed, in 2009, over 40 million prescriptions or refills were written for youths under nineteen years of age: 24.3 million for stimulants, 9.6 million for antidepressants, and 6.5 million for antipsychotics (Mathews, 2010).

Industry/Psychiatry

Only recently have academics and journalists described the role of the pharmaceutical industry in these trends without being dismissed as antiestablishment radicals with a grudge against profitable industries. The industry did not merely bring new drugs to market, it made every effort to ensure that physicians would view whatever latest drug or drug class was being promoted as indispensably beneficial and would prescribe them readily for the widest range of patients' complaints and presenting problems. This involved "disease mongering"—broadening the boundaries of treatable problems and creating anxieties about the seriousness of ordinary ailments (Moynihan, Heath, & Henry, 2002)—as well as purchasing the hearts and minds of practitioners and those leaders and organizations who could influence the ideas and behavior of practitioners. Psychiatry, which already embodied the medicalization of deviance and distress, wholeheartedly embraced its partnership with the drug industry, to the point, we think, of becoming virtually indistinguishable from it.

During the first decades of the twentieth century, in order to present their products as more scientifically-based, drug manufacturers began to voluntarily relinquish the option to advertise drugs directly to the public. This made direct marketing to physicians indispensable, and the appearance of science in marketing grew correspondingly. Amphetamine, first developed in the 1920s as an oral anti-asthma drug, was actively promoted the next decade by the Smith, Kline and French firm among "neuropsychiatrists" for the treatment of mild depression, from whence it spread to general medicine. "By the 1930s," writes historian Nicholas Rasmussen (2006), "leading firms like Smith Kline and French had learned to involve themselves in the medical research literature to a remarkable extent, from conceiving and designing clinical studies that targeted particular medical audiences, to overseeing their execution by competent or even eminent researchers, to managing their writing, illustration, and publication in top journals" (p. 301). Thus began the "remarkable extent" to which the pharmaceutical industry is involved in the design, conduct, and dissemination of clinical trial research today.

Over the century, the drug industry has developed and employed systematic drug-detailing techniques to convince individual doctors to prescribe its latest products. The basic techniques—gifts, flattery, and persuasion—have not changed much since the 1930s. Today, however, drug manufacturers can target virtually every practicing physician in the United States with laser-like precision and maximum efficiency. Using computerized databases purchased from a plethora of commercial medical information firms and from professional organizations such as the American Medical Association, drug firms closely monitor the effects of their promotional strategies on drug sales or prescriptions at national, regional, and even local pharmacy levels. It is no exaggeration that an entire multinational pharmaceutical firm can adapt or customize its marketing strategies down to a single prescriber if necessary (Fugh-Berman, 2008).

To support these techniques, the industry proceeds by mass infusion of money, dozens of billions of dollars each year (Gagnon & Lexchin, 2008). The money facilitates the professional activities (studies, travels, hostings, communications, disseminations) of students, clinicians, educators, researchers, legislators, policymakers, drug regulators, journal editors and reviewers, hospital administrators, and consumer advocates—as long as the endpoint of the activity is perceived as favorable to the industry's products or completely neutral (by which we do not mean objective). The money comes in myriad forms, such as salaries, prizes, awards, donations, reimbursements, unrestricted educational funds, research grants, endowments, equipment grants, seed grants, travel allowances, and bribes. This fuel keeps the drug industry's views, interests, and agenda active or quiescent in the mind of every player and potential player in the mental health system. (A more detailed analysis of drug-industry funding appears in the next chapter.) Thus, by the early 1990s, the multinational pharmaceutical industry had cemented an intricately complex, multilevel partnership with the profession of psychiatry, both at the level of psychiatric institutions and educational centers and at the level of individual practitioners, and with national, state, and local opinion leaders in the mental health movement. With every passing year, as more patented drugs sold, more profits accrued to the industry, and more funds were plowed back into making friends, influencing people, and generating "evidence," the partnership grew in breadth and depth.

As discussed especially in chapter 5, starting sometime after 2005, signs of a backlash against this alliance appeared. Rumblings were heard from some newspapers, some legislators, and some outspoken members of various professional groups. In 2008, for the first time, the crusading US Senator Charles Grassley asked the American Psychiatric Association to disclose precisely how much of its annual budget came from the drug industry. The APA (2008) divulged that 28 percent (approximately $14 million of its budget the previous year) were industry contributions, primarily paid in advertising in APA journals and funds for continuing medical education (CME) courses offered by the APA.

As public acceptance of industry control begins to decline, psychiatric associations are beginning to clean house, for example by reducing the number of industry-funded symposia offered as CME at their annual meetings (Carlat, 2009). For the foreseeable future, however, if psychiatry wishes to maintain itself as the flagship mental health profession, it has little choice but to maintain its financial and intellectual dependence on the pharmaceutical industry. The APA's ability to attract substantial industry funding outside of membership dues to promote its image and its activities has been unique among all the mental health professions. This is not difficult to understand. In the absence of scientific demonstrations of the validity of its particular medical approach, all psychiatry can unequivocally show is the popularity of psychoactive drugs that physicians prescribe after opinion leaders in psychiatry show them the way. But the popularity of drugs is a double-edged sword. Though it has propelled biological psychiatry to undreamed heights, a number of recent trends suggest that it may eventually engulf the profession—render psychiatry obsolete, in other words—in a rising wave of industry-promoted and consumer-directed medication choices.

Drugs for Everything

With the allowance by the Food and Drug Administration (FDA) of direct-to-consumer advertising of prescription drugs in the United States beginning in full force in 1997, psychoactive drugs became yet another consumer product advertised to the public in a myriad of artfully produced television, magazine, newspaper, and internet ads. In all of these, the message that doctors are somehow in control is unfailingly transmitted ("Ask your doctor . . ."), but its repetition has finally served to underscore its absurdity. Advertisers and "drug reps," not doctors, are now the actual middlemen between people and their drugs, just as they were a century ago, in the wild era of "patent medicines" (Young, 1961).

Daily, with the full blessings of medical and educational authorities, millions of parents give their prepubescent children psychoactive drugs—some of which, like amphetamines (e.g., Adderall), were banned only twenty years earlier in the United States and whose use or distribution without a medical prescription can elicit draconian penalties. [2] The boundary between licit and illicit psychoactive drug use is vanishing: celebrities like Michael Jackson, Heath Ledger, and Anna Nicole Smith "accidentally" die from ingestions of duly prescribed medications, and experts in mental health, law, and ethics call for the prescription of psychoactive drugs to the healthy for cognitive enhancing or "neuroenhancement" (Greely et al., 2008). Several factors are interacting in complex ways to produce these trends. They include the increased role of consumer preferences and choices, the reverberation of popular discourse, direct-to-consumer advertising campaigns, and the pronouncements of experts. This is not unlike factors such as consumer preferences, the price of fuel, and advertisements interacting to influence individual purchases of consumer goods such as automobiles.

Moreover, the once-hallowed market approval of a drug by a powerful regulatory agency like the FDA has become, from the viewpoint of pharmaceutical firms, the last obstacle to promoting drugs aggressively with only the barest connection to the indication and age group for which the FDA approved the drugs. Doctors who might claim to practice "evidence-based psychiatry" routinely prescribe drug cocktails (combinations of two or more psychiatric drugs) whose effects no published controlled study has ever probed (Bhatara et al., 2004).

As for the published studies themselves—as David Healy has suggested and as we explore ahead, "There is probably no other area of medicine in which the literature is so at odds with the raw data" (cited in Leo, 2006, p. 31). And, the most vulnerable—children covered by Medicaid because of low income—are four times more likely to receive antipsychotic drugs and for less severe "conditions," than children with private insurance (Wilson, 2009). According to most available estimates, about two-thirds of all money spent to purchase psychotropic drugs (and mental health and substance abuse treatment in general) in the United States is spent by government programs, prominently Medicaid and Medicare (e.g., Donohue, 2006).

"The Care We Provided Was Appropriate . . ."

National headlines were made in 2007 by the heartbreaking case of Rebecca Riley, a four-year-old child found dead on her parents' bedroom floor from a drug overdose. The Riley parents were unemployed, and the family was almost wholly supported by Social Security benefits. Starting at age two, Rebecca was diagnosed as suffering from attention-deficit/hyperactivity disorder and bipolar disorder, almost entirely on the basis of the accounts of her behavior given by her mother to Kayoko Kifuji, a child psychiatrist employed by Tufts-New England Medical Center. Dr. Kifuji also prescribed to Rebecca (and her two slightly older siblings, also diagnosed with bipolar disorder by Dr. Kifuji) the antipsychotic quetiapine (Seroquel, $3 billion in US sales that year), the anticonvulsant depakote, and the antihypertensive drug clonidine (used in child psychiatry for its sedative properties, often prescribed in tandem with the stimulant methylphenidate, or Ritalin). Rebecca also was given two over-the-counter cold remedies (both of which were, a year later, in an unrelated action, "voluntarily" withdrawn by drug manufacturers for use in very young children). None of the three prescribed drugs were FDA-approved for psychiatric use with children because the FDA had never considered any evidence of even their short-term, superficial behavioral benefits for children.

Yet, immediately after Rebecca's death, her medication regimen was defended by Tufts-New England Medical Center, whose spokesperson stated: "The care we provided was appropriate and within responsible professional standards" (WCVB TV, 2007). As recounted in a series of grim reports, Rebecca's father had a confirmed history of abusive behavior. Both parents were chronically unemployed and seemed intent on declaring the whole family mentally ill to increase their financial support from state agencies. Moreover, they appeared to ignore Rebecca's complaints during her last painful hours of life. This shielded Dr. Kifuji from criminal prosecution, and in separate trials the Riley parents, Michael and Carolyn, were convicted of first- and second-degree murder, respectively (Wen, 2010). Dr. Kifuji continues to practice as a child psychiatrist. Kaitlynne Riley, Rebecca's older sister by two years, away from her parents and Dr. Kifuji since her sister's death, was said to have "recovered" from her bipolar disorder, symptom-free and drug-free (Diller, 2010).

In another case, Nada Stotland, then president of the American Psychiatric Association, commented on the simultaneous prescription of the antidepressant Prozac, the tranquilizer Xanax, and the sleeping pill Ambien by a psychiatrist to a tormented twenty-seven-year-old man, Steven Kazmierczak, who eventually went off the drugs and then went on a shooting rampage at Northern Illinois University, where he had formerly been a student. Although some observers might interpret Kazmierczak's actions as evidence that the drugs were helping him, others could point to the unusual reactions occasionally reported as triggered by combinations of psychoactive drugs and by the rebound and withdrawal reactions triggered by medications stopped abruptly. Stotland was quoted as stating: "It is not unusual for doctors to prescribe anti-anxiety agents and sleep medication along with antidepressants, since [antidepressants] can cause anxiety and interfere with sleep" (CNN, 2008).

That very young children could be psychiatrically diagnosed and medicated so arbitrarily and that national psychiatric authorities could state matter-of-factly that the drugs they prescribed to treat anxiety and depression "can cause anxiety and interfere with sleep" in effect meant that society had given psychiatry a blank check. As the biological wing of psychiatry and the mental health movement had ascended during earlier decades, new catch phrases and slogans justified the ancient human rituals of taking and giving drugs. Everywhere, chemical imbalances, neurotransmitter malfunctions, and impaired neural circuits were corrected, balanced, modulated, or stabilized by evidence-based treatments. These vague, medical-sounding phrases cloaked people's unquenchable desires for psychoactive drugs in the explanatory language of people's need for essential treatments provided by medically informed experts.

The Chickens Are Coming Home to Roost

Starting in the fall of 2005 and still continuing as these lines are written, a series of articles appeared in the major American psychiatric and medical journals, reporting the results of three exceptionally large NIMH-funded studies evaluating the effectiveness of state-of-the-art psychiatric drug treatments for schizophrenia, depression, and bipolar disorder. The three studies, reportedly costing taxpayers over $100 million, provided what a *Boston Globe* journalist described as "the most realistic look ever at the state of psychiatric medicine" (Allen, 2006). The studies showed unambiguously that drugs do not make most people considered psychiatrically impaired significantly better for any sustained period of time. Since the studies appeared, mainstream popular and professional reactions suggest that the demonstration has been absorbed, digested, and recycled like every such negative finding over the past sixty years: it appears to have made only a tiny dent in the myth of psychiatric progress.

New Antipsychotics: A Bust

The first article appeared in the September 18, 2005, issue of *The New England Journal of Medicine*. Its lead author, Jeffrey Lieberman, chairman of the Department of Psychiatry at Columbia University, and the coauthors read as a list of the "Who's Who" of schizophrenia drug treatment in the United States (Lieberman et al., 2005). The article was the first of many reporting on the results of a psychiatric mega-study, Clinical Antipsychotic Trials of Intervention Effectiveness, since known by its acronym, CATIE. The general aim of the study was to compare five different antipsychotic drugs in the treatment of nearly 1,500 patients diagnosed with psychosis and schizophrenia and recruited from fifty-seven different sites. Four of the drugs were second- or third-generation antipsychotics (olanzapine, quetiapine, risperidone, and ziprasidone), approved by the FDA between 1994 and 2002. The fifth was perphenazine, a nearly forgotten antipsychotic introduced in the late 1950s, almost never prescribed today.

To place the findings of this study in some context, one should note that schizophrenia is one of the few conditions that psychiatry can be said to "own"; nothing better exemplifies the application of psychiatric knowledge than treating schizophrenia. It is widely held that psychiatry came of age in the 1950s when it stumbled upon chlorpromazine (named Thorazine in the United States) and similar drugs that suppressed the agitation of asylum inmates. Since then, the drugs, first named neuroleptics and eventually antipsychotics, have been given to hundreds of millions of people throughout the world and are consecrated as having ushered in the "psychopharmacological revolution"—the very subject of this chapter and the next. Although schizophrenia is considered to affect about 1 percent of the population, during the first decade of the twenty-first century, antipsychotics ranked among the five top-selling classes of *all prescription drugs* in America. This was because most of their prescriptions were for problems outside schizophrenia and bipolar disorder, the drugs' approved indications by the FDA, and because their manufacturers had accurately gauged that third-party payers would spend hundreds of dollars monthly for individual courses of treatment prescribed by appropriately primed physicians.

In CATIE, each entering patient was randomly assigned to receive one of the drugs and was followed for up to eighteen months or until he or she dropped out of the study or was switched to another drug. Notably, the primary outcome reported in the 2005 article was not a measure of the drugs' intended benefits. The researchers did not convey effectiveness by the usual means used in clinical trials: ratings of what the researchers believe disturbs the participants or marks their behavior as abnormal (psychiatric symptoms), or of the participants' reports about their ability to fulfill conventional social, occupational, and interpersonal roles (degree of impairment) over the course of the study. Instead, researchers emphasized only *how long subjects remained on their assigned drug.*

This simple outcome reported in the first CATIE report would suggest that the benefits of antipsychotic drugs are so well established that only a crude proxy measure is needed to demonstrate that they actually improve the diagnosed problem in the population studied. (If that were the case, of course, the CATIE trial would have been unnecessary.) The measure is deceptive, however, because the actual benefits of giving people psychoactive drugs are difficult to ascertain objectively, especially if the drugs are given to people who do not want to take them for long. Typically, antipsychotics are subjectively experienced as producing sedation, heavily clouded cognition, emotional dampening, and abnormal involuntary movements (Moncrieff, Cohen, & Mason, 2009). Moreover, people with diagnoses of psychotic disorders are relentlessly pressured or coerced to take and stay on antipsychotic medications, regardless of their feelings about doing so—which takes away much of the validity of the outcome measure in this CATIE study. Finally, as we discuss later, researchers in psychiatry have invested precious little creativity in determining how to assess the complex effects of psychoactive drugs taken daily over months and years. Yet for all its limitations the outcome measure was self-evidently practical, as a person who stops taking a drug cannot benefit from any of the drugs' potentially desirable effects.

In any case, the proxy measure in this CATIE study painted an unfavorable portrait of the drug's effectiveness: by study's end, an average of 74 percent of patients on each drug (range, 69 to 84 percent) had "discontinued their assigned treatment owing to inefficacy or intolerable side effects or for other reasons" (Lieberman et al., 2005, p. 1209). Patients on olanzapine (Zyprexa) did stay longer on that drug, but they were also more likely to gain significant weight and show abnormalities in glucose and lipid metabolism. Trilafon (perphenazine), the obsolete antipsychotic selling for about 3¢ a dose, lost only slightly more patients from its group than Zyprexa, selling for three hundred times as much and ranked just two years earlier as the world's most prescribed antipsychotic (between 1996 and 2002, its first six years on the market, Zyprexa's gross sales were $13 billion, and it has gone on to gross over $45 billion as of this writing).

New Antidepressants: If at First You Don't Succeed . . .

In January 2006, the *American Journal of Psychiatry* published one of the largest studies ever conducted on the drug treatment of depression (Trivedi et al., 2006). Also characterized by its acronym, STAR*D (for Sequenced Treatment Alternatives to Relieve Depression), this study recruited over 4,000 participants (the Trivedi et al. article reported on a first wave of 2,900 followed for fourteen weeks of planned treatment). Unlike carefully screened subjects in shorter clinical trials, most participants in STAR*D resembled ordinary patients who would ordinarily end up treated with antidepressants in outpatient doctors' offices. They were recruited only when they sought care from over forty different outpatient general medical and psychiatric clinics across the United States.

All patients in STAR*D were first treated with Celexa (citalopram), a selective serotonin reuptake inhibitor (SSRI) approved in 1998 by the Food and Drug Administration to treat major depressive disorder (MDD). Celexa was chosen by the investigators because it is the most serotonin-selective of the SSRIs. Dosage was flexible and individually tailored by each patient's own doctor, based on ongoing feedback from the patient. The results, then, were expected to be more representative of ordinary practice situations than the results from controlled clinical trials, which normally used fixed doses and rarely last beyond eight weeks. Also, to provide a relatively unambiguous outcome measure that would be immediately relevant to anyone, *remission* (or virtual disappearance of symptoms, rather than relative improvement compared to a placebo-treated control group, as in controlled clinical trials) was employed in STAR*D to determine the outcome. In sum, here was what appeared as a fairly "realistic" test of an already extremely popular drug treatment. The findings: a bit more than one quarter of the participants (29 percent) receiving a full course of SSRI drug treatment for depression (which lasted on average about eighty-three days), were reported by Trivedi and colleagues to have experienced a remission, while 47 percent were said to have shown a "response."

Two months later, on March 23, 2006, a second article from the same study was published in the *New England Journal of Medicine* (Rush et al., 2006).

It reported on a subsample of 727 left over from the original 2,900 participants. The subsample was made up of still depressed individuals who had immediately agreed to undertake a second course of drug treatment, to last another fourteen weeks, despite their failed attempt with Celexa. These subjects had then been randomly assigned to receive one of three other antidepressants: Effexor (venlafaxine) or Wellbutrin (bupropion) in extended release forms, or Zoloft (sertraline). Slightly less than half of the people in each antidepressant group also received concomitant psychotropic drugs, described as trazodone (for sleep), anxiolytics (excluding alprazolam), and sedative-hypnotics. (This raises the question: what drugs, or drug combinations, were actually being tested?) By the end of that continuation study, an average of 21.2 percent of the patients in each group (varying from about 18 to 27 percent, depending on the measure used by the investigators) had experienced a remission (with no statistically significant difference between any of the groups). However, more patients dropped out of the study for intolerance of the drugs than experienced a remission. More than half of people in each group experienced adverse effects of greater than "moderate" intensity. About half of the people in each drug group experienced adverse effects for more than half of the time they remained on treatment, including about one quarter who reported experiencing them 90 to 100 percent of the time.

The mainstream media universally put a positive spin on the disappointing findings, as illustrated by this comment from the medical newsletter *MedPage Today* (Osterweil, 2006): "STAR*D investigators demonstrated that in the treatment of major depression, patience and persistence can pay off."

The STAR*D Reassessment

Despite STAR*D's lackluster reports, the findings should have painted an even worse portrait of antidepressants' effectiveness. "Publication bias" is the name given to the practice of skewing, hiding, suppressing, twisting, or cooking data in order to inflate the apparent value—the "efficacy"—of marketed drugs. In a series of publications and in a blog, psychologist Ed Pigott (2011a; 2011b) has conducted his own review and reanalysis of the STAR*D trial findings, as have other researchers (Cohen, 2010; Leventhal & Antonuccio, 2009; Pigott, Leventhal, Alter, & Boren, 2010). These authors have reported a disturbing pattern of publication bias, including the following examples, most of which involve deviations from the prespecified STAR*D research protocol.

- Patients who dropped out of the first antidepressant treatment step without completing a second Hamilton Rating Scale for Depression (HRSD) were to be counted as *treatment failures*. Instead, these patients were simply excluded from analyses, thus inflating the reported success rates.

- Patients with an HRSD score below 14 points were to be considered too mildly depressed for inclusion in the study. Instead, they were included. An additional 324 patients lacking an initial HRSD score were later included. In all, 931 of 4,041 patients (23 percent) failed to meet the prespecified eligibility criteria but nonetheless were included in the analyses, again inflating the drugs' reported efficacy.
- Also contrary to the STAR*D research protocol, the authors switched to using a proprietary assessment measure, the Quick Inventory of Depressive Symptoms–Self Report (QIDS-SR) as the sole measure to report outcomes in the key summary article from STAR*D. This switch inflated published remission and response rates. In the QIDS-SR, a patient reporting, "I feel sad more than half of the time" or "Most of the time, I struggle to focus my attention or to make decisions" *and* "I rarely eat within a 24 hour-period, and only with extreme personal effort or when others persuade me to eat" would earn a score of 5 on the QIDS-SR—qualifying that patient as *remitted*. More than 90 percent of such remitters had at least one residual symptom (as a group, remitters showed a median of three symptoms), usually sleep disturbance, appetite or weight disturbance, sad mood, fatigue or decreased energy, and decreased concentration.
- As of mid-2011, despite over a hundred articles having been published from the STAR*D findings, eleven prespecified research measures collected to evaluate outcomes at entry and exit from each treatment step and every three months of follow-up still had not been reported.

These deviations from protocols, presentations of ad hoc findings as the prespecified outcomes of interest, and uses of explicitly excluded strategies to inflate apparent drug efficacy show how unwilling elite researchers and their institutional collaborators are to telling it like it is. The STAR*D investigation stands out from others due to its breadth and scope, but some of its reports provide more of the same endless psychopharmacological spinning that debases countless studies in the field by doing everything possible to avoid challenging the ideological, intellectual, and clinical status quo. Whether the investigators were deceiving themselves or deceiving others or both, the published STAR*D findings exemplify the sad but stark fact that an undetermined portion of psychopharmacological studies—especially those conducted by researchers who have made a successful career of promoting psychiatric drugs—cannot be trusted unless their findings are checked and rechecked (though the original data may never be available).

"Mood Stabilizers": Still Unbalanced

Findings from the third study to consider, the largest ever of the treatment of bipolar disorder (known as manic depression since the 1890s), first appeared in the February 2006 issue of the *American Journal of Psychiatry* (Perlis et al., 2006). The study was named the Systematic Treatment Enhancement Program for Bipolar Disorder (STEP-BD). Manic depression refers to alternating periods of depression and mania. Although as bipolar disorder it has been extensively researched and discussed in the psychiatric literature and although that moniker has fully penetrated popular discourse, very little seems to be known about the condition. In a 2006 editorial in the *American Journal of Psychiatry* entitled "What Is Bipolar Disorder?" psychiatrist Alan J. Swann could only answer the question by saying it was "recognized as a potentially treatable psychiatric illness that has substantial mortality and high social and economic impact." Swann continued, "Every aspect of its definition, boundaries, mechanisms, and treatment, however, is subject to debate. In fact, there is no objective measure that can determine if one has bipolar disorder or does not have it" (p. 177). Naturally, as we have discussed earlier in this book, lacking objective measures to define or even detect the condition objectively should pose considerable problems for evaluating its treatment. The condition came to prominence in the 1970s when some psychiatrists claimed (and still do) that ordinary lithium salts were a specific *and* preventive treatment for it, conjuring the image of lithium-deficient madpersons transformed by a mineral supplement. When later studies showed that people taking lithium experienced mania or depression virtually as often as patients not taking any drug and when lithium toxicity showed itself to be insidious and potentially fatal, lithium begin falling out of favor (Healy, 2008). For the pharmaceutical industry, lithium also carried the enormous disadvantage of not being patentable, which may have doomed the intensive commercialization of that substance. Older and newer anticonvulsant drugs used in the treatment of epilepsy and other seizure disorders, but also for a variety of behavior problems in adults and children, started to replace lithium as the name and the presentation of manic depression changed to bipolar disorder, starting with *DSM-III* in the early 1980s. These drugs have been viewed since the early 1990s as the best available treatment for bipolar disorder.

Experts justified the shift to prescribing anticonvulsants by analogizing an episode of mania to an epileptic seizure. In seizure disorders, anticonvulsants seem to stop the "kindling" of seizures in the brain of many affected persons and reduce the likelihood of future seizures. Some psychiatrists hypothesized that anticonvulsants could similarly suppress an episode of mania while reduce the likelihood of future manic episodes. Rigorous demonstration of this claim was lacking, especially since studies of anticonvulsants used comparisons with poorly performing lithium. Like lithium, however, anticonvulsants are powerful depressants of the activity of the central nervous system (a property that explains their anti-seizure action, just like benzodiazepines). As such, they typically tranquilize and sedate their users. Also, relative to placebo, tranquilizing drugs will almost inevitably produce "improvement" on virtually any of the short-term symptom rating scales used in psychiatric drug trial research, because such scales contain many items related to nervousness, insomnia, agitation, and spontaneous verbalizations of variously offending or disturbing thoughts—all of which "respond" to sedative drug effects.

Moreover, the rebranding of anticonvulsants as "mood stabilizers" by clever pharmaceutical company executives gave a tremendous boost to marketing these drugs, as well as the bipolar diagnosis itself (Healy, 2006). The new name implied that anticonvulsants could directly "raise" depressed mood. Although it has no official standing in any drug nomenclature, "mood stabilizer" is an instantly recognizable designation of some psychiatric drugs today, and it appears in dozens of reports published each year. Its popularization must rank as one of the great marketing feats of the past decades.

As in STAR*D, the STEP-BD investigators tried to emulate real-world treatment conditions. They employed a best-available treatment protocol, including individually tailored monitoring of a broadly representative sample of almost 1,500 patients given anticonvulsants, typically with other drugs such as antidepressants, antipsychotics, lithium, and benzodiazepines (only 10 percent of the patients were prescribed a single drug). The patients' treatment and response were then monitored for up to twenty-four months. As with the contemporaneous CATIE and STAR*D concerning psychosis and depression, respectively, STEP-BD constituted perhaps the largest group ever of people diagnosed with bipolar disorder and followed so carefully for such a length of time.

The main findings of STEP-BD were also eerily consistent with those of its two large sister studies. By study's end, less than one-third of the sample (31 percent) were reported to have experienced a remission of their manic or depressive episode with no recurrence during the rest of the study period.

While writing this book, we did not compare the study protocols of CATIE and STEP-BD with the published findings, nor have we crosschecked the published methodologies across separate articles to assess the coherence and consistency of the findings. Yet, given what has been uncovered regarding STAR*D and given previous statements from other established research-ers—that their own co-investigators in other landmark federally-funded studies have tried to suppress disturbing findings of drugs' dangers (see, for example, one account by Vedantham, 2009)—readers should exercise due caution in accepting any claim of drug efficacy put forth in our drug-soaked culture (Healy, 2012).

Psychotropic or Placebo?

The findings from CATIE, STAR*D, and STEP-BD were actually not too surprising to knowledgeable observers, because they were almost identical to findings from countless short-term (six to twelve weeks) clinical trials that make up the contemporary psychiatric treatment literature since the 1980s. For example, dropout rates in some short-term olanzapine (Zyprexa) trials that led to that drug's market approval by the FDA in 1996 showed that 73 percent of subjects had left the study after four weeks, a rate the FDA reviewer called "overwhelming" (cited in Jackson, 2003). The average CATIE dropout rate was 74 percent. As to the rate at which subjects responded positively to drugs, during the first treatment phase of STAR*D, 47 percent of recruited subjects were rated as responders, much like the average 50 percent responder rate among antidepressant-treated subjects estimated by the Food and Drug Administration in 2006 from its database of 189 randomized, short-term placebo-controlled clinical trials of antidepressants involving over 53,000 patients (Stone & Jones, 2006).

When a drug manufacturer wishes to market its product, the very best of these trials are submitted to the FDA so that claims of efficacy and safety can be verified. FDA regulations require only two multisite randomized controlled trials that have produced positive results, *regardless of how many negative trials were conducted*. Randomized controlled clinical trials became the standard test for drug makers to demonstrate the efficacy (and some of the safety) of drugs for specific *DSM* disorders, which would grant an FDA approval to market drugs for these indications. In a randomized controlled trial, "Patients should be randomized to matching groups; be tested using both the active therapy and a control, or placebo; should not know which group they are in, nor be aware of whether they are getting an active drug or a placebo. They must be blinded from the doctor who might influence the treatment" (Nesi, 2008, p. 121). These precautions are essential in principle, but the actual conduct and reporting of clinical trials (whether for antipsychotics, antidepressants, or stimulants) has always left much to be desired, as review after review has observed (e.g., Jaddad et al., 1999; Larkin, 2010; Thornley & Adams, 1998). This problem has been magnified as the drug industry increased its already considerable involvement in funding, designing, conducting, and disseminating results of clinical trials of its own products.

For the FDA, moreover, "efficacy" has only meant demonstrating *some kind of effect*, or so-called proof in principle. Cure, or extended recovery, or remission has never been the anticipated outcome in the clinical trials evaluated by the FDA. On the contrary, therapeutic effects from psychoactive drugs have always been expected to be relatively small, and the problems being treated have always shown large, spontaneous variations across and within individuals. That is why phase III trials (the multisite, randomized controlled trials) had to be quite large in order to show *some kind of effect* (Healy, Langmaark, & Savage, 1999). If a drug were clearly efficacious, this could be shown in very small trials (think of an antibiotic treating a bacterial infection), and the results of efficacy should be easily replicable. Clinical trials of some of the century's best-selling prescribed psychotropics, the SSRIs, never, ever demonstrated anything near this level of efficacy. The SSRIs showed weak, marginal effects in comparison to placebo.

In 2002 and again in 2008, Irving Kirsch and colleagues reanalyzed all data they obtained using Freedom of Information laws from the FDA's evaluations of the forty-seven RCTs funded and submitted to it by the makers of the six most widely prescribed antidepressants approved by the FDA between 1987 and 1999. Nearly 5,200 individuals had participated in these trials, including 3,300 randomized to receive drugs and 1,800 to receive placebo. The reanalysis found that 82 percent of the response of medicated patients was duplicated in placebo-treated patients. This occurred despite the FDA allowing researchers to replace people on some of the drugs who were not improving after two weeks into the trial. Moreover, in most trials, tranquilizers were also prescribed to the participants whose insomnia and agitation increased (probably as an adverse effect of the SSRIs). Despite these methodological breaches (which might serve to explain why *only* 82 percent of the drug response was duplicated by placebo), on the chief outcome measure, the patient's score on the Hamilton Depression Rating Scale (HAMD), the mean difference between drug and placebo groups was 1.8 points (the version of the scale most often used in the trials has a maximum 50-point score). In their later reanalysis, Kirsch and colleagues (2008) did observe that among people with the highest HAM-D scores (suggesting the most severe depressive symptoms), the outcome difference (just about 4 points on the HAM-D) favored the drug-treated groups. But this was shown to reflect a *waning of the placebo effect* among such people, *not* an increased efficacy of the SSRIs. In other words, drug response scores among the most severely depressed were similar to scores among the less depressed, but placebo response scores were not (perhaps because when one feels quite bad it is much harder to summon a positive outlook).

Obviously, the very small average difference between groups could not in itself mean a clearly superior gain for most patients who take SSRIs. On a large enough sample of people, however, given the laws of probability, it could show *statistical* significance. In this case, statistical significance meant that the 3 percent *smaller uselessness* of SSRIs compared to placebo would be quite unlikely to result from chance and should be observed almost every time drugs are compared to placebo. Because of this mathematically conclusive but probably clinically negligible difference, the FDA followed its rule that the manufacturers had provided evidence, in at least two clinical trials for each drug, of the drugs' efficacy to treat whatever was treated in the clinical trials.

As noted, the high placebo response rates were obtained despite a number of strategies deliberately designed to reduce placebo responses from the participants (Cohen & Jacobs, 2007). First, almost every study used placebo-washout or placebo-lead-in periods, wherein all subjects are abruptly discontinued from any drugs they might be taking and placed on a pill-looking placebo. The idea is to identify people who are likely to improve early when they believe that they are receiving a genuine treatment—and to exclude these people from those who will then be randomized for the "start" of the "actual" study. For example, in the forty-seven SSRI trials reviewed by Kirsch and colleagues, any subject whose HAM-D score improved 20 percent or more during this early period was excluded from the study. But since the point of a trial is to compare the efficacy of active drugs to placebo, it is by no means clear what the rationale could be for excluding people who tend to respond to placebo early on. To be fair, those who respond to drugs early on should also be excluded.

Second, all studies employed inert rather than active placebos. An inert placebo might contain yeast, sugar, or lactose. An active placebo might contain caffeine, benztropine, or diphenhydramine. Why use one or the other? Certain drug effects, such as dry mouth, dizziness, sleepiness, or increased heart rate can serve as early cues to patients and clinicians about which treatment condition patients are in. This would "break the blind," threatening the trial's internal validity (the confidence to draw conclusions about what is causing what). One way around this problem is to use active placebos: substances that give some physical sensations to people, who might therefore think that they are receiving the "real" medication, but which do not produce the sort of psychoactive effects of the tested drug.

Results from some antidepressant trials in the 1970s and early 1980s showed that active placebos did indeed produce greater placebo response than inert placebos (Fisher & Greenberg, 1993a, 1993b). It therefore seemed likely that the subtle physical sensations produced by active placebos had tricked subjects into thinking that they were taking "real" medication, thus possibly amplifying the subjective feeling of improvement that they would communicate to the clinician raters during their brief structured encounters. This would translate as higher scores of these subjects on rating scales—the major outcome of the clinical trials. A different dynamic would occur in a study comparing a drug to an inert placebo. Here, noticeable physical sensations are more likely to be experienced by those taking the drug, which would give clinicians a cue about which treatment condition subjects are in, and might tilt clinicians' expectations toward observing improvement in drug-treated patients.

Reviews and reanalyses of these earlier trials (Moncrieff et al., 2004; Petovka et al., 2000) have not settled the matter of the precise role of inert versus active placebos, and one author suggests ignoring this issue altogether because the studies are too old (Quitkin, 2003). But the issue remains profoundly relevant: if mere sugar pills produce equivalent or nearly equivalent responses in the most sophisticated controlled trials of antidepressants today, wouldn't active placebos do at least as well and probably much better? That is, wouldn't active placebos *lay waste* to antidepressants' effectiveness nearly every time? This question has no known answer, because as of this writing in late 2011, one still cannot find a single major randomized controlled trial comparing a modern SSRI antidepressant with an active placebo. By contrast, in neurology, controlled trials of pain treatments routinely use active placebos. This fact alone should bracket clinical psychopharmacology as a studiously unscientific enterprise. Let us restate the point differently and explicitly.

Pain researchers, who know that pain often responds to placebo, appear truly *interested* to discover whether new analgesics work better than placebo. Thus pain researchers stack the deck against their proposed analgesics by using placebos that superficially create a sensation to trick the patient into thinking that an analgesic may have been taken. The hurdle that must be overcome by the proposed analgesic is thus raised higher. By contrast, psychiatric researchers, who also know that depression often responds to placebo, appear *uninterested* to discover whether modern psychiatric antidepressants work better than placebo. Thus psychiatric researchers stack the deck against *placebo*. The hurdle that must be overcome by the proposed antidepressant is thus lowered. From either a scientific or clinical perspective, the absence of *rigorous* comparisons between drugs and active placebos in psychiatry makes no sense. It may nonetheless be easily understood when ideological or commercial imperatives—for example, or the compulsive need to suggest that genuine illnesses are being targeted by specific treatments or the compulsive need to demonstrate a profit every quarter to satisfy mutual fund investors—shape the pursuit of knowledge.

In controlled trials designed to minimize placebo response, inert placebos given to subjects who meet the *DSM*'s Major Depressive Disorder criteria benefit up to half of subjects, exactly as antidepressant drugs are shown to benefit subjects: by steady reductions in depression rating scale scores, from the very start of the trial and every week thereafter (Walsh et al., 2002). Nor are placebo effects confined to the treatment of depression and anxiety with antidepressants and anxiolytics (Shear et al., 1995). For example, in March 2009, Eli Lilly and Company announced results from a phase II clinical trial of its new investigational antipsychotic, named LY2140023, against its block-buster drug olanzapine (Zyprexa). The press release stated: "In Study HBBI, neither LY2140023 . . . nor the comparator molecule olanzapine, known to be more effective than placebo, separated from placebo." As a result, "neither drug performed better than the placebo" (Eli Lilly and Company, 2009, p. 1). Over the last two decades, placebo response rates have steadily increased in trials of antipsychotic drugs, in parallel with a steady decrease in drug response rates. In some trials, 50 percent of participants (diagnosed with schizophrenia and experiencing an acute psychotic episode) taking inert placebo pills show at least a 20 percent improvement on their psychosis rating scale score relative to baseline, the criteria sometimes used in the past to demonstrate efficacy of antipsychotic drugs (Kemp et al., 2008). Various factors may account for this steady diminishing of drug-placebo differences, ranging from the extra attention given clinical trial participants to differences in scoring methods used in foreign study sites, which are increasingly used today for drugs to be approved in America. Official discussions of the trend, however, conform to a predictable line: drug response is a true and worthy "signal," while any placebo response is a distracting, confusing, confounding "noise" (Kemp et al., 2008).

How and why placebos produce such results in comparison to drugs whose psychoactive effects sustain them through years of animal and clinical testing (see next chapter) remains an utterly fascinating question. By themselves, the cost-savings and reduction in adverse effects implied by the possible amplification of the placebo effect could justify reorienting but a small part of the stupendous research activities in psychopharmacology toward understanding and harnessing placebo effects. Yet it is obvious that the psychopharmacology field as a whole has been much less interested in answering the placebo question than in disposing of it methodologically. This is not astonishing, as using placebos in the practice of medicine is a most controversial topic. Using placebos is at odds with the image that medicine has projected of itself—that of a scientific profession having discovered and devised, based on the scientific method, effective and specific treatments for genuine diseases. Within psychiatry, more than other branches of medicine, in which placebo effects may constitute most of clinical practice, systematically understanding the role of placebos would threaten the entire profession.

Because the placebo is unpretentious and nameless, its competitors—compounds that have passed the FDA-approval hurdle and been given branded identities as genuine medications—can claim placebo's benefits, and any deception basically remains unexposed. One might view the placebo effect in many different ways: as a vital human capacity for self-restoration, a complex form of self-deception, and anything in-between. Either way, it is difficult to dismiss it as "no treatment" or "nothing." One can dismiss placebo effects as noise only if one is resolutely committed to finding uses for a commercially-funded investigational drug—a different aim than being resolutely committed to finding out what people say helps them, or what helps people despite what they say helps them.

Here is Charles Medawar and Anita Hardon's social view of the placebo effect:

> All sorts of human beliefs, motivations and styles of organization make medicines work as they seem to do. These factors are typically invisible, go largely unrecognized and have no other name. They go largely incognito . . . The fact that they have no collective name underlines that their impact is generally unrecognised and therefore poorly understood. Probably the main reason is that the word placebo has come to stand for *all* the non-drug factors that affect treatment outcomes. It does not seem an appropriate word: it does not take into account many non-pharmacological factors on treatment outcomes. (2004, p. 175)

231

How much are expectations of patients amplified when virtually all authoritative discourse about a drug consists of statements that it has positive effects on those who receive it from their doctor? The felt effectiveness of a medicine has to do not only with the relationship between user and drug. Doctors' and patients' experiences and history, their values, statuses, and roles, their faith and hope—not to mention suggestion from their peers and from advertising, drug company sponsorship of doctors' events, the names given to drugs—these and other factors must also count as important, interacting determinants in drug "effectiveness," as they introduce themselves in still largely unknown ways into the clinician-patient relationship.

It is sobering to realize that the technique of testing a drug in a double-blind trial against a placebo, a so-called dummy pill, is at present the only existing scientific guarantee that the drug does not work somehow through suggestion, hope, and belief. Today, without such a trial, a mere chemical compound could not become a "medication," as bestowed by FDA approval (and this, for conditions ranging from migraine to Parkinson disease to multiple sclerosis). Without comparing the tested drug to something that can elicit improvement from the patient merely by appearing to be a genuine medication, one cannot confidently determine the true effects of the tested drug. This makes the placebo especially necessary when testing treatments for conditions with a substantial rate of spontaneous or developmental improvement, such as depression and anxiety or a first episode of psychosis. But the nature of the placebo effect remains largely unknown (Benedetti, 2009). Something or a combination of many things does appear to be *there*, and it begs explanation. Of course, we cannot yet rule out that the placebo effect may turn out to be another colossal reification, much like mental illness, an idea whose concrete reality is assumed merely because it has a name and because alternative explanations for its associated features have not been widely understood or disseminated.

But even if we stick to the placebo effect as traditionally defined in drug trials (the measurable therapeutic changes induced by pharmacologically inactive or inert substances), we may consider the conclusion reached by psychologists Seymour Fisher and Roger Greenberg. After one of the most insightful, restrained, and evidence-informed reviews in the entire literature on antipsychotics, stimulants, antidepressants, and anxiolytics, these two authors stated, "that when proper controls are introduced [in research studies] the differences in therapeutic power between the active drugs and placebos largely recede" (1997, p. 382). It is sobering for anyone to reflect that merely introducing "proper controls" in scientific research would doom the modern psychopharmacologic enterprise.

New Cost, New Hype, Old Myths

In an editorial accompanying STEP-BD's first publication, psychiatric researcher J. Raymond DePaulo, Jr. (2006) observed that "the results are so similar to those observed in lithium treatment studies of 20 to 35 years ago that the question of whether today's best available treatments for bipolar disorder are better than older treatments begs for an answer" (p. 175). But the study actually did answer the question—in the negative. DePaulo omitted to mention that a few earlier, long-term observational lithium studies had themselves suggested that lithium was no better than lithium's predecessors—shock treatments and barbiturates—and even, in some investigations, no better than no drugs at all (Harrow et al., 1990). DePaulo did generously allow for the possibility that "modern pharmacological treatments may be no more beneficial than older ones, despite their added cost" (p. 175). And, one might add, despite their added hype.

Indeed, exaggerated publicity intended to excite public interest has characterized the portrayal of psychiatric drug treatments these past few decades. Who has not heard that drugs have revolutionized the treatment of mental illness, that newer medications are safer and more effective than older ones, that they can make their users "better than well," and that drugs have removed the stigma of psychiatric labeling? It has even been said that drugs can be so helpful that *not* forcing them on certain disturbed people constitutes negligence or worse. In sum, experts and their followers have stated that psychiatric medications have brought society immeasurably closer to solving the problem of mental illness once and for all.

With unremitting support from many partners in the mental health movement, such claims were transformed into robust cultural beliefs or myths. The power and purpose of myths to give meaning to our lives and societies cannot be understated. In the age of science, myths are often portrayed as scientific truths. Myths unify people by expressing themes that resonate with people's longings. When experts and laypersons continually reaffirm a myth, they convey their wish to belong to the group of believers. They may also convey that, as far as they are concerned, debate about the essential truth of the myth has ended and that one need only be concerned with technical details arising from the application of its essential truth.

That is how CATIE, STAR*D, and STEP-BD were greeted. Three large, exemplary studies conducted by the clinical and research elite of American psychiatry and funded by the world's largest mental health research institute, the NIMH, to the combined tune of almost 100 million dollars, demonstrated dismal results, if not failure, of the paradigmatic biological treatments for the paradigmatic mental disorders. Yet, as far as one can tell, no prominent mental health authority (neither an investigator from one of the studies or a NIMH official) suggested re-evaluating the routine drugging, these past fifty years, of madness and misbehavior, or launching an intensive analysis of the practical uses of placebo effects in the drug treatment of all manners of mental distresses. Quite the contrary, experts and commentators only lamented the heavy burden of mental disorders and stoked the ever-so-great imperative to

233

find newer, better drugs or biological treatments. In the world of mad science, the myth of treatable mental illnesses must go on.

To illustrate the persistence of probably wrong-headed thinking despite the facts, we turn again to NIMH director Thomas Insel. In 2009, Insel thus summarized the findings from the CATIE, STAR*D, and STEP-BD studies:

> Given that these trials used evidence-based treatments of well-documented efficacy that were administered with optimal clinical standards, the results show the significant limitations of current pharmacological interventions. This point bears emphasis. These limited outcomes, in terms of recovery and remission, are not due to suboptimal delivery of care. Instead, with optimal care using today's medications, too many people will not recover. (p. 129).

Insel nonetheless went on to announce a new program of research to uncover the "molecular pathophysiology" underlying mental disorders by focusing research on brain circuits, genes, and personalized medicine focusing on individual moderators of treatment outcomes such as "genetic traits, imaging results, plasma proteins, or clinical features" (p. 131).

The connections between the uses of drugs and the sort of biological thinking exemplified by Insel's new call to action obviously need to be restated. Chemical substances with powerful effects on thinking, feeling, and behaving ushered an era of biological theorizing about madness as the consequence of chemical imbalances in the brain. In turn, that biological thinking was used to promote the usefulness of psychoactive drugs to treat mental distress and misbehavior of every stripe and variety. Then, the mental health system was entirely reorganized to encourage drug use among the distressed and strict compliance with one's prescribed medication regimen thereafter. After decades of this arrangement, the drugs ("evidence-based treatments of well-documented efficacy") are formally acknowledged by authoritative experts citing authoritative evidence to have little of the usefulness so long attributed to them. Yet the same experts and institutions who touted drugs' benefits with certainty, tolerating no dissent and suppressing alternative viewpoints, today urge their constituencies to adopt even more far-flung biological thinking strung together by bits of medical technology and corporal components. We believe that these experts should pause to identify what may have gone wrong and what future errors might be avoided, but we do not think this appears anywhere in the official agenda.

In the following chapter, we develop the argument that the effort to develop a scientifically-based drug treatment of specific mental disorders has mainly consisted of the recycling of perennial human drugging practices. We also propose that despite all the hoopla, an understanding of psychiatric medications as *psychoactive substances capable of producing complex mental and physical states regardless of why they are taken by people or prescribed by doctors* appears wholly sufficient to explain drugs' observed therapeutic effects (and adverse effects) in "mental disorders" (Jacobs & Cohen, 1999; Moncrieff, 2008; Moncrieff & Cohen, 2009). The notion of drugs specifically targeting identifiable or soon-to-be-identified pathological substrates of mental disorders remains a hypothesis supported by an exceedingly tiny amount of evidence. To paraphrase psychiatrist Peter Breggin and co-author Ginger Breggin (1994), to respond to any drug (that is, to like it, to find it helpful for some purpose, to want to keep taking it), a human being does not need a chemically imbalanced or an electrically short-circuited brain; *just a brain will do.* If so, then the modern psychiatric discipline of clinical psychopharmacology, having mostly tied its scientific fortunes to the validity of biological psychiatric theorizing, rests on the flimsiest of foundations and needs to be reconstructed, from scratch.

Notes

1. First isolated from opium at the start of the 1800s, morphine was massively used for the first time during the Austro-Prussian War of 1866 and found to be an unsurpassed painkiller. About a dozen years later, some physicians began to see it as causing a state of hellish chemical servitude they called *morphinomania.* By the end of the 1800s, morphine was condemned as a "main scourge of humanity" (Chast, 1995, p. 112).
2. We remain astonished at encountering parents who would balk at serving their nine-year-old child a single cup of coffee but who would feel less unease to give that child a daily dose of prolonged-action amphetamine, for several months.

References

Allen, S. (2006, March 6). Beyond guesswork: Treatments often fail, but new studies might help doctors find drugs and therapies that work. *Boston Globe.* Retrieved from: http://www.boston.com/yourlife/health/mental/articles/2006/03/06/beyond_ guesswork/

American Psychiatric Association. (2008, September 2). APA responds to Senate request for records [News release]. Retrieved from www.psych.org/MainMenu/Newsroom/NewsReleases/2008NewsReleases/APAPresident-Responds.aspx

Bachman, C., & Coppel, A. (1989). *Le dragon domestique—deux siècles de relations étranges entre l'Occident et la drogue* [The domestic dragon: Two centuries of strange relations between the West and drugs]. Paris: Albin Michel.

Benedetti, F. (2009). *Placebo effects: Understanding the mechanisms in health and disease.* Oxford and New York: Oxford University Press.

Bhatara, V., Feil, M., Hoagwood, K., Vitiello, B., & Zima, B. (2004). National trends in concomitant psychotropic medication with stimulants in pediatric visits: Practice versus knowledge. *Journal of Attention Disorders, 7*(4), 217–226.

Breggin, P. R., & Breggin, G. (1994). *Talking back to Prozac: What doctors aren't telling you about today's most controversial drug.* New York: St. Martin's.

Carlat, D. (2009). APA votes to phase out industry-funded CME. Retrieved from http://carlatpsychiatry.blogspot.fr/2009/03/apa-votes-to-phase-out-industry-funded.html

Centers for Disease Control and Prevention. (2006). *Health, United States* (Table 92). Retrieved from http://www.cdc.gov/nchs/hus.htm

Chast, F. (1995). *Histoire contemporaine des médicaments* [Contemporary history of medications]. Paris: Éditions La Découverte.

CNN. (2008). Shooting reopens debate over drug, violence link. Retrieved from http://edition.cnn.com/2008/HEALTH/02/25/antidepressants.violence/

Cohen, D. (2010). Psychopharmacology and clinical social work practice. In J. R. Brandell (Ed.), *Clinical social work: Theories and methods*, 2nd ed. (pp. 763–810). Thousand Oaks, CA: Sage.

Cohen, D., & Jacobs, D. (2007). Randomized controlled trials of antidepressants: Clinically and scientifically irrelevant. *Debates in Neuroscience, 1,* 44–54.

DeGrandpre, R. (2007). *The cult of pharmacology: How America became the world's most troubled drug culture*. Durham, NC, and London: Duke University Press.

DePaulo, J. R. Jr. (2006). Bipolar disorder treatment: An evidence-based reality check. *American Journal of Psychiatry, 163*(2), 175–176.

Diller, L. (2010, March 27). Wholesale sedation of young children medically, morally indefensible. *The Patriot Ledger* (Quincy, MA). Retrieved from http://wickedlocal.com/hull/news/opinions/x905411678/COMMENTARY-Wholesale-sedation-of-young-children-medically-morally-indefensible

Donohue, J. (2006). Mental health in the Medicare Part D drug benefit: A new regulatory model? *Health Affairs, 25*(3), 707–719.

Eli Lilly and Company. (2009, March 29). Lilly announces inconclusive phase II study results for mglu2/3 at the International Congress on Schizophrenia Research. [News release]. Retrieved from http://newsroom.lilly.com/releasedetail.cfm?releaseid=373650

Fisher, S., & Greenberg, R. P. (1993a). A meta-analysis of antidepressant outcome under "blinder" conditions. *Journal of Consulting and Clinical Psychology, 60,* 664–669.

Fisher, S., & Greenberg, R. P. (1993b). How sound is the double-blind design for evaluating psychotropic drugs? *Journal of Nervous and Mental Disease, 181,* 345–350.

Fisher, S., & Greenberg, R. P. (1997). What are we to conclude about psychoactive drugs? In S. Fisher & R. Greenberg (eds.), *From placebo to panacea: Putting psychiatric drugs to the test* (pp. 359–383). New York: Wiley & Sons.

Fugh-Berman, A. (2008). Prescription tracking and public health. *Journal of General Internal Medicine, 23*(8), 1277–1280.

Gagnon, M. A., & Lexchin, J. (2008). The cost of pushing pills: A new estimate of pharmaceutical promotion expenditures in the United States. *PLoS Medicine, 5*(1), e1.

Greely, H., Sahakian, B., Harris, B., Kessler, R. C., Gazzaniga, M., Campbell, P., & Farah, M. J. (2008). Towards responsible use of cognitive enhancing drugs by the healthy. *Nature, 456* (7223), 702–705.

Harrow, M., Goldberg, J. F., Grossman, L. S., & Meltzer, H. Y. (1990). Outcome in manic disorders: A naturalistic follow-up study. *Archives of General Psychiatry, 47,* 665–671.

Healy, D. (2006). The latest mania: Selling bipolar disorder. *PLoS Medicine*, 3(4), e185.

Healy, D. (2008). *Mania: A short history of bipolar disorder*. Baltimore: Johns Hopkins University Press.

Healy, D. (2009). Trussed in evidence? Ambiguities at the interface between clinical evidence and clinical practice. *Transcultural Psychiatry*, 46, 16–37.

Healy, D. (2012). *Pharmageddon*. Berkeley: University of California Press.

Healy, D., Langmaak, C., & Savage, M. (1999). Suicide in the course of the treatment of depression. *Journal of Psychopharmacology*, 13, 94–99.

Hegarty, J., Baldessarini, R., Tohen, M., Waternaux, C., & Oepen, G. (1994). One hundred years of schizophrenia: A meta-analysis of the outcome literature. *American Journal of Psychiatry*, 151, 1409–1416.

Hughes, S., & Cohen, D. (2009). A systematic review of long-term studies of drug treated and non-drug treated depression. *Journal of Affective Disorders*, 118, 2–9.

IMS Health. (2012). Top therapeutic classes by U.S. dispensed prescriptions. Retrieved from http://www.imshealth.com/deployedfiles/ims/Global/Content/Corporate/Press%20Room/Top-Line%20Market%20Data%20&%20Trends/2011%20Top-line%20Market%20Data/Top_Therapy_Classes_by_RX.pdf

Insel, T. R. (2009). Translating scientific opportunity into public health impact: A strategic plan for research into mental illness. *Archives of General Psychiatry*, 66, 128–133.

Jackson, G. E. (2003, March 3). An analysis of the olanzapine clinical trials: Dangerous drug, dubious efficacy. Retrieved from http://psychrights.org/states/Alaska/CaseOne/30-Day/ExhibitD-Olanzapine.htm

Jacobs, D. H., & Cohen, D. (1999). What is really known about psychological alterations produced by psychiatric drugs? *International Journal of Risk and Safety in Medicine*, 12, 37–47.

Jadad A. R., Boyle, M., Cunningham, C., Kim, M., & Schachar, R. (1999). *Treatment of attention-deficit/hyperactivity disorder*. Rockville, MD: Agency of Healthcare Research and Quality.

Kemp, A. S., Schooler, N. R., Kalali, A. H., Alphs, L., Anand, R., Awad, G. . . . Vermeulen, A. (2008). What is causing the reduced drug-placebo difference in recent schizophrenia clinical trials and what can be done about it? *Schizophrenia Bulletin*. Retrieved from schizophreniabulletin.oxfordjournals.org

Kirsch, I., Moore, T. J., Scoboria, A., & Nicholls, S. S. (2002). The emperor's new drugs: An analysis of antidepressant medication data submitted to the U.S. Food and Drug Administration. *Prevention & Treatment*, 5, article 23. Retrieved from http:// www.journals.apa.org/prevention/volume5/pre0050023a.html. Accessed July 15, 2002.

Kirsch, I., Deacon, B. J., Huedo-Medina, T. B., Scoboria, A., Moore, T. J., & Johnson, B. T. (2008). Initial severity and antidepressant benefits: A meta-analysis of data submitted to the Food and Drug Administration. *PLoS Medicine*, 5(2), e45.

Larkin, C. (2010, April 20). Pfizer's Geodon trial had "significant" violations. *Business Week*. Retrieved from www.businessweek.com/news/2010-04-20/pfizer-s-geodon-trial-had-significant-violations-update2-.html

Leo, J. (2006). The SSRI trials in children: Disturbing implications for academic medicine. *Ethical Human Psychology & Psychiatry*, 8, 29–41.

Leventhal, A. M., & Antonuccio, D. O. (2009). On chemical imbalances, antidepressants, and the diagnosis of depression. *Ethical Human Psychology & Psychiatry, 11*, 119–214.

Lieberman, J. A., Stroup, T. S., McEvoy, J. P., Swartz, M., Rosenheck, R. A., Perkins, D. O. . . . Hsiao, J. K. (2005). Effectiveness of antipsychotic drugs in patients with chronic schizophrenia. *New England Journal of Medicine, 353*, 1209–1223.

Mathews, A. W. (2010, December 28). So young and so many pills: More than 25% of kids and teens in the US take prescriptions on a regular basis. *Wall Street Journal.* Retrieved from http://online.wsj.com/article_email/SB10001424052970203731004576046073896475588-lMyQjAxMTAxMDIwNDEyNDQyWj.html?mod=wsj_share_email

Medawar, C., & Hardon, A. (2004). *Medicines out of control?* London: Askant Publishers.

Moncrieff, J. (2008). *The myth of the chemical cure.* London: Routledge.

Moncrieff, J., & Cohen, D. (2009). How do psychiatric drugs work? *BMJ, 338*, b.1963.

Moncrieff, J., Cohen, D., & Mason, J. (2009). The subjective effects of taking antipsychotic medication: A content analysis of Internet data. *Acta Psychiatrica Scandinavica, 120*, 102–111.

Moncrieff, J., Wessely, S., & Hardy, R. (2004). Active placebos versus antidepressants for depression. *Cochrane Database Systematic Reviews, 1*, CD003012.

Moynihan, R., Heath, I., & Henry, D. (2002). Selling sickness: The pharmaceutical industry and disease mongering. *BMJ, 324*, 886–891.

Nesi, T. (2008). *Poison pills: The untold story of the Vioxx drug scandal.* New York: St. Martin's Press.

Nierenberg, A. A., Ostacher, M. J., Huffman, J. C., Ametrano, R. M., Fava, M., & Perlis, R. H. (2008). A brief review of antidepressant efficacy, effectiveness, indications, and usage for major depressive disorder. *Journal of Occupational and Environmental Medicine, 50*, 428–436.

Osterweil, N. (2006, March 22). Antidepressant switch or add-on produces more remissions. *MedPage Today.* Retrieved May 19, 2006 from http://www.medpagetoday.com/Psychiatry/Depression/tb/2916

Patten, S. B. (2004). The impact of population treatment on population health: Synthesis from two national sources in Canada. *Population Health Metrics, 2*:9. Retrieved from http://www.pophealthmetrics.com/content/2/1/9

Perlis, R. H., Ostacher, M. J., Patel, J. K., Marangell, L. B., Zhang, H., Wisniewski, S. R., Ketter, T. A. . . . Otto, M. W. (2006). Predictors of recurrence in bipolar disorder: Primary outcomes from the Systematic Treatment Enhancement Program for bipolar disorder (STEP-BD). *American Journal of Psychiatry, 163*, 217–224.

Petovka, E., Quitkin, F. M., McGrath, P. J. et al. (2000). A method to quantify rater bias in antidepressant trials. *Neuropsychopharmacology, 22*, 559–565.

Pieters, T., & Snelders, S. (2005). Mental ills and the "hidden history" of drug treatment practices. In M. Gijswijt et al. (eds.), *Psychiatric cultures compared. Psychiatry and mental health care in the twentieth century: Comparisons and approaches* (pp. 381–401). Amsterdam: Amsterdam University Press.

Pigott, H. E. (2011a). STAR*D: A tale and trail of bias. *Ethical Human Psychology and Psychiatry, 13*, 6–28.

Pigott, H. E. (2011b, April 21). The STAR*D scandal. Retrieved from: http://www.madinamerica.com/madinamerica.com/Pigott.html

Pigott, H. E., Leventhal, A. M., Alter, G. S., & Boren, J. J. (2010). Efficacy and effectiveness of antidepressants: Current status of research. *Psychotherapy & Psychosomatics, 79*, 267–279. doi: 10.1159/000318293

Quitkin, F. M. (2003). Reply to "Active placebos versus antidepressants for depression" by J. Moncrieff, S. Wessely, & R. Hardy in The Cochrane Database of Systematic Reviews, 2002. Retrieved 27 June 2006 from: http://www.cochranefeedback.com/ cf/cda/ citation.do?id=9048#9048

Rasmussen, N. (2006). Making the first anti-depressant: Amphetamine in American medicine, 1929–1950. *Journal of the History of Medicine and Allied Sciences, 61*(3), 288–323.

Rush, A. J., Trivedi, M. H., Rush, A. J., Wisniewski, S. R., Stewart, J. W., Nierenberg, A. A., Thase, M. E., Ritz, L., Biggs, M. M., Warden, D., Luther J. F., Shores-Wilson, K., Niederehe, G., & Fava, M., for the STAR*D Study Team. (2006). Buproprion-SR, sertraline, or venlafaxine after failure of SSRIs for depression. *New England Journal of Medicine, 354* (12), 1231–1242.

Shear, K., Leon, A., Pollack, M., Rosenbaum, J., & Keller, M. (1995). Pattern of placebo response in panic disorder. *Psychopharmacology Bulletin, 31*, 273–278.

Stagnitti, M. N. (2007, February). *Trends in the use and expenditures for the therapeutic class prescribed psychotherapeutic agents and all subclasses, 1997 and 2004.* Statistical Brief No. 163. Rockville, MD: Agency for Healthcare Research and Quality. Retrieved from http://www.meps.ahrq.gov/mepsweb/data_files/publications/st163.pdf

Stone, M. B., & Jones, M. L. (2006, November 17). *Clinical review: Relationship between antidepressant drugs and suicidality in adults.* Food and Drug Administration, Center for Drug Evaluation and Research. Retrieved from www.fda.gov/OHRMS/DOCKETS/ AC/06/briefing/2006-4272b1-01-FDA.pdf

Swann, A. J. (2006). What is bipolar disorder? *American Journal of Psychiatry, 163*, 177–179.

Szasz, T. (1974). *Ceremonial chemistry: The ritual persecution of drugs, addicts, and pushers.* Garden City, NY: Anchor Books.

Thornley, B., & Adams, C. (1998). Content and quality of 2000 controlled trials in schizophrenia over 50 years. *BMJ, 317*, 1181–1184.

Tierney, J. (2010, April 11). Hallucinogens have doctors tuning in again. *New York Times.* Retrieved from www.nytimes.com/2010/04/12/science/12psychedelics.html

Trivedi, M. H., Rush, A. J., Wisniewski, S. R., Nierenberg, A. A., Warden, D., Ritz, L., Norquist, G., Howland, R. H., Lebowitz, B., McGrath, P. J., & Shores-Wilson, K. (2006). Evaluation of outcomes with citalopram for depression using measurement-based care in STAR*D: Implications for clinical practice. *American Journal of Psychiatry, 163* (1), 1–13.

Vedantham, S. (2009, March 27). Debate over drugs for ADHD reignites: Long-term benefit for children at issue [Electronic version]. *The Washington Post.* Retrieved October 19, 2009, from www.washingtonpost.com/wp-dyn/content/article/2009/03/26/AR2009032604018.html

Walsh, B. T., Seidman, S. N., Sysko R., et al. (2002). Placebo response in studies of major depression: Variable, substantial, and growing. *JAMA, 287*, 1840–1847.

WCVB TV. (2007, February 6). Parents charged in death of daughter, 4. *The BostonChannel.com.* Retrieved from http://www.thebostonchannel.com/news/10943835/detail.html

Wen, P. (2010, March 26). Father convicted of 1st-degree murder in death of Rebecca Riley. *The Boston Globe*. Retrieved from http://www.boston.com/news/local/breaking_news/2010/03/hold_for_verdic_1.html

Wilson, D. (2009, Dec. 12). Poor children more likely to get antipsychotics. *New York Times*, A1, A11.

Young, J. H. (1961). *The toadstool millionaires: A social history of patent medicines in America before federal regulation*. Princeton, NJ: Princeton University Press.

7

From Drugs to Medications— and Back

Introduction

Since time immemorial, humans have used substances that noticeably alter mood, consciousness, and behavior. Today we call these substances psychoactive or psychotropic drugs[1]. The main psychoactive compounds in use throughout the world roughly until the last decade of the nineteenth century were alcohol, coffee, tea, tobacco, opium, cannabis, coca, iboga, kola, khat, as well as countless species of mushrooms. People used these and other psychoactive drugs to work, to relieve pain, to induce sleep, to stay awake, to fraternize, to endure sadness and loss, to experience euphoria or joy, to reach or heighten states of transcendence and spiritual contemplation, and to perform religious rituals (Meyers, 1985). These manifold uses indicate that psychoactive drugs touch directly and deeply on what it means to live as a human being. Put another way, psychoactive drugs have helped many human beings to bear, to make meaning of, to celebrate, or to temporarily escape their circumstances. Observing the universality of psychoactive drug use among humans, Andrew Weil (1970) wondered whether it reflected an inborn drive to alter one's consciousness.

If psychoactive drug use did not provide the user or the user's group with some perceived benefit in enduring or enjoying life, it seems hardly possible that it would continue, century after century, regardless of migratory patterns or the nature and pace of social and cultural changes. This is an especially compelling consideration, given that the dangers of psychoactive drug use were never lost on their users. As far as we can determine from observations of indigenous peoples around the world, use of psychoactive drugs in premodern societies typically involved communal preparations, elaborate precautions, and rituals that served simultaneously to elevate and restrain drug taking (Naranjo, 1979). In our contemporary society, precautions against much of psychoactive drug use still involve informal rites of passage in families and peer groups, legal drinking ages, as well as formal sanctions, such as laws against impaired driving and public inebriety. Increasingly, however, precautions have involved the transfer of authority and responsibility for psychoactive drug use onto the physician and the addiction specialist. The consequences of this shift have transformed users' motives to use drugs into diseases or disorders, the use of drugs into a treatment, and the user of drugs into a patient. Of the utmost importance, the physician writes a prescription that allows licit access to various psychoactive drugs. (As more and more "healthy" people want to use certain psychoactive drugs available only by prescription, the rationale for the medical prescription system might be strained beyond credibility, but we are getting ahead of our story.)

Precisely because of psychoactive drugs' fluid but obvious appeal, rulers, healers, and priests throughout history have never ceased to promote or repress particular drugs, and (by definition) their users (Tracy & Acker, 2004; Porter & Teich, 1997). Psychiatrist Thomas Szasz (1974) has most consistently and clearly made this case. He has argued that using forbidden drugs is the simplest way by which some individuals can affirm their autonomy vis-à-vis authorities. As societies encountered foreign drugs and as social customs and conventions changed, certain psychoactive drugs became socially and legally accepted, rejected, and accepted again, in cycles of varying durations. Almost every psychoactive drug legally banned in America today was, at some point over the last century, freely available for purchase or import or prescribed or dispensed by physicians to their patients. This includes heroin, cocaine, LSD, and methamphetamine. The latter drug is still available by prescription as Gradumet, a brand-name drug indicated for ADHD while considered the "gravest drug threat" by 57 to 80 percent of state and local law enforcement agencies in most of the United States (US Department of Justice, 2010).

Separating Medications from Drugs

The major turning point occurred at the end of the nineteenth century, when the opium derivative morphine, first greeted by physicians as an unequalled painkiller, became demonized. This transformation probably marked the beginning of the linguistic and conceptual separation of "dangerous drugs" from "psychoactive medications." With time, the first phrase came to designate disapproved substances traded illicitly and about which almost no one cared to distinguish "use" from "abuse." The second phrase came to designate approved substances that eventually became dispensed under medical supervision and government regulation. Progress in chemistry and pharmacology refined these "medications" as they were brought to market using techniques of mass production, with the goals of treating, preventing, and combating mental disease (Chast, 1995).

No intrinsic material property will ever distinguish a "drug" from a "medication" because the difference rests not on pharmacology but on social, legal, and medical norms and linguistic usage. Those who establish these norms, however, have either tacitly or explicitly supported the opposite view—that "drugs" differ intrinsically from "medications"—shielding the norms from scrutiny. As a result, as both Szasz (1974, 2001) and DeGrandpre (2007) amply document, *views and prejudices about drugs have been conflated with chemical properties of drugs*. Such a grave confusion could only lead to contradictions and inconsistencies. Amphetamines and methamphetamine, classified legally as controlled Schedule II addictive substances and characterized as "scourges" in the field of drug abuse, are simultaneously prescribed by physicians as essential treatments to children and adults said to suffer from attention deficits. Similarly, some individuals, groups, and states advocate or permit access to "medical marijuana" while supporting or enforcing the ban on marijuana. Regularly, the Drug Enforcement Administration (DEA) hounds physicians for prescribing "excessive" doses of perfectly licit narcotic painkillers (Rosenberg, 2007). As for tobacco, it occupies several roles simultaneously: ordinary agricultural product freely grown with state subsidies; the world's deadliest drug; illegal drug when used in certain public spaces; addictive psychotropic drug when the FDA wishes to regulate smoking; or approved medication when its ingredient nicotine is prescribed as an aid to quit smoking (Cohen, 1995).

These ambivalences and inconsistencies are reflected in what American authorities have been warning the public about at the start of the second decade of the twenty-first century, though they acknowledge it is not a new problem: prescription drug abuse. The title of a White House call to action uses the appropriate rousing words: *Epidemic: Responding to America's Prescription Abuse Crisis,* and the opening words announce the "Nation's fastest growing drug problem" (Executive Office, 2011, p. 1). Here, the dangerous drugs are not obtained illegally, they are legal remedies found in our home pharmacy cabinets. Their nonmedical or idiosyncratic use constitutes the current public health scourge (Janofsky, 2004). No less than 10 percent of state and local law enforcement agencies now view diverted uses of controlled prescription drugs as their "gravest drug threat" (U.S. Department of Justice, 2010). The National Institute on Drug Abuse (2011) defines *prescription drug abuse* as "the intentional use of a medication without a prescription; in a way other than as prescribed; or for the experience or feeling it causes" (p. 1).

In addition to wildly inflating the population of potential and actual abusers, prescription drug abuse blends two perspectives that authorities have taken pains to keep separate: the imagery and logic of the war on illegal drugs with the imagery and logic of the medical prescription of approved medicines. Even more than mere drug abuse, prescription drug abuse opens a fruitful terrain for drug experts and drug warriors, in which public health and repressive measures can mix in any manner and quantity and in which patients and prescribers can come under equal scrutiny. Presently, the drugs of concern are opiates, sedatives, and stimulants dispensed under prescription. In principle, however, there is no barrier to extending the concern to antidepressants, antipsychotics, and anticonvulsants, the paradigmatic *psychiatric* or *psychotherapeutic* drugs of the past half century.

Escaping and Entering Normality

With the arrival of Prozac, introduced to the US market in late 1987 and prescribed a few years later to over ten million people, the *New York Times* was announcing in a front-page article the rise of a "legal drug culture" (Rimer, 1993), as if such cultures had not always existed in this country and elsewhere. Testifying to the enduring but unarticulated social ambivalence toward psychoactive substances, the author took pains to distinguish the use of medications from that of drugs. Similar distinctions were being made across the Atlantic shortly after the arrival of Prozac to France. In a magazine article, psychiatrist Marc Bourgeois asked rhetorically whether "the proportion of 11% of users of psychotropics [is] scandalous?" Bourgeois answered reassuringly: "These are not drugs, but of course approved medications" (1994, p. 9).

Undoubtedly, most of the millions of citizens using antidepressants prescribed by their doctors would not have thought that they were "altering their consciousness." Still, during the early 1990s, media-amplified evaluations by some users and promoters of Prozac and the SSRIs (e.g., "I am free to be me," "I am better than well"; Kramer, 1993) did sound eerily like the benefits claimed by some users of illicit psychoactive drugs. There was, however, an important difference, as French sociologist Alain Ehrenberg (1995) was one of the first to note: the stated goal of using Prozac was *admission to*, not escape from, ordinary consciousness; it was "fitting in," not "dropping out." The modern user of prescribed psychoactive drugs wished to *function* better. The search for ecstatic highs morphed into the hope of "cosmetic psychopharmacology."

The Psychoactive Effects of Psychiatric Drugs[2]

We may now more fully consider the notion, repeated several times so far in this book, that prescribed psychiatric drugs should first and foremost be considered as psychoactive drugs. This notion rests on the conclusion that the usual explanations for how psychiatric drugs are supposed to work in the treatment of problems called psychiatric disorders can barely account for the only pertinent effects that can be attributed with any certainty to these drugs: their *psychoactive* effects (Moncrieff & Cohen, 2009).

Most people have a reasonable understanding of the psychoactive effects of substances that are typically used for recreational purposes, such as alcohol and cannabis. Besides the pleasant or often euphoric effects that lead people to use them, most people understand that these drugs modify how they think or reason, how they speak, how vigilant or forgetful they become, how they experience emotions, and, certainly, how they behave.

Most people understand that these drug-induced changes can be quite subtle and relatively easy to hide from observers who do not know them, just as they can be dramatic and obvious. Most people understand that drug-induced changes from recreational drugs can be persistent, if the drug use is persistent. Most people come to recognize and anticipate some effects from these drugs and use them to reach certain ends that might not be considered purely recreational, such as falling asleep more easily, ignoring unpleasant circumstances, completing necessary but annoying tasks, or acting more or less sociably. People also understand that, however pleasurable drug effects might be initially, they might become unpleasant with persistent use or in different circumstances. Similarly, people know from their experience and that of others that with prolonged use, users of recreational drugs often experience difficulty trying to cease using these drugs, even when their effects have become unpleasant.

A similar understanding applied to *prescribed* psychoactive drugs—popularly called psychiatric medications—is mostly absent, however, because there are virtually no authoritative summary descriptions in psychopharmacology textbooks of how these drugs alter our normal thoughts, emotions, and behavior. This state of affairs results from the single-minded effort in psychiatry over the past half century to portray psychiatric drugs as conventional medical remedies (targeting physiological abnormalities) and those who take psychiatric drugs as conventional medical patients (affected by physiological abnormalities). This has been called the "disease-centered model," wherein drugs' therapeutic effects are believed to stem principally from their action on (presumed) disease states or physiological pathways to such states (Moncrieff, 2008). This disease-centered model, as we argue throughout this book, has numerous weaknesses, especially so with respect to understanding and predicting the effects of psychiatric drugs, both in humans and in animal tests (Moncrieff & Cohen, 2005).

We know, however, that drugs used in psychiatry have *psychoactive* effects because people prescribed these drugs have described such effects, because healthy volunteers given only one or two doses of such drugs have described such effects, and—importantly—because countless experiments with animals from many species unmistakably show that these drugs alter normal animal behavior (make animals more or less active, more or less indifferent, more or less exploratory, more or less avoidant, more or less aggressive, and so on).

The nature of these drug effects appears to depend largely on the particular drug ingested. Each drug seems to trigger a particular sort of altered consciousness, inextricably linked to some altered physiology, and this global effect, though varying somewhat from user to user and often based on how much of the drug is ingested, seem relatively easy to identify when drugs are first investigated in human users and when the investigators are appropriately curious and open-minded about what they expect to observe.

Accumulated observations with psychiatric drugs confirm that certain psychiatric drugs have pleasant, initially desirable, euphoric effects. This is the case notably with stimulants (such as amphetamines and methylphenidate, or Ritalin) and benzodiazepines (such as alprazolam, or Xanax, and clonazepam, or Klonopin). For these reasons, many people interested in experiencing such effects chemically seek out these drugs and may use them "excessively." These drugs, though prescribed by physicians, are therefore widely available on the black market. Other psychiatric drugs, however, rarely or simply do not produce euphoric sensations. On the contrary, they are reliably observed or reported to produce strongly unpleasant, undesirable, or "dysphoric" sensations. This is the case with antipsychotic or neuroleptic drugs, the tricyclic antidepressants, lithium, and many anticonvulsants. To a lesser but still unmistakable degree, it is also the case with modern antidepressants (usually the SSRIs), as one can tell from the few investigations that note that their subjective effects are judged rather negatively by normal volunteers as well as by diagnosed patients (reviewed by Moncrieff, 2008; Goldsmith & Moncrieff, 2011). Of course, it is crucial to realize that even if these latter groups of drugs do not easily produce euphoric, generally pleasant effects and even if they have almost no value on the black market (i.e., extremely few people seek them out for recreational purposes), *this does not mean that they are not psychoactive drugs.*

All psychiatric drugs in common use affect how people think, how they feel, and how they behave. Antipsychotic drugs produce states of psychological indifference, clouded cognition, stunted emotions, and sedation. Anticonvulsants, today part of the standard maintenance treatment of bipolar disorders, show a panoply of dysphoric effects, ranging from strong sedation and cognitive slowing to anxiety and agitation (Cavanna et al., 2010). Antidepressant drugs include a large range of substances with effects ranging from mild sedation to severe, mania-like agitation. It remains difficult to characterize them in psychological or subjective terms, as their psychoactive effects have not been seriously investigated up to now. A study by Goldsmith and Moncrieff (2011) examined comments by nearly five hundred users of fluoxetine (Prozac) and venlafaxine (Effexor) posted on a website and categorized the most frequent described effects as sedation (about 26 percent), activation (about 25 percent), and reduced libido (about 20 percent). Benzodiazepines typically produce sedation, relaxation, and indifference. Their deleterious effects on memory are notable. Stimulants typically produce euphoria, wakefulness, increased concentration, and a feeling of endurance—characteristics which combine to give stimulants a privileged place as performance enhancers in several societies.

With only the above cursory observations, one can see that drugs can affect people with and without a psychiatric diagnosis in similar ways, but we can also see how the psychoactive effects of psychiatric drugs can be useful to people undergoing psychological crises or who are misbehaving (and therefore whom others wish to control). This possibility and its implications have been termed the drug-centered model of psychotropic drug action, as an alternative to the disease-centered model (Moncrieff & Cohen, 2005, 2006, 2009).

Cohen and Hughes (2011), for example, suggest that by inducing much-needed sleep, all drugs with sedative effects can trigger positive changes in well-being. All drugs with stimulating or activating effects may help people complete unfinished frustrating tasks or bring about people's exposure to social situations that provide opportunities for reinforcement and practice of social skills. Emotional blunting, observed with most classes of psychoactive medications but especially with antipsychotics, lithium, and anticonvulsants, may help people distance themselves from sources of stress in their environment. Conversely, it is possible to see how the persistent production of such effects over time, whether of an activating or deactivating sort, may turn into frank disablement. For example, where psychological indifference and cognitive clouding can help an individual and his or her relatives during an acute emotional crisis, it can also impair a person from functioning normally. Where wakefulness and increased activity can help someone focus efficiently on a task, it can lead them to be impetuous or aggressive in unpleasant environments. Where decreased vigilance and increased relaxation can help one during informal social gatherings and before bedtime, it can be deleterious if these effects persist while driving or when having to perform at the office or simply when having to make a decision.

It is extraordinary that such considerations regarding the obviously useful or impairing effects of chemically triggered psychoactive states, depending on one's psychological problems, situation, or circumstances have not been taken seriously in modern psychopharmacology. Given that psychiatric medications modify thinking, feeling, and behaving, it follows logically that these effects interact with the thoughts, the feelings, and the behaviors that are said to constitute the symptoms or the diagnostic criteria of mental disorders as described in the *DSM* and other diagnostic manuals. One nonetheless can peruse dozens of manuals of psychopharmacology without encountering any mention, let alone clear acknowledgment, of this possibility. Still, during the introduction of the first modern psychotropics during the 1950s, several clinicians and researchers, regardless of their theoretical orientation, became quite interested in these psychoactive effects and how to distinguish them (e.g., Cole, 1960). In the case of antipsychotics, for nearly two decades, the production of psychic indifference and abnormal involuntary movements became accepted as the very mechanism of action in psychosis (review by Cohen, 1997a, 1997b; Jacobs & Cohen, 1999; Moncrieff, 2008).

The fact is that these psychoactive effects are simply not controlled nor are they accounted for in interpretations or discussions of the results of clinical trials of psychiatric drugs—which are supposed to investigate how these drugs affect symptoms. In other words, we do not know, from the results of countless clinical trials, how sedation, activation, or reduced libido (to use only commonly reported subjective effects of antidepressants) would lead to the conclusion that antidepressants effectively reduce symptoms of depression. Because of the lack of controls for psychoactive effects, no one is really in a position to assert that psychotropic medications have, in reality, *any other pertinent action in the treatment of psychological distress over and above their common psychoactive effects.*

There have been no discoveries of any sort that indicate how psychotropic medications might, in fact, be modifying any (still unknown) physiological processes hypothesized by psychiatrists and psychopharmacologists to cause psychological distress and misbehavior. Therefore, the failure to investigate rigorously and creatively how psychoactive effects of psychiatrically prescribed drugs—including the effects of tolerance, dependence, and withdrawal—affect psychological and behavioral states called mental disorders seems like a remarkable form of scientific denial.

The Lure of the Magic Potion

It is instructive to review with a twenty-year hindsight how the enormous publicity generated around claims that Prozac could "transform" personality or around narratives of persons affected by Prozac led many social commentators to claim that society had entered a "new era" of widespread personal transformation by means of drugs. The expression "cosmetic psychopharmacology," coined somewhat ironically by American psychiatrist Peter Kramer in his 1993 bestseller *Listening to Prozac*, quickly took hold during that decade (Farr, 1994; Rothman, 1994).

Cosmetic psychopharmacology promised the design of drugs targeting specific neuronal receptors, a specificity of action expected to produce desired effects with few or no unwanted effects. As a result, it was claimed, people would be able to modify their personalities regularly: they would improve their intelligence, their memory, and their concentration—shape their brain at will (Restak, 1994). Twenty-some years later, the Prozac revolution stands not as a genuine clinical or scientific breakthrough but instead as a stupendous advance in the marketing of drugs (and of psychiatric diagnoses to market even more drugs). The Prozac revolution appears merely as a modern version of the ever-alluring myth of the magic potion.

Optimistic scenarios of the implications of the Prozac revolution seemed to ignore history. Cosmetic psychopharmacology, described by the Prozac faithful as an advance unique to late-twentieth-century psychotropics, had a longer past. Already in the 1880s, as he accustomed himself to using cocaine daily for five years, Sigmund Freud enthused that the drug was transforming his entire personality for the better, made him more "normal," gave him abundant energy for work, and produced not a single unwanted effect (Byck,

1976). In contrast with the official history of antidepressant drugs as "discovered" in the early 1950s by dedicated biochemists, as early as 1937, the Smith, Kline and French pharmaceutical firm was creating the first antidepressant, by mailing a pamphlet to ninety thousand doctors (the majority of American general practitioners as well as neurologists and psychiatrists), to promote amphetamine, stating that "the main field for Benzedrine Sulfate will be its use in improving mood" (cited in Rasmussen, 2006, p. 311). From that time until well into the 1960s, the amphetamines (Benzedrine, Dexedrine) were actively promoted in medical journals and prescribed by doctors across America and the world for conditions and ailments including depression, fatigue, and being overweight (Breggin & Breggin, 1994; Pickering & Stimson, 1994). Only fifteen years before these drugs became strictly controlled substances considered by medical and legal authorities to have limited medical value and high potential for abuse and dependence, readers of a medical textbook were reminded how, "Gradually, as experience with amphetamines has ripened, they have become firmly established as versatile and helpful remedies, given to millions of people, and under such conditions as to offer remarkably low potential for causing harm or unwanted effects" (Leake, 1958, p. 18). The use of amphetamines as performance enhancers by athletes, pilots, drivers, and soldiers had of course already been well-established and discussed before then (Rosen, 2008).

In truth, during the 1990s on both sides of the Atlantic, commentators raised concerns about the challenges for individuals and society of an anticipated wave of post-Prozac substances. "If one can modify mental perceptions without endangering self or others," asked Ehrenberg (1995, p. 34), "will our societies be made up of 'normal' individuals permanently assisted by psychic products?" For French psychoanalyst Pierre Fédida (1995, p. 95), a seemingly omnipotent psychopharmacology triggered "the anguish of a loss of psychic identity," in which the individual "would conserve his appearance, while being dispossessed of all that constitutes him genuinely." For medical historian David Rothman (1994, p. 36), the use of Prozac fed what he termed a typically American illusion, "the possibility of a single act of redemption, of victory without struggle or suffering."

Despite some of these fears, however, whatever future scenario these authors envisaged rested on rosy renderings of the history of psychopharmacology, especially concerning the discovery of the antipsychotics and the invention of most of today's psychiatric pharmacopeia. The psychiatric discourse on the *progress* represented by these accomplishments was accepted lock, stock, and barrel by virtually every commentator on the Prozac phenomenon.

Even as enthusiasm about the SSRIs waned significantly, as it did at the start of the twenty-first century (Scott, 2008), knowledgeable observers could not bring themselves to call the enterprise a scientific failure. Sharon

Begley (2010), in a cover story in *Newsweek*, "The Depressing News about Antidepressants," summarized the research showing that placebos produce equivalent outcomes, minus the adverse effects. Calling the drugs "basically expensive Tic Tacs" and citing experts acutely aware of the "disconnect between the scientific evidence and public impression," especially concerning the serotonin-deficit theory of depression "built on a foundation of tissue paper," Begley nonetheless expressed sympathy for those who would keep patients in the dark. She characterized the truth-propaganda disconnect as a "moral dilemma." After all, patients who suffer from what Begley termed "a devastating, underdiagnosed, and undertreated disease" and who find their medications helpful "need to believe in their pills." But it isn't a "belief in pills" that Begley was promoting, more than a belief in what patients and the public *have been told by organized psychiatry and the mental health establishment about pills* as specific treatments for depression. Psychiatry, in short, is too big to fail.

It seems to us, on the other hand, that clinical psychopharmacology—the medically sanctioned use of psychoactive drugs for the treatment of medically legitimated distress and misbehavior (termed *mental disorders*)—has always been a pseudoscientific enterprise. We argue in the rest of this chapter that what has been passed off as the "psychopharmacological revolution" of the 1950s has consisted, at bottom, of the taming of madness via the remote chemical control of madpersons and the strengthening of psychiatry's medical self-image. The wholesale application of biological language to old psychiatric practices and perennial personal problems constitutes merely the latest pseudomedical façade to the edifice of psychiatry. Besides psychiatric physicians' singular ability to forcibly medicate and incarcerate, their indispensability as mental health practitioners rests on an exceedingly simple and obvious fact: they alone provide access to licit psychoactive medications. And all this, we and a growing chorus of observers can now affirm with support from abundant evidence, was made possible—indeed, was actively encouraged or manufactured—by psychiatry's enthusiastic enlistment as a satellite branch of the multinational pharmaceutical industry and the co-optation of the FDA as an agency aiming, not merely to protect the public, but rather to advance the drug industry's interests and reinforce mainstream cultural notions that nonspecific psychoactive drugs (demons) are, in the hands of medical prescribers, conventional medical remedies (angels) targeting specific mental disorders.

To make this case, we first address the idea that tremendous, rapid advances in the fields of molecular biology and pharmacogenomics may have provided psychopharmacology with a secure scientific basis.

Progress in Molecular Biology?

The development of molecular biology seems to represent a radical break contrasting a current era of "rational drug design" from a previous one of chance discoveries. Molecular biology has enabled the amazing feat of designing a molecule introduced into the body from the outside to bind itself on a particular type of cell membrane receptor, thus triggering changes within and around the cell and throughout the pathways comprised of similar cells that communicate with each other. Paradoxically, this feat merely confirms that in the domain of brain-behavior interactions, we are taking our first baby steps. As philosopher of science Isabelle Stengers observed, "Between the richness of the psychic effects of a drug and the hypothesis that it disturbs the effects of a type of neurotransmitter, there exists a gulf that no contemporary theory can cross" (1995, pp. 134–135).

The future of all medications is often said to depend on biotechnologies. These techniques consist of mapping and then mastering the genetic code and functioning of a bacterium, a cell, or a whole living organism in order to make it produce various substances at will. A well-known example is the synthesis of human insulin from bacteria. However, not even a miracle of genetic engineering could contribute to the design of psychiatric drugs that do not merely sedate, stimulate, render indifferent, or provide nonspecific subjective relief for emotional distress or mental disorder. This is because there are no demonstrated biological anomalies for any drug to target to "cure" the mental disorders in question.

Such biological targets, a sine qua non for rational drug design, would be identified from a detailed knowledge of the cellular and molecular biology of a disease. Nothing of the sort exists in the case of psychiatric "diseases" and drugs. Not only does the field lack basic biological understanding of any presumed disease process, psychiatric researchers that we cited earlier in the book—who have committed their careers to developing this biological understanding—state flatly that *nothing biological* has been reliably associated with any *DSM* diagnosis that aids to make the diagnosis or to predict how someone will respond to drug treatment. There are no biomarkers for psychiatric disorders—no biological signs that can be used reliably to measure the presence, change, improvement, or worsening of the condition that one might deem "pathological." To be sure, every month, investigators propose new biological measures in the literature as candidate biomarkers, but none survives for long. Most telling, none is used in any clinical trial testing a drug for the treatment of any psychiatric condition.

Comparing Psychiatric Progress with Neurological Progress

We repeat: no distinct biological determinism has been demonstrated in any mental disorder. For decades this was occasionally acknowledged, but discreetly, deep in textbooks and professional articles, rarely by experts in popular discourse. According to a survey of a probability sample of the US population, conducted by the American Psychiatric Association (2005), 75 percent of people believe that mental disorders result from "chemical imbalances." But, already, chemical imbalances are passé, at least according to the director of the NIMH.

Given the belief that mental disorders are brain disorders, a good way to assess the concrete scientific fruits of the decade of the brain for psychiatry and for understanding mental disorders is to compare what Thomas Insel as the director of the National Institute of Mental Health, and Story Landis as the director of the National Institute of Neurological Disorders and Stroke state about progress in their respective fields. Neurological disorders, by definition, are diseases of the brain. Mental disorders are *claimed* to be diseases of the brain. Both Insel and Landis were invited by the Dana Foundation to summarize, in one thousand words, what the massive investments into research in their respective fields had produced.

Insel (2010) wrote: "If scientists introduced mental disorders as brain disorders in the Decade of the Brain, researchers in the past 10 years have *demonstrated* the importance of specific brain circuits" [emphasis added]. The caveat: "Unlike neurological disorders, which often involve areas of tissue damage or cell loss, mental disorders have *begun to appear more like* circuit disorders." As evidence for his statement, Insel writes that "specific brain pathways are involved in major mental disorders." Also, "deep brain stimulation *has shown promise* as a treatment for depression and obsessive-compulsive disorder." Due to laser technology, "for the first time, researchers can conduct specific *tests of theories* about brain circuits and behavior." About schizophrenia, Insel states that "The disorder *might result* from excessive loss of synapses in a critical cortical pathway." He reasserts: "recent research *suggests* that mental disorders are really developmental brain disorders, caused by disruptions in the circuitry map of the developing brain." Finally, he concludes: "The answer for psychiatry will likely be the same as the answer for the rest of medicine: Basic discoveries regarding genes and proteins will point the way to molecular and cellular mechanisms, which in turn will yield new targets for treatment and prevention."

In her assessment of progress in neurological research, Story Landis (2010) states that "in the past decade, the list of gene defects that contribute to neurological disorders grew at an extraordinary pace, leading to almost an embarrassment of riches." She gives a specific example: "Classification for ataxias by genetic profile has replaced the clinical classification based on time of onset, rate of progression, and subtleties of the clinical exam." At least six additional Parkinson's-related genes "appear to underly the disease in as much as 35 percent of patients with Parkinson's disease." For some diseases, Landis writes, "An inexpensive genetic test can now bring [patients' odysseys in search of a diagnosis] to a rapid and conclusive end." Then, Landis counters with the sobering assessment that "to date this translation has proved to be much more difficult than we had imagined. For example, in 1987, researchers discovered that mutations in the dystrophin gene cause Duchenne muscular dystrophy [a fatal disease in affected boys usually before the age of twenty]. Despite two decades of research and the availability of both mouse and dog models, the only treatment currently in use is corticosteroids."

We note Insel's assertion that the long-held view of mental disorders as conditions characterized by "loss of cells" should now give way to one of conditions characterized by "disruptions in the circuitry map." In essence, Insel states that the dominant neurobiological hypothesis of mental disorder *has been abandoned*. Will the 75 percent of Americans who believe in "chemical imbalances" be informed that circuitry has dethroned chemistry? Does it matter to anyone? Yet it indicates an important scientific event: the failure of research to support the biochemical paradigm. Touting a new conduction paradigm, however, Insel gives no example of any "circuit disorder," nor of any mechanisms underlying any such disorder. The transformation brought about by the decade of the brain, we have grounds to conclude from Insel's exhibit, is mainly metaphorical.

Landis names actual discoveries of genetic markers that definitively *replace clinical diagnosis* of various neurological disorders—something psychiatry can still only dream of concerning its "brain-based" disorders. Yet, progress notwithstanding, Landis sounds an important cautionary note: in one specific disorder, the identification of no less than a *causative* gene resulted in no improvement in palliative, let alone curative, treatments. The gap between neurology and psychiatry, even between hoped-for psychiatry and actual neurology, appears quite large.

The Promise and the Reality

In the general area of drug development, however, molecular biology has enormously helped researchers to screen for molecules that would resemble one or more aspects of currently (commercially) successful drugs, so that these can be copied. This was the case with the various SSRIs and the second-generation or atypical antipsychotics, designed to copy the initial leader in their class. The sophistication and efficiency of the screening tools have increased exponentially, so that the stock of potentially testable molecules (designed by computer) is nearly infinite. As one or another neurotransmitter pathway becomes more intently discussed (in the literature by key opinion leaders hired as consultants by drug companies) as a potential target for drug action in one or another mental disorder, scientists can use supercomputers to model molecules that could bind themselves to the desired target. Also, as gene-to-behavior and environment-to-gene pathways and interactions are increasingly understood, the effects of drugs on the expression of genes are also beginning to be better understood.[3] In principle, this knowledge might help to reduce the risk of *harm* from drugs based on individuals' genetic profiles. But, to repeat, no radical innovation based on genetic knowledge is leading the way to find any *curative* compounds in psychiatry, because there is simply no idea about what specific part of the body, if any, needs fixing when people suffer or misbehave.

None of the products derived from current biotechnologies are psychiatric medications, and the number of FDA approvals for psychiatric drugs over the past decade has significantly declined (Cutler et al., 2010), as has, in general, the number of new molecular entities (drugs never used before in clinical practice) approved by the FDA, from thirty-one in 2004 to seventeen in 2008 (Dorsey et al., 2010). That number had risen back to thirty in 2011, but included only a single drug approved for a mental disorder (FDA, 2012). The tendency in psychiatry has mostly consisted in recycling existing drugs for expanded uses. To illustrate, a drug evaluated by the FDA for approval for the treatment of sleepiness in narcolepsy in the mid-2000s was merely an old stimulant on the European market for more than forty years (Provigil, or modafinil). The second-to-last antipsychotic approved by the FDA in late 2007 was paliperidone (Invega), the major active metabolite (a byproduct formed during metabolism) of risperidone—itself on the market since 1994 and whose patent of exclusive marketing to its manufacturer, Janssen, was expiring.

In the spirit of providing the illumination that often comes from visiting old exhibits of the future, here is how a *Newsweek* article by Sharon Begley published in 1994 announced imminent drug breakthroughs. The author described the use of five "new mind drugs"—though none were new at the time. In the article, beta blockers, largely used around the world to lower blood pressure, were renamed "anxiolytics"; Ritalin, on the United States market since the late 1950s, was promoted to increase concentration in adults (part of the intriguing shift to "adult ADD" starting in the mid-1990s); dexfenfluramine, another stimulant long available in Europe as a diet pill, was renamed a "mood stabilizer"; phenytoin (Dilantin), one of the oldest antiepileptic drugs on the market, was dubbed a "stress reducer"; and phenelzine, prescribed sporadically since the 1950s as an antidepressant, was presented as an innovative treatment for "hypersensitive patients." What happened to these drugs? Of the five, dexfenfluramine was later withdrawn from the market for toxic cardiac effects, and phenytoin and phenelzine are barely used.

To Begley's list one might add the antipsychotic clozapine, prescribed modestly in Europe since the end of the 1960s, but launched in North America in 1990 as a "revolutionary new treatment for schizophrenia," with a publicity campaign that included a *Time* magazine cover (July 6, 1992) and a story displaying a photograph of a young man diagnosed with schizophrenia dancing wildly and happily at a party. In reports to the FDA between 1998 and 2005, however, health professionals named clozapine as a suspected cause in nearly 3,300 deaths—more than any other prescribed psychoactive drug (Moore, Cohen, & Furberg, 2007).

Several observers of the rise of Prozac in the 1990s predicted that the psychopharmacologist would soon hold the keys to understanding the brain and to shape it at will. Another analogy seems more fitting during the second decade of the twenty-first century: facing the somewhere around 100 trillion glia, neurons, receptors, and synapses in the brain, the psychopharmacologist resembles the astronomer facing the cosmos.

The Complex Life Cycle of Medications

Most medications have a long, complex, and unpredictable lifecycle. Although modern psychoactive medications are implicitly and explicitly portrayed as pure substances whose indications for prescription are intrinsic to their chemical structure, no such medication appears to have ever existed. Psychoactive drugs, let us note, are prescribed in the absence of demonstrated physical pathology. Thus, how and why drugs end up being prescribed for one clinical indication in psychiatry rather than another is the result at least as much from trial and error and marketing as from clinical necessity (Cohen et al., 2001; Horwitz, 2010).

The Elusive Costs of Developing Drugs

To transform a molecule into a medication approved by the FDA for marketing and prescription takes several years. Of thousands of molecules screened in the laboratory, only a handful start the journey to approval. The most widely cited estimate of the average cost of the process to approval for a single drug—what is commonly referred to as research and development (R & D)—was $802 million in 2000, updated to $1.32 billion in 2006 (cited in Light and Warburton, 2011, p. 3), and again to $1.8 billion in a 2010 NIMH report ("From Discovery to Cure," 2010). However, Donald Light and Rebecca Warburton have demonstrated that the $802 million estimate constitutes a hodge-podge of unverifiable early development costs, costs of "profits foregone" by choosing to invest in R & D (about half of the $802 million estimate), largely inflated costs of clinical trials, exaggerated time for R & D, and other questionable strategies, such as using mean rather than median costs. Despite this, the R&D estimates are immediately 100 percent deducted from taxable profits for the companies involved, a convenient federal incentive for them to exaggerate the actual costs.

Light and Warburton's analysis deserves close reading. They suggest that "based on independent sources and reasonable arguments, one can conclude that R&D costs companies a median of $43.4 million per new drug, just as company supported analysts can conclude they are over 18 times larger, or $802 million" (2011, p. 14). They conclude that, "Readers should appreciate the constructed nature of R&D cost estimates and always ask very closely about where the data for an estimate come from, how they were assembled and whether they can be verified" (p. 14). Our view is that this caution also applies to claims of drug effectiveness and safety as we will describe below.

The FDA Obstacle Course

For a new molecule (one that has not already been approved by the FDA for any indication), the approval process includes overlapping phases involving many players. Each phase is well-outlined in the literature, but only the latter phases—large, randomized controlled clinical trials (RCTs) in humans—have been examined by scholars in any depth. Under the legally enforced principle that drugs are proprietary products and that competitors in the drug industry may unfairly benefit from a company's disclosures of its commercial practices, most of the activities during the early phases of drug development remain shielded from serious scrutiny. The components of the various phases, and regulatory agencies' expectations about them are well-known in theory, but how the phases are orchestrated in practice is not. Over the last decade, however, more glimpses have been obtained as confidential documents have been unsealed or leaked during lawsuits against drug companies.

Animal Tests and Phase I Human Tests. The first step in drug development consists of preclinical testing. Computers simulating the precise chemical structure of the chosen molecule allow investigators to make predictions about its affinity for certain receptors in the body and its resemblance to other molecules with known effects. Then, testing on several animal species (rodents, cats and dogs, occasionally primates) is undertaken to rule out the drug's potential to cause obvious physical damage, including genetic or chromosomal mutations, birth defects or malformations, and cancer.

Preclinical studies may be conducted in the manufacturer's own facilities or contracted out to private research labs and university departments. Typically, the initial work is conceived in a university laboratory receiving government funding. Breakthrough pioneering work is inherently unpredictable, and few drug companies are willing to invest in such uncertainties, especially, as in the case of mental disorders, if there is no understanding of how the "disease" works and thus no established path to breakthrough drugs. Thus, once a potentially useful substance is discovered or identified in a university lab, the drug firm, betting on the potential clinical value of the particular substance, enters into a commercial agreement with a researcher and/or the university to pursue its development. After having amassed the required data indicating that the drug is not likely to cause gross physical damage to animals and outlining general neurochemical and behavioral effects of the molecule as determined through in vitro and in vivo tests on animals, the sponsor might then apply to the FDA to begin testing it on humans.

If the FDA agrees and the sponsor decides to undertake human testing, phase I of clinical trials may begin. The aim now is to determine the major parameters of the drug's effects in humans. Starting with tiny doses, the drug might be administered to approximately twenty to a hundred younger, healthy men. Close medical monitoring is necessary, since the first administration in humans—despite the extensive animal studies that preceded it—may lead to completely unforeseen effects. An example was revealed in March 2006 when six volunteers receiving the first-ever injections to humans of TGN1412, tested as a potential remedy for autoimmune diseases, became desperately ill and suffered multiple organ failures. Five of the six recovered only after a full month in intensive care. Doses up to 500 times as high as those received by this first group of volunteers had been given to animals, with no sign of toxicity whatsoever (Wood & Darbyshire, 2006).

Testing for "abuse liability" might take place during phase I. At the urging of the FDA, the sponsor might be asked to determine whether the substance is pleasurable to take, whether experienced users ("abusers") of illicit substances report some equivalence of effect with the new substance, or whether ordinary participants in clinical trials diverted it to friends. This reflects one of the rare instances of interest in specifically *psychoactive* effects by any responsible authorities. A clear indication that a new drug intended for prescription creates euphoria in a few users or is diverted by a few clinical trial participants to their relatives or friends would certainly delay if not doom its prospects of obtaining FDA approval as a prescription medication. Yet, that a drug creates dose-dependent dysphoria (unpleasant emotions or behavior such as depression, agitation, restlessness, or anxiety) in more than a few users would evoke absolutely no concern among regulators unless the effects are clearly and repeatedly described as dramatic or observed frequently in the trials' reports submitted to the FDA. The implied reasoning is that these unpleasant effects are most likely manifestations of the subjects' pre-existing psychiatric disorders and need not be considered from the start as attributable to the drugs.[4]

Banishing the Psychoactive. Based on the results of animal trials, it is likely that a distinctive profile of the psychoactive drug has begun to emerge: the drug has either energized, or sedated, or paralyzed, or rendered animals indifferent, or inhibited some learning and memory tasks, or increased or decreased various species-like or un-species-like behaviors in contrived settings. At present, it is impossible to imagine a drug with no noticeable behavioral effects in animals being viewed as a potentially useful psychiatric medication and thus proceeding to human testing. Despite these definite observations that drugs intended for psychiatric use have clear behavioral effects in animals, no systematic search of equivalent psychoactive effects in humans takes place during the drugs' clinical trials. Neither drug firms nor the FDA have developed (or publicized) methodical procedures to test, in human volunteers, emotional, cognitive, and behavioral effects—which psychoactive drugs produce and are expected to produce, *by definition.* The case of Strattera (atomoxetine), a claimed "nonstimulant" approved by the FDA for the treatment of ADHD in 2002, is illustrative. Records and data released by the FDA show that atomoxetine was administered to nearly three hundred healthy volunteers during phase I studies. Yet in several hundred pages of FDA evaluation summaries, neither the drug firm nor the FDA reviewers who pored over these data made a single comment on anticipated *psychoactive* effects besides those related to the potential abuse of the drug. This bears restating: No exploration of Strattera's effects on mood, attention, memory, or any other emotional or intellectual quality in healthy humans was reported in the FDA review of the sponsor's application for marketing (Cohen, 2011).

In any case, based on a combination of animal and phase I observations, on the resemblance of the tested substance to others on the market, and on whether its use can be justified by marketable theoretical considerations such as dopamine, serotonin, or other still-undiscarded hypotheses related to the anticipated indication, a testable clinical indication in humans has been proposed, worded by means of the *DSM* psychiatric disorder. This is obligatory because federal regulations define a drug as something intended for the prevention or treatment of "disease." A drug cannot be approved by the FDA because it has potent or potentially useful stimulant or sedative effects—it must be judged efficacious for a recognized disease or disorder: for example, Attention Deficit-Hyperactivity Disorder, General Anxiety Disorder, or Schizophrenic Disorder. (There are exceptions to this rule, as for example when the FDA approved risperidone for the treatment of "irritability" associated with autistic disorder in 2006.)

In this connection, it is noteworthy that the FDA has explicitly recognized that psychiatric diagnoses have no validated physiopathology. A consumer queried the FDA on whether it agreed with a statement by Health Canada, the Canadian government's drug regulatory agency, that "For mental/psychiatric disorders in general . . . there are no confirmatory gross, microscopic or chemical abnormalities that have been validated for objective physical diagnosis." In its reply to the consumer, the FDA's Center of Drug Evaluation and Research agreed that "psychiatric disorders are diagnosed based on a patient's presentation of symptoms that the larger psychiatric community has come to accept as real and responsive to treatment. We have nothing more to add to Health Canada's response" (cited in Pringle, 2009, p. 1). This statement by the FDA explains why any discussion by the sponsor of the expected or presumed biological mechanisms by which the tested psychiatric drug might reduce symptoms of the mental disorder of interest in the clinical trial is itself reduced to an absolute minimum in the sponsor's application for drug approval. For example, Cohen (2011) observed that in approximately 695 pages making up the FDA-released evaluation of Strattera, the presumed biochemical rationale of Strattera as a treatment for the proposed indication, ADHD, was discussed in *two sentences*, with no references.

Phase II Trials. Phase II consists of relatively small trials, lasting about two to eight weeks, usually including anywhere from fifty to three hundred people diagnosed with the *DSM* condition for which the sponsor hopes to market the future medication. Thus phase II trials attempt to establish that the drug will, indeed, improve the officially designated symptoms of an officially designated psychiatric condition. To determine for which disorder the drug will be tested is, as we have mentioned earlier, probably based on a combination of factors, none of which appears in the literature as decisive. It is possible to suggest that the decision is not an inherently complicated clinical matter (although it may be a risky marketing matter). For example, looking at a number of previous drug approvals, it may be that drugs having revealed a distinctive behavioral profile of sedative effects (and a molecular activity profile somewhat consistent with that of other sedative drugs on the market) will likely be tested for the treatment of *DSM* disorders characterized by symptoms of anxiety or agitation, for which sedating drugs are often found useful. Similarly, drugs having revealed a distinctive profile of deactivating effects will likely be tested for *DSM* disorders characterized by delusions, loss of control, and severe agitation.

Phase II studies vary greatly in methodological rigor and are usually "open," meaning that if the studies involve control groups of participants receiving a comparison drug or placebo, investigators know who these participants are. To measure outcomes, rating scales that usually list the appropriate *DSM* symptoms of the particular disorder—as well as other symptoms of general psychological distress (especially anxiety, agitation, and depression)—are used. From the sponsor's perspective, phase II trials must succeed to justify the next phase of testing, phase III, because this is where the most examined trials will take place. It appears that less than one-tenth of substances that enter phase I trials make it to approval. Over half of the failures apparently result from an inability to demonstrate efficacy during phase II trials: that is, superior response of patients on the drug compared to placebo, even in open trials (Hurko & Ryan, 2005).

Controlled Trials out of Control. Phase III trials are often called "pivotal" trials because they employ what experts in medicine widely consider the gold standard design: the randomized, controlled clinical trial (RCT). In RCTs for most psychiatric drugs, eligible participants (about five hundred to three thousand people in total, recruited from multiple sites in different cities and, increasingly, different countries) are randomly assigned to receive either the drug or an alternate treatment, usually an inert placebo. Because random assignment is the strongest way to ensure similar groups and thereby minimize important threats to the methodological (logical or internal) validity of a study, RCTs are believed to produce the highest-grade evidence to determine how much observed change in participants is due to the treatment rather than to any confounding variables.

The validity of the RCT rests on several assumptions, one of which is that participants in the trial are all *the same* on the key reason why they have been enrolled in the trial (i.e., they all have the same "mental disorder" to be treated). The point of the RCT is to determine the specific influence of a treatment on the outcome of the trial; therefore one needs to rule out the influence of other factors (within and outside the participants) that could cloud this determination. Thus, FDA clinical trials of psychoactive drugs always specify that the participants meet the specific diagnostic criteria necessary for mental disorder X, as determined by a structured *DSM* psychiatric diagnostic interview and confirmed by experienced clinical psychiatrists. Yet that participants meet the *DSM* criteria for the disorder in question does not in any way guarantee the sameness of their problem. The issue is not merely one of the "heterogeneous presentation" of a disorder, just as one person with lung cancer might differ from another person with lung cancer. At issue here is the *nature* of the problem. The sadness or despondency experienced by one person's unemployment and by another's realization of a spouse's infidelity might both meet the *DSM*'s diagnostic criteria for "Major Depressive Disorder" or its synonyms, but they are worlds away in cause, meaning, and experience (Jacobs & Cohen, 2010). The *sameness* that characterizes lesions or infections in physical disorders cannot exist in the case of psychological problems that are only diagnosed based on an individual's *subjective view* of their own circumstances and predicament, a view that develops and differs according to circumstances (including the very circumstances of a clinical trial). If this is the case, the whole point of conducting a psychiatric drug RCT and randomizing participants in separate groups in order to ensure that *only* treatment (drug or no drug) differs between groups so that only treatment can be implicated in the outcomes is exposed as nonsensical. This foundational issue is not, to our knowledge, ever discussed in the psychiatric clinical trial literature, so strong is the tacit acceptance of *DSM* disorders as conventional medical diseases, impersonal and invariant medical disorders, *the same* in every person.

A well-known refinement of the RCT involves double-blind placebo-control, wherein neither researchers nor participants are supposed to know who is receiving an active drug and who an identical-looking but inert placebo. This precaution is meant to counter the potentially enormous impact of researcher and participant expectations on the outcome. But the actual effect of the precaution is rarely if ever tested or reported in modern psychotropic drug trials, possibly to avoid knowing that patients and clinicians can guess correctly (apparently, more than 80 percent of the time in older trials of benzodiazepines or antidepressants) which treatment they are receiving (Even et al., 2000). Blindness in psychotropic drug trials is therefore a completely relative notion, which means that the scientific value of the RCT in the enterprise must also remain a relative notion. This bears repeating: although the whole preapproval drug-testing process culminates with phase III randomized controlled trials with their obligatory double-blind feature, the breach of blindness in these trials may be routine and widespread, tainting impartiality of the raters (assuming such impartiality can exist in the sponsor-controlled clinical trial environment) and rendering the whole exercise no different than phase II open trials. For example, Benson and Hartz (2000) compared RCTs and merely "observational" studies of nineteen different treatments (excluding psychotropic drugs) but found estimates of treatment effects from the lesser-grade studies to be neither larger nor qualitatively different than those from RCTs. In sum, the RCT, erected as a massive stone guardian of the medical validity of testing *psychoactive* drugs for *mental disorders* by the FDA and the drug industry, has feet of clay.

Besides their larger size and supposedly more rigorous design, phase III trials are essentially similar to phase II trials in length (about two to eight weeks) and outcome measures (a predefined average percentage improvement on rating scale scores in the drug-treated group that should exceed any improvement seen in the non-drug-treated group and not be attributable to chance, as determined by statistical tests).

Finally, phase IV trials (also known as post-marketing surveillance trials) might be undertaken after the drug has received market approval from the FDA. Regularly, the FDA requires the sponsor to promise to conduct such trials as a condition for approval. Phase IV trials serve as an explicit recognition that the premarketing clinical trial process is inherently limited as the types and numbers of patients studied, the durations of treatment, and the overall conditions of use differ greatly from the real-world patients, durations, and conditions of use expected once the drug hits the market. Only after several years or decades of such use might one expect a more realistic safety profile to be established. The three major drug studies discussed in chapter 6 (CATIE, STAR*D, and STEP-BD) may all be considered phase IV trials. As of 2006, 71 percent of phase IV trials that sponsors had promised the FDA to conduct as a condition of the approval of their drug had not yet started (Avorn, 2007).

On the Market

We mentioned earlier that choosing the tested indication for a drug (e.g., the "disease" that it will be officially approved for) may be a more risky marketing than clinical issue. This is because, years before the possibility of market approval, the drug maker must anticipate future therapeutic needs in the field—or, if necessary, create such needs—so that the medication appears to clinicians and the public to arrive just in time to allay a serious problem and that a respectable return on investments (or better, blockbuster status for the drug, usually defined as $1 billion or more in yearly sales) is obtained. After having received a brand name, the psychotropic medication will now be the subject of a promotional blitz targeted to all persons, groups, and institutions who might have some interest in its use. A key part of this campaign involves formulating a simple way to understand how the drug works and why it is so essential (Nesi, 2008). From these strategies are born or reborn invented phrases such as "chemical imbalance," "mood stabilizer," and "treatable medical condition." The money spent on this marketing will greatly exceed the sums invested in all the phases of preclinical and clinical testing that led to the drug's approval by the FDA and any subsequent studies once on the market (Gagnon & Lexchin, 2008).

The drug will be placed in a therapeutic class corresponding to the disorder for which the FDA approved it for prescription (such as antipsychotic, antidepressant, anxiolytic). This classification may at first matter to doctors, pharmacists, patients, and journalists, as it will be the first and perhaps the only formally advertised indication for that drug. Quickly, however, this classification will mean little in practice, as nearly all psychotropic drug classes end up prescribed for all groups of disorders (Bezchlibnyk-Butler & Jeffries, 2005). Rapidly, by means of the tools and techniques of pharmaceutical promotion, the drug's uses will expand in the form of off-label prescribing (use of the drug for different problems than its official label specifies), which constitutes the principal means for psychotropic drugs to reach blockbuster status. A couple of years after Neurontin (gabapentin) was approved by the FDA as an adjunctive treatment for epileptic seizures, 90 percent of its prescriptions were for conditions such as ADHD, bipolar disorder, migraine, and depression (Fullerton, Busch, & Frank, 2010). In its heyday, Prozac, initially approved in 1987 for depression, then bulimia and obsessive-compulsive disorder, became prescribed for more than a dozen other conditions, in and out of psychiatry. As Eli Lilly's patent on selling Prozac neared expiration, the company resubmitted Prozac to the FDA for approval as a treatment for Late Luteal Phase Dysphoric Disorder (later renamed Premenstrual Dysphoric Disorder in the *DSM-IV*). Prozac re-emerged in 2000 as Sarafem. Lilly then changed the coating on the Prozac pill so that it would only dissolve fully in the intestine, keeping it longer in the body, and changed its name to Prozac Weekly, which the FDA approved in 2001.

Once on the market, the observation of undesirable or absence of desirable effects not previously detected (or detected during the drug's journey to FDA approval but suppressed from publication) can transform the medication into a public health hazard and limit its use—if patients are lucky. A drug might be available only by prescription for years and then become available for purchase over-the-counter. Immediately, its price, its indications, its usual dosage, and how the public perceives its risks and benefits will dramatically change (Mahecha, 2006).

From Chemical Straitjacket to Happy Pill

Different years have been proposed as marking the start of the twentieth century's so-called psychopharmacological revolution. According to Frankenburg (1994), it's 1931, year of the first studies of *rauwolfia serpentina*, a plant whose extract, reserpine, had a meteoric rise and fall as a treatment for mental illness in the 1950s. According to Strassman (1995), modern biological psychiatry started in 1943, when Albert Hoffman discovered the hallucinogenic lysergic acid diethylamide (LSD). The year 1949 has also been proposed, when psychiatrist John Cade first published his account of administering lithium salts to the inmates of his mental hospital in Australia. Most everyone else, however, has chosen 1952 as the start of the revolution, when the first observations were made public in France that a drug called chlorpromazine could subdue agitated inmates in insane asylums.

Striking Effects on Madmen and Their Keepers

Chlorpromazine was the first to be baptized "neuroleptic" ("that seizes the nerve"). Without putting the subject to sleep, the drug induced a state that its pioneer observers termed "psychic indifference" and which sometimes progressed to a stupor. The unique emotion dampening and behavior subduing effects of neuroleptics (still unequaled by any other drug class) radically changed the internal organization of the asylums and the relations between inmates and their keepers (Cohen, 1997b; Freyhan, 1955).

Over a ten-year period, neuroleptics began to replace impaludations, (a method of treating psychosis by injecting blood infected with malaria), sleep cures, barbiturate comas, insulin comas, electrically-induced seizures, and lobotomies, treatments that had been vogue since the end of the 1910s but had done little to change a popular perception of madness as incurable or of psychiatry as only vaguely related to medicine. In the 1950s, by enabling psychiatrists to prescribe pills to suppress psychosis, chlorpromazine allowed psychiatry to officially accede to the rank of a medical discipline. According to the late French psychiatrist Edouard Zarifian, "There is no medicine without prescriptions. To be medical, psychiatry needed drugs" (1995, p. 74).

Within a year of chlorpromazine's introduction, however, psychiatrists began describing how its tranquilizing action seemed inseparable from newly-appearing neurological impairments, notably parkinsonism and various types of abnormal involuntary movements termed dyskinesia, akinesia, and akathisia. Intriguingly, as a group these movements closely resembled the sequelae of encephalitis lethargica, an epidemic that swept through the world between 1915 and 1926. Pierre Deniker, the French psychiatrist credited with Jean Delay for the first psychiatric uses of chlorpromazine without other drugs, stated he and his colleagues had long realized that, although the neuroleptics were new drugs, their adverse effects were not: "All the side effects of neuroleptics had already been described between 1920 and 1935 as a sequelae of encephalitis" (Deniker, 1989, p. 255). Such realizations, however, did not raise concerns for the simple reason that psychiatrists were not surprised that their treatments could cause damage, even extremely serious damage. Indeed, since the very beginnings of hospital psychiatry, an "effective" treatment was one that could disable the person receiving it. Psychiatrists were completely familiar with the amnesia provoked by electroshocks, the occasional deaths or anoxia produced by prolonged hypoglycemia from insulin coma, and the emotional blunting and loss of volition following lobotomy, a procedure some of them openly described as "partial euthanasia" (see Constans, 1992).

Consider the reminiscences of Heinz Lehmann, who introduced chlorpromazine to North America in 1953, on the sorts of interventions that he used in his Montreal hospital in the 1940s:

> "Our two major therapies were insulin-induced hypoglycemic coma and electric shock therapies . . . Paraldehyde and the barbiturates were about our only means to quell agitation and violence in addition to seclusion and restraint . . . 70% to 80% of [patients] relapsed" (1993, p. 294).

Lehmann therefore experimented with procedures "that would be impossible to repeat today" (p. 295). In an earlier paper, he mentions, among others, "brain biopsies" done on "randomly selected psychotic patients"; "carbon dioxide treatment"; the use of "very large doses of caffeine. . . of course with no results"; nitrous oxide "to the point where there was complete loss of consciousness"; injections of sulphur in oil and typhoid antitoxin, both of which only produced high fevers; injections of "turpentine into the abdominal muscles which produced—and was supposed to produce—a huge sterile abscess and marked leucocytosis" (1989, p. 263). Lehmann's candid accounts, which are here obviously truncated and deserve to be read in full, illustrate how, in devising treatments for their forgotten and socially devalued wards, asylum doctors had little incentives, desires, or training to choose treatments causing least harm.

Most retellings of the revolution brought about by neuroleptics completely ignore that it was only in comparison to these other extremely damaging yet consecrated treatments that neuroleptics were first appraised, and this, *inside* the twisted world of the asylum (Breggin, 1983; Cohen, 1997b). The ease of administering pills and the indisputable gains in bringing order to the asylum carried the day over any strictly medical considerations. Within ten years after the first psychiatric use of chlorpromazine, about thirty similar drugs had been brought to market. The damaging effects of neuroleptics came to preoccupy psychiatry only thirty years later, when an epidemic of tardive dyskinesia (and its legal consequences in the United States in particular) had to be faced and when the modest *therapeutic* gains from neuroleptics were discussed unambiguously in professional journals and meetings (Cohen & McCubbin, 1990). Until that occurred, neuroleptics were universally lauded as the decisive psychiatric advance of the century.

In 1994 a team of four American research psychiatrists analyzed 368 studies spanning the century (published between 1896 and 1992) that reported on clinical outcomes for individuals diagnosed with schizophrenia (or dementia praecox, as it was known or recorded until the 1920s–1940s) and who had received whatever treatment was in vogue during their time (Hegarty et al., 1994). These authors found that overall, 46 percent of patients were rated as improved with antipsychotics, 42 percent with convulsive treatments (electric, insulin, or cardiazol shocks), and 28 percent with lobotomy. The small difference between drugs and shock, considering the reputation held by neuroleptics as uncontrovertible advances over all existing treatments against psychosis, is quite revealing. Moreover, Hegarty and colleagues also found that 29 percent of patients were rated as improved with "nonspecific" interventions, which they defined as "placebo trials, psychotherapy, hydrotherapy, fever therapy, and nonneurological surgery" (p. 1411). This 29 percent might be considered a *baseline* improvement rate in psychotic disorders, regardless of—or despite—any intervention. If so, one would be justified to subtract it from each of the other totals, to get a better sense of their net value, just as in a two-group clinical trial one may deduct placebo response rates from drug response rates to approximate the net response from drugs.

Also, when Hegarty and colleagues examined the twenty studies published just before the end of their review (1986–1992), they calculated an improvement rate (36.4 percent) that they termed "statistically indistinguishable from that found in the first half of the century [35.4%]" (p. 1412). Hegarty and colleagues' investigation provided a unique long-term view showing—just as the twenty-first century CATIE study—that a full generation of antipsychotic drug treatment of schizophrenia did not appear to be any more effective than interventions in vogue during the pre-drug era.

Enter the "Atypicals"

Starting in the early 1990s, forty years after chlorpromazine, a new generation of antipsychotic drugs, called "atypicals" by their promoters, made its appearance. The occasion allowed many psychiatrists to finally rail openly against classical neuroleptics, now portrayed as ineffective and exceedingly toxic, and to express the hope that the newer drugs would solve the problem of psychosis. The atypicals—so called because their makers claimed (1) that their biochemical actions were much broader than those of the older drugs, (2) that they effectively suppressed psychotic symptoms yet did not cause the typical neurological impairments of the older drugs, and (3) that they actually helped reverse the apathy observed in treated patients—were greeted enthusiastically as a new dawn in the treatment of schizophrenia.

One by one, except for clozapine, the five atypical antipsychotics introduced between 1994 and 1999 became blockbusters, their off-label use flourishing due to extremely aggressive marketing. In most cases, this occurred despite early signs that the drugs increased risks of inducing weight gain and metabolic complications such as diabetes. A few dissonant analyses and observations (e.g., Geddes et al., 2000; Cohen, 2002) also showed that the perceived therapeutic progress rested on strained tests or ignoring evidence and common sense, but these were drowned out. One advertisement for Risperdal (risperidone) in the *American Journal of Psychiatry* went as far as to claim that the drug was as harmless as a placebo pill (appeared in April 1994, p. A11).

The atypicals experienced an unprecedented surge in use, spreading to children and older persons and to any diagnosis in which the existing drugs seemed less than satisfactory. We have mentioned that Zyprexa (olanzapine), first approved in 1995 for the treatment of acute schizophrenic episodes, had grossed $45 billion dollars by 2011, becoming one of the world's most profitable medications. However, the publication of the CATIE study in late 2005 and of several other large and non-industry-funded studies around the same time confirmed that these new antipsychotics were neither more effective nor better tolerated than the drugs they had so quickly replaced.

Most observers agreed that, among children and adolescents (targets for off-label prescriptions in the United States during the two decades straddling the centuries), aggressive or hostile behavior probably accounted for most antipsychotic prescribing (Patel et al., 2005). Yet one controlled study of a classic antipsychotic (haloperidol), an atypical antipsychotic (risperidone), and an inert placebo among three groups of youths with intellectual disabilities who showed "challenging aggressive behavior" found that "aggression declined dramatically in all three groups by four weeks, with placebo showing the greatest reduction (79%) (vs. 57% for combined drugs)" (Tyrer et al., 2007). Here again, demonstrations of clinical gains under real-world conditions lagged far behind the claims that drug manufacturers and their proxies made even before their drugs had passed the FDA approval hurdle.

It is still too soon to know the full story of the atypical antipsychotic debacle and to understand how the owners of the drug treatment of schizophrenia,— tens of thousands of highly educated medical practitioners—swallowed drug industry propaganda that the exceedingly complex problem of schizophrenia could be solved by the industry's latest drugs. Jeffrey Lieberman (2006), the lead CATIE investigator and a previously unabashed proponent of the atypicals, summed up the affair:

> The claims of superiority for the [atypicals] were greatly exaggerated. This may have been encouraged by an overly expectant community of clinicians and patients eager to believe in the power of new medications. At the same time, the aggressive marketing of these drugs may have contributed to this enhanced perception of their effectiveness in the absence of empirical information. (p. 1070)

It is tempting to let this quote speak for itself. Still, Lieberman not only described presumably rational psychiatrists "eager to believe in the power of new medications" and embracing "greatly exaggerated" claims *"in the absence of empirical information,"* but doing so fifty years after the arrival of the first antipsychotic, during the flowering of clinical psychopharmacology as the foundational, "evidence-based" activity of psychiatry.

"Beautiful Picture, Isn't It?"

In 1962, researchers showed that antipsychotics bound to neuronal receptors that normally attracted the neurotransmitter dopamine. The drugs were blocking dopamine's flow through its habitual neuronal pathways. Thus was born the "dopamine hypothesis," according to which an excess of dopamine activity causes schizophrenic psychosis. This hypothesis (modified and refined) remained dominant, though it has never enjoyed any directly supporting evidence. In other words, no dopamine abnormality in the brains of never-medicated people diagnosed with schizophrenia has ever been confirmed reliably (Tandon, Keshavan, & Nasrallah, 2008).

As we've discussed, the search for new drugs (for physical disorders) uses animal models to test possibly curative compounds on animals with the disease or to analyze biological causes. The ease with which animals can be studied and sacrificed is the obvious perceived advantage here. "Depressed mice" or "psychotic monkeys," however, can hardly serve as adequate models for depressed or psychotic states in humans (even putting aside the definitional and diagnostic problems covered throughout this book). In psychiatric drug studies, therefore, "animal models" typically consist of observing drug effects on various instinctive or conditioned animal behaviors that only have a tenuous connection to the problems purportedly treated in people. Many animal tests merely screen for drugs that will produce similar effects to those produced by commercially successful drugs on the market, which is how "me-too" drugs appear.

One reason for the focus on neurobiology in the absence of definitive findings may be the extent to which descriptions of biomedical facts over the last two decades have become tied to technological advances that dazzle observers with their appealing images of brain function. Finding that the brains of different people seem to function differently has provided endless fascination for those who see in these differences confirmation that biology "explains" everything disordered in humans. That taxi drivers or musicians show different brain activity on certain spatial or musical tasks than other people seems merely interesting. That depressed people occasionally show different brain functioning than other people, however, "proves" that they're diseased. This logic is erroneous, because subtle physiological difference might arise from experience or learning; it might be a consequence, not a cause, of the person's problem diagnosed as a psychiatric disorder. And such a difference does not mean "disease" unless the meaning of disease is—as we have been suggesting—distorted beyond recognition.

Other advances in molecular biology, especially the ability to label drug molecules with radioactive tracers, allowed scientists to deepen their knowledge on the micromechanisms of neurotransmission and to chart a drug's distribution in the brain. Whereas five to ten substances were identified as neurotransmitters in the 1960s, more than one hundred are identified today, and their multiple functions are only beginning to be revealed. For example, in the 1970s, psychiatrists used to write generally about "dopamine receptor blocking." Dopamine cells are now known to possess five different families of receptors, each of which seems to have quite different functions. For serotonin, at least five subfamilies of receptors have been cloned for only a single of the fourteen families of receptors for that neurotransmitter already identified. But receptor pharmacology, the Holy Grail of psychiatric drug development in the 1990s, is passing on. The post-genomic focus is on proteins and genes whose expressions appear to affect physiological processes that, in some theoretical or in some animal model, might be related to the core physiopathology that—the whole field has committed itself to assume—underlies the *DSM* disorder for which the drug is tested. Moreover, the latest insights within conventional psychopharmacology suggest that current thinking about the importance of neuronal transmission be reevaluated to consider "the other brain," that is made up by glia, the once-thought-inconsequential neural glue that holds the brain together (Fields, 2009).

The notion of chemical imbalance evaporates when reproducible evidence must be provided about the exact nature of pathophysiology in the serotonin or dopaminergic system. The enormously complex play, interplay, and counterplay of the cascades of alterations triggered by drugs binding to receptors and subreceptors has no connection to the claims made for years in advertisements, oft-repeated by journalists, that certain "drugs restore the balance of the serotonin system," as if this balance was actually known or charted (Leo & Lacasse, 2008). Furthermore, as each newly identified neurotransmitter has been immediately considered as a possible player in depression, anxiety, or psychosis, the number of biochemical hypotheses of these problems increased radically during the 1980s, though few lasted for more than a few years. It is difficult to overemphasize how much value these hypotheses, and the new brain imaging technology, had for marketing drugs. Psychiatrist and historian David Healy (2008) put it this way: "When in the 1990s neuroscience threw up colorful images of the brain, marketers found these invaluable for purportedly showing the cleaner effects of SSRIs compared to older antidepressants. There was little neuroscientific value to the images—but they provided wonderful marketing copy" (p. 226). In Healy's view, the monoamine hypothesis of depression—positing a lowering of neurotransmitters that drug treatment corrected—was abandoned by the science of psychopharmacology as early as 1970, but "the serotonin hypothesis was resurrected within the marketing departments of SSRI companies, because it was marketing copy par excellence" (p. 226).

In practical terms the discovery of neuroleptics gave birth to modern biological psychiatry and provided a springboard to develop the neurosciences generally. Yet do we understand psychosis? The inescapable answer is no. Neuroscientifically, after decades of intensive research, it remains completely mysterious why about 1 percent of young people develop "schizophrenia." Scientists merely repeat, mantra-style, that schizophrenia results from an interplay of genetic, biochemical, and environmental factors. A recent review purports to identify no less than seventy-seven distinct "facts" about schizophrenia, yet its authors cannot mention a single universal biological abnormality, let alone specify a single necessary or sufficient cause (Tandon et al., 2008). The authors nonetheless conclude their article by emphasizing the importance of *calling* schizophrenia a *disease.*

At the level of the day-to-day management of very disturbed persons, the discovery of neuroleptics marked a change: the management began to operate from inside patients' bodies even if their keepers and clinicians were physically distant. Centuries ago, controlling the madman meant restraining his body at close proximity, for inside the madman resided a wild beast thought to require restraints and beatings. Later, with electroshock and insulin coma, the "treatments" were directed more specifically toward the brain, but their administration still required close contact between the inmate and the clinician/keeper, a contact that even elicited psychodynamic interpretations of why inmates were terrorized to receive shocks (Dunham & Weinberg, 1960, pp. 181–182). Giving a pill to swallow makes control more efficient because it involves still less contact: hundreds of patients could be treated daily in a single institution. Finally, with the development of long-acting injectable neuroleptics by the late 1960s, a single intramuscular injection every four to six weeks sufficed to maintain the patient under the medication's effect. Between injections, no need to see the patient, to talk with him, to know what he did—he was, after all, deinstitutionalized and others were taking care of his "social integration into the community." Taking in these linear developments, one of us speculated fifteen years ago that the administration of antipsychotic drugs would take a logical next step: subcutaneous implants allowing continuous, unmonitored drug administration for months or years (Cohen, 1996). It should come as no surprise that this option has been studied seriously (Irani et al., 2004; Metzger et al., 2007).

The Other Opium of the Masses

Tranquilizers and sedatives such as the barbiturates and chloral hydrate were widely used prior to the neuroleptics (Lopez-Munoz et al., 2005). Starting in the mid-1950s, two other classes of psychoactive drugs were named: the antidepressants—originally, some anti-tuberculosis medications but mostly modifications of neuroleptics—and the "minor tranquilizers" or "anxiolytics," originally identified because of their muscle-relaxing properties.

The first modern anxiolytic was meprobamate, introduced in 1955 into clinical practice under the brand names Miltown and Equanil. Within five years, it was the most widely used prescription drug in the United States and many other countries. Then came chlordiazepoxide (Librium) in 1960, and diazepam (Valium) in 1963 (Ban, 2006). These two drugs and their cousins, known as benzodiazepines, became hugely popular in primary care medicine, and their prescription increased 100 percent in most Western countries between 1965 to 1970, compared to about 20 percent for other classes of psychotropics (Lader, 1978). The drug industry's promotional efforts, extending a variety of techniques of mass marketing to doctors, has been proposed to explain much of this success (Smith, 1981). Valium appeared in more medical advertisements than any other drug and—cause and effect relation according to some (Krupka & Vener, 1985)—climbed to the rank of number one prescribed drug in the world by 1970.

Observing this phenomenon, sociologists began to produce accounts of the social control function of a growing "medical-industrial complex." They proposed hypotheses that have remained fruitful: tranquilizers medicalize the daily hassles of modern life (especially for women), pacify those people with legitimate grounds for making social and political claims, and distract professionals from discerning any social determinants of psychological distress (Koumjian, 1981). Crowning the 1970s as the "era of benzodiazepines," British psychiatrist Malcolm Lader (1978) designated these drugs as "opium of the masses."

As with other tranquilizers in previous decades, however, a consensus emerged within the medical profession in the 1980s that benzodiazepines carried a risk of dependence with prolonged use (including a withdrawal syndrome when stopped abruptly). These concerns about unwanted effects of benzodiazepines stabilized, then decreased their use in most Western countries, as health authorities enacted various measures (such as triplicate prescriptions, with copies sent to state justice agencies to monitor "unorthodox" scripts) to dissuade doctors from prescribing them. Recently, a spike in prescriptions of Valium was observed in Great Britain, but a comment from Professor Steve Field, chairman of Britain's Royal College of General Practitioners, nicely illustrated the change in attitudes since Valium was number one: "In my own practice we have reduced dramatically the amount of prescribing we do of these kinds of drugs, because they are horrifically addictive, and people can get hooked on them within just a few days" (cited in Donnelly, 2010, para. 8). Similarly, in Louisville, Kentucky, Seven Counties Clinic decided to stop writing all prescriptions for its three thousand patients on Xanax (alprazolam), and some of these patients have been switched to clonazepam (Klonopin), described as "a longer acting benzodiazepine that does not kick in as quickly and is thought to pose less risk of addiction." One doctor stated that on clonazepam, "They don't get the high that's associated with Xanax, nor the withdrawal associated with it" (Goodnough, 2011).[5] The benzodiazepines too followed the path of stigmatization, or the Seige cycle.

The rise of a medical and social debate about tranquilizers and sleeping pills did not mean that doctors abandoned these drugs. Probably because of their quick onset of relaxing effects, benzodiazepines have remained a staple for people in acute distress (especially over losses of spouses, relatives, jobs, and status) who want rapid tranquilization or sleep but not stupor. The drugs provide more than respectable revenues to their manufacturers and are also actively traded on the black market. Importantly, about one quarter of older persons who were introduced to benzodiazepines a generation ago still use them regularly, and fully 40 percent of these users view themselves as "dependent" (Voyer et al., 2010). They generally have no difficulty obtaining benzodiazepines from doctors, who are in effect maintaining these users' dependence. Alprazolam (Xanax), considered one of the most addictive benzodiazepines, vigorously traded in the illicit drug trade, and the subject of extremely little advertising to doctors today, was the sole psychoactive drug appearing among the top fifteen most frequently dispensed (i.e., sold or delivered by pharmacies) prescription drugs in the United States in 2008 (41.5 million prescriptions, up from 33.5 million in 2004; IMS National Prescription Audit, 2010).[6]

Starting in the late 1980s, the backlash against benzodiazepines prompted industry-influenced "key opinion leaders" to encourage general practitioners to alter their prescription of a psychotropic drug (usually to a woman in distress), away from benzodiazepines and toward the new SSRI antidepressants exemplified by Prozac. Precisely as occurred previously and would occur again, the new disorder of concern—depression—was presented as widespread and damaging, and the new class of drugs promoted as effective and harmless—*and* without the bothersome effects (dependence) that were stigmatizing the existing drugs. Perhaps something else a bit more encompassing did happen, as Pieters and Snelders (2009) aptly summarized: "The age of anxiety and blaming society gave way to the age of depression and blaming your own brain" (p. 71). But the new fashion probably would not have occurred without at least two other overlapping events: the arrival in 1980 of the third edition of the *Diagnostic and Statistical Manual of Mental Disorders* of the American Psychiatric Association, and an ever-deepening involvement of the pharmaceutical industry in every facet of psychiatric thinking, research, and practice.

The Waltz of Drugs and Diagnoses

By the 1970s psychiatrists were prescribing about fifty different psychoactive drugs to their patients but could not claim that they had any validated diagnoses. As has been discussed previously in this book, there is still no clinical, radiological, electrical, or other physical test or exam that can reveal, during life or after death, reliable markers in the body of a purported condition called a mental disorder—except of course for drug intoxications and organic psychoses still inexplicably called "mental disorders" in the *DSM*. Thus, how was psychiatry to ensure that diagnoses did not remain merely subjective judgments about distressing thoughts or behaviors, robbing the profession of its medical aspirations?

As we have seen in chapter 4, the *DSM-III* listed criteria for each diagnosis, defined each mental disorder as distinct from others, and added eighty new diagnoses to the previous edition of the *DSM*. The new manual was adopted fairly quickly by other professions sharing the treatment turf. This was a truly significant event because psychology, social work, and counseling had evolved precisely by adopting nonmedical perspectives on deviance and distress. Their embrace of the *DSM-III* began to perfect a theoretical, financial, and bureaucratic integration of the mental health industry, with psychiatry at the top (Kutchins & Kirk, 1988).

More relevant for our discussion of psychoactive drug use, by modifying its diagnostic manual, psychiatry and its institutions of leadership, research, and treatment strengthened their already close association with the pharmaceutical industry into a full-fledged *partnership*. The whole question of classification and diagnosis did not concern clinicians when conversation (psychotherapy) was the prototypical treatment. With the arrival of new drugs and the regulatory requirement that drugs must be effective to treat a "disease," clinicians were directed to classify presenting problems as specific diagnoses, so that their prescribing would resemble prescribing in other branches of medicine (Eisenberg, 1995; Klerman, 1978).

Drug treatment fit beautifully with the *DSM-III*, which presented on the surface a descriptive, symptom-based approach to diagnosis. Mental illnesses became mental "disorders," defined as "not culturally sanctioned" distressing or impairing "symptoms" that resulted from undefined physical, behavioral, or psychological dysfunctions (though the dysfunctions could not be ascertained independently of the symptoms). These symptoms constituted the criteria to make a diagnosis. In turn, the criteria were—in a perfect lateral move— used to compose the items in rating scales that would help to evaluate patients' states in clinical drug trials. Each mental disorder named in the *DSM-III* was automatically assumed to be a clinical entity, the pathophysiology of which was unknown but assumed to be elucidated with future research.

The technological advances we briefly described earlier, which allowed researchers to trace drug molecules until they reached cell membrane receptors, stimulated the development of speculative animal models and of molecules synthesized to bind more tightly to receptors. As psychiatrist Edouard Zarifian remarked, pharmacologists and neurobiologists "formulate hypotheses on the causes of a disorder and, once they have invented a molecule, explain to the doctor the effects that they are expected to observe" (1994, p. 88).

Thus, during most of the century no one seemed to complain of "panic attacks" and doctors could not name this problem when they saw it, nor did they easily assimilate it within the realm of anxiety. But two drugs (imipramine, an old tricyclic antidepressant and alprazolam [Xanax], a new benzodiazepine anxiolytic) began to be promoted as specific treatments for *DSM-III*'s new panic disorder in the early 1980s. According to Kramer (1993), psychiatrists had to re-create anxiety in theoretical terms. Several authors have described the symbiosis between drug makers and the diagnosis: the Upjohn drug company apparently funded the entire effort, culminating the creation of the diagnosis of Panic Disorder in *DSM-III* with the sole intention of obtaining approval to market Xanax as specific treatment for . . . panic disorder (Elliott, 2003; Lane, 2007). Almost instantly, panic disorder acquired an incontestable "reality." This made psychologist David Jacobs (1995) observe how remarkable it was that problems without distinct boundaries, created with the pragmatic aim of drug treatment, came to be promoted as if medicine possessed discriminating data on their pathophysiology.

In the background, psychiatric epidemiology was reporting an increase in the prevalence of mental disorder, notably depression. In 1984, using *DSM-III* criteria, the vast Epidemiological Catchment Area Survey of the National Institute of Mental Health estimated the prevalence of depression during a person's life to be 6 percent, the highest rate ever reported (Robins & Regier, 1991). Ten years later, another national survey using *DSM-III-R* criteria reported the rate as 17 percent, and for all mental disorders, 48 percent (Kessler et al., 1994).

At the level of populations, psychological distress waxes and wanes and is affected by political and economic instability (Cross-National Collaborative Group, 1992). Nonetheless, this new increase seemed *inflationary*, reflecting medicalization and the promotion of antidepressant drugs. According to business journalist James Krohe (1994), who wrote in the midst of the Prozac craze, "Depression is the latest product—and the most promising—of the wellness industry" (p. 24). In the workplace, concern about depression began to replace concerns about alcohol and substance abuse, creating new possibilities for counselors and administrators. Krohe described a web of phone hotlines, support groups, conferences and seminars for health administrators, free anonymous screening programs, infomercials, and public interest TV shows launched "to catch the two out of three depressed Americans who are not seeking treatment—almost 7.5 millions people who, in their misery, persist in confusing treatable depression with life" (p. 24). The National Depression Screening Day was inaugurated in 1991 on a college campus, subsidized by the maker of Prozac. By 1995, "In each of the 50 states and the District of

Columbia, people can be tested for free to see if they are depressed or are at risk of so becoming" (Screening the Public, 1995, p. A42).

Its territory greatly enlarged, mental disorder became banal. Abnormality became, well, normal. Validly distinguishing whether someone truly had a mental disorder became somewhat irrelevant, given that half the population of the United States was designated as diagnosable with a chronic, recurrent, unpredictable mental disorder. Indeed, how could one even distinguish disorder from nondisorder if the former was characterized by impossible-to-detect variations of neurotransmitter circuits? Pieters and Snelders (2009) have also alluded to what they call this "democratization of mental disorders." They recall that a drug company once advertised depression as "the most democratic of all disorders. It can affect everyone at any moment, for shorter or longer duration, without a recognizable course" (p. 71).

Two decades earlier, self-styled antipsychiatrists were claiming that everyone was sane, or everyone was insane. Their goal had been to abolish boundaries between sanity and madness, pushing society toward their ideal of equality. In some fashion, that goal was realized with the arrival of the SSRI antidepressants of the late 1980s and the widespread popular acceptance that despair, deviance, and distress were actually symptoms of medically treatable mental disorders. The drugs and the *DSM* seemed to have energized a new societal project of moral leveling, in which everyone is equal because everyone is diagnosable and treatable. Society and government could not be changed, but *neurochemistry* certainly could (Greenberg, 2010).

Does Cure Prove Anything?

By focusing on the many symptoms of disorders finely chopped by the *DSM* and by invoking variations in neurotransmitter functioning that were becoming more easily imaged and presumably targeted by drugs, psychiatry could cease pursuing an elusive goal required for unquestioned membership in the realm of scientific medicine: to validate traditional diagnostic entities according to cellular models of disease. The new psychiatric diagnoses and their symptoms multiplied the possibilities to observe, in any behavior the least bit disturbing to a person or their network, a symptom calling for drug treatment. Mere descriptions of the habitual neuronal effects of drugs were recast as *demonstrations* that symptoms hid specific neurochemical imbalances. The way was open to *validate a diagnosis by medicating a complaint.*

American journalist James Wright (1994) illustrated the sway of this logic when he indicated that American policymakers who wished to provide equal insurance coverage for mental health as for physical health claimed that "the simple fact that pharmacology gives results is proof that mental illness are bona fide illnesses." Wright asked approvingly: "But if a successful chemical treatment constitutes the distinctive sign of an illness, why are not all conditions treated by means of cosmetic psychopharmacology considered as illnesses? And why shouldn't they be?" (p. 25). Scientific demonstration of the existence of disease had been turned on its head, replaced with circular definitions. What is an illness? Whatever a medication treats "successfully."

The *necessity* of a medication was indicated by its positive results. In turn, these were demonstrated by the medication's widespread use, especially by an increasing chorus of users' appreciative testimonies. Consumers wanted and were incited by marketing to ask for antidepressants, drugs only available from physicians. As a result, scientific constraints on psychiatrists were loosened. They were again freed from justifying why one scientific/clinical model is worthier than another. Comforted by their patients' narratives of relief, improvement, or recovery, psychiatrists could view the whole point of their enterprise as prescribing drugs in response to patients' complaints. Predictably, such use of drugs bred dependence on drugs, and an avalanche of well-publicized clinical trials demonstrating contrived improvements for other complaints isolated remaining skeptics. Other interventions besides prescription grew more unfamiliar, and trying them would trigger uncomfortable discussions about the point of looking at distress as medical pathology.

If consumerism does indeed drive prescription, if patients receive just what they ask for, how then can we distinguish psychopharmacology from quackery? For philosopher of science Isabelle Stengers (1995), modern medicine is defined by the awareness of a single fact, itself stemming from the scientific repudiation of Anton Mesmer's "magnetic treatment" at the end of the eighteenth century. The fact is this: "*Cure proves nothing*" (p. 121, italics in original). Then, as now, reports by people that they felt better or cured as a result of exposure to some intervention (then, magnets, trees, or objects "magnetized" by Mesmer; today, psychoactive drugs consecrated by clinical trials and FDA approval) cannot constitute proof that the people suffered from genuine diseases or that magnets or drugs are genuine treatments. Stengers adds a corollary to her fact: "The aim pursued by medicine (cure) does not suffice to distinguish between rational practice and quackery" (p. 121). In other words, the physician's intention to cure the patient also cannot distinguish medical practice from that of the charlatan who merely seeks profit or aggrandizement. Yet, in psychiatry, as exemplified by the success of Peter Kramer's *Listening to Prozac*, it was precisely the personal testimony of symptom relief, the narrative of transformed personality—in sum, the tale of the "cure"—that was put forth as the irrefutable proof of the validity of psychopharmacology.

What Psychoactive Drugs Seem to Do

The long history of drugs and medications amply demonstrates the richness of their effects on users as well as on the experts and authorities charged with regulating drugs. No discovery in neurobiology is necessary to grasp that psychoactive drugs have powerful effects that people might find desirable or undesirable or both. With a high enough dose, a psychoactive drug will affect virtually all people who take it. Yet its effects can vary slightly or greatly between individuals and are often unpredictable in any one person or even in the same person at different times. Depending on a person's state of distress, for example, a drug effect might be experienced positively, and the person might decide that the drug is beneficial to him or her. Is there any reason to think that this person is reacting in a way that indicates underlying *pathophysiology*? We believe not.

We have argued so far that a great deal of the measurable success of a prescribed psychotropic medication appears to rest on a placebo effect—admittedly an inadequate concept insofar as it refers to something that can include suggestion from oneself, suggestion from other people and institutions, spontaneous remission of one's troubles, as well as active self-improvement through deliberate and unknown methods triggered by the mere fact of having ingested what one believes to constitute a genuine treatment. But, in a complementary though not similar line of thought, we have also argued that another ingredient seems necessary for the success of a psychoactive drug, and that is, of course, a psychoactive effect. We have argued that psychoactive effects of prescribed drugs are ubiquitous, but that clinical trials and conventional psychiatric investigations have rarely if ever focused on the nature of such psychoactive effects, and especially how psychoactive effects as reported by users are related to the occasional evaluations of therapeutic benefits reported by users or inferred by clinicians. Thus we conclude that very much remains to be discovered about the nature of the varied psychoactive effects produced by the panoply of psychiatric medications on the market today. We venture what we consider to be reasonable observations, but their limitations will be immediately apparent.

In the case of nonconsenting or disturbing individuals (for example, children, psychotics, and the demented elderly in nursing homes), the aim of drugging is simply the control of outward behavior that bothers or offends other people or hampers the smooth functioning of institutions. In these cases, the finality of the prescription is to please these other people, and the favored psychoactive and behavioral effects for the conditions displayed by such individuals therefore usually consist of some form of compliance, reduced spontaneity, on-task-performance (stimulants), sedation or drowsiness, or indifference (neuroleptics). How the drug users themselves might appreciate the drug is of secondary concern, if at all.

The aim of drugging obviously differs in the case of consenting, consumerist adults, but here the situation gets increasingly murky and difficult to understand. The SSRIs, exemplars of the modern consumerist medications, may have succeeded partly because in the social, cultural, and economic context since their FDA approval, their most marketed psychoactive effects seemed to consist of a mild arousal believed to enhance the competitive capacities of citizens in the West, "exhausted by work, scared by unemployment, anxious about the future, [and] spellbound by the media" (Ramonet, 1995, p. 13). But with hindsight, the picture must be much more complex, as the SSRIs appear to produce sedation as much as they produce activation and arousal, and the latter are not seen by users as improving but rather as impairing function. And what to make of another important psychophysiological effect of SSRIs, the suppression of libido or sexual desire (the prevalence of which might suggest classifying the SSRIs primarily as sex-drive reducers)? It is tempting to speculate how such an effect might have dovetailed with many adults' anxiety-laden experiences of sexuality in the age of AIDS and on-demand online pornography.

But neither placebo nor psychoactive effects can fully account for how Valium, Prozac, and Zyprexa became blockbuster drugs that dramatically altered or reinforced professional practices, popular perceptions, and pharmaceutical profits. Another ingredient has been necessary, especially in the age of science. We have referred to it repeatedly throughout this book, and we turn presently to examine it in more detail, paying special attention to its intertwining with research in psychiatry. This ingredient is the marketing of drugs by the pharmaceutical industry. The topic has been covered admirably in scholarly, insider, and journalistic accounts over the past decade (e.g., Critser, 2005; Elliott, 2010; Healy, 2012; Moynihan & Cassels, 2005; Petersen, 2008), and we have little original analysis to add to these, except to reinforce the notion that it is today no longer possible to discern where psychiatry and psychiatric science begin and where drug industry marketing ends.

Paradisio Promotion

Since the passage in 1951 of the Humphrey-Durham amendment to the Pure Food, Drug, and Cosmetic Act of 1938, getting certain psychoactive drugs inside people's bodies has required a physician's prescription (Abood, 2011). Accounts of pharmaceutical marketing agree on one thing: the pharmaceutical industry has magnificently honed its ability to make physicians "decide" to prescribe its products. Given the time, effort, and money spent by the industry to promote drugs, this should surprise no one.

As noted earlier, Canadian accountant Marc-André Gagnon and emergency physician Joel Lexchin (2008) analyzed several databases and proprietary expenditure reports to generate a startling estimate of the US pharmaceutical industry's total spending to push pills in 2004: $57.5 billion. This gargantuan amount is in addition to the $31.5 billion that the industry said it spent that year on clinical trials and tests for its products. With total sales of pharmaceuticals in the US that year totaling $235.4 billion, promotional spending therefore made up 24.4 percent of sales (nearly double the spending on research and development). In 2011, sales of antipsychotics, antidepressants, stimulants, and anticonvulsants in the United States were reported to total $43.0 billion (IMS Health, 2011). Using 24.4 percent of sales for promotional spending as our yardstick gives the sum of nearly $10.5 billion spent by the industry to promote only these four classes of drugs in America. Using Gagnon and Lexchin's breakdown of the categories and proportions of marketing expenses for all pharmaceutical products, table 7-1 gives one idea how the $10.5 billion might have been spent to promote antipsychotics, antidepressants, stimulants, and anticonvulsants.

Table 7-1
Estimate of Promotional Spending on Four Classes of Prescribed
Psychotropic Drugs, USA, 2011

Type of promotion	Spending (in $ billions)	% of total spending
Detailing by sales representatives	3.73	35.5
Drug samples	2.9	27.7
Unmonitored promotion	2.6	25.0
Direct-to-consumer advertising	.73	7.0
Continuing medical education	.37	3.5
Journal advertising	.11	~1.0
E-promotion, mailings	.05	~0.5

The billions of dollars spent each year obviously show how industry marketing can operate on a gigantic scale. The marketing of no other treatment or intervention comes close to drugs in terms of the support that these products enjoy and in terms of the creative energies continually invested to make everyone view them as indispensable. The success of the enterprise hereby appears not as natural or self-evidently justifiable. Rather, it appears to require these billions of dollars to ensure that, first, prescribers cooperate, and second, the public asks for or is willing to accept drugs, to keep the American psychiatric drug enterprise moving along smoothly each year. But the figures suggest that at least (and probably much more than) three-quarters of all promotional spending targets physicians or health care professionals. One might conclude that it has been relatively easy to turn the public into a willing participant, a willing believer.

How Industry Marketing Shapes Everything

The monies spent on drug marketing operate in myriad ways. One way is via free or subsidized continuing education courses offered to physicians by key opinion leaders. Communication companies earned over $1 billion in 2004 to deliver industry-sponsored continuing medical education. Industry-sponsored courses find subtle but effective ways to highlight sponsors' drugs and are associated with increased prescriptions of those drugs (Elliott, 2004; Wazana, 2000). The US Senate expressed concern over drug firms' influence on continuing medical education and its impact on off-label drug prescriptions. The Committee on Finance (2007) of the US Senate describes how pharmaceutical firms have "too much influence" over the content of "supposedly independent educational programs." At least one quarter of all accredited CME providers fail to ensure independence of content. The courses are described as forms of "veiled advertising."

Pharmaceutical companies' money is used for lobbying at all levels of government and making donations to political parties and to senators' and congressmen's re-election campaigns. The money influences legislators and government agencies to approve drugs and create favorable conditions for the industry (such as deducting opportunity costs to develop drugs that fail to gain approval). In addition, the drug industry agreed with the provisions of the Prescription Drug User Fee Act, which requires drug manufacturers to pay substantial user fees to the FDA's Center for Drug Evaluation and Research to finance the process of government approval of the manufacturers' drugs, in return for speedier approval times. In 2011, users fees were expected to add up to $707 million, fully 65 percent of the budget of the FDA department responsible for evaluating the efficacy and safety of prescription drugs and about 25 percent of the total FDA budget (Dutton, 2011). It is easy to understand how such fees, presented as natural payments for services rendered, make the FDA a stakeholder in the commercial success of the pharmaceutical industry.

Looking at lists of the recipients of funds from some drug companies' charitable foundations (which some states have been requiring be disclosed and federal legislation has mandated as of 2011), one gets a sense of the intimate penetration of drug company money into the widest-ranging activities and to countless groups, organizations, and individuals (Cohen, 2008). These funds paid for scholarships; fellowships and research awards for medical students, young researchers, and established senior researchers; consulting and teaching opportunities for clinicians; endowed chairs for professors in academia; large research project and other centers within academia and university-affiliated hospitals; mental disorder screening initiatives and events in universities, workplaces, and communities; continuing education courses for health care professionals on "diseases" in the public eye for which particular drugs are now being advertised; professional and consumer magazines and newsletters; diagnostic task force committee members; grand rounds in hospital departments; breakfasts and lunches in medical schools, clinics, and hospitals; encyclopedias, books, prescription guides, and subscriptions to journals; funds (and sometimes lent personnel) for operation, research, and promotion of small, medium, and large nonprofit interest and advocacy groups that can be counted on to propagate a pro-drug message to their constituencies. In this connection, for example, the National Alliance for Mental Illness, widely considered the nation's leading family and patient advocacy organization and therefore obligatorily represented in any mainstream policy forum, received no less than 81 percent of its 2009 funding from drug firms, becoming, for all practical purposes, more of an advocate for drug companies rather than for families of patients (NAMI's Pharma Funders, 2010).

Table 1 shows that visits to doctors by drug reps constitutes the key marketing vehicle in the drug industry. The amount devoted to drug reps is consistent with estimates of their number in the United States, with about 85,000–100,000, or one rep for every six to ten doctors (Oldani, 2004; Greene, 2004; Fugh-Berman & Ahari, 2007). A *Time Magazine* guest column entitled "Attack of the Pharma Babes" emphasized the personal attractiveness and seductiveness of many drug reps (Haig, 2007). In a first-rate account of the tactics drug reps use with physicians and of the psychology of gift-giving in these relationships, physician and ethicist Carl Elliott (2006) writes:

> When an encounter between a doctor and a rep goes well, it is a delicate ritual of pretense and self-deception. Drug reps pretend that they are giving doctors impartial information. Doctors pretend that they take it seriously. Drug reps must try their best to influence doctors, while doctors must tell themselves that they are not being influenced. Drug reps must act as if they are not salespeople, while doctors must act as if they are not customers. And if, by accident, the real purpose of the exchange is revealed, the result is like an elaborate theatrical dance in which the masks and costumes suddenly drop off and the actors come face to face with one another as they really are. Nobody wants to see that happen.

Drug marketing via individual detailing influences physicians to prescribe drugs essentially by offering them gifts, such as free drug samples. The importance of drug samples, again indicated by the amount of money that drug companies spent on them, lies in the simple fact that the sample introduces a drug into a doctor's office for the first time. This will influences both patients' and doctors' brand choices, and later generate sales. The return on this investment can be substantial, with studies suggesting that up to $10 in sales can result for every $1 spent on samples (Chew et al. 2000; Adair & Holmgren, 2005; Backer et al. 2000). Contrary to common sense, small and relatively inexpensive gifts (such as pens, pads, and meals) may be a powerful form of influence: in some studies, the more small gifts a doctor received, the more the doctor believed that they had no influence on his prescribing (Reist & VandeCreek, 2004; Dana & Loewenstein, 2003; Oldani, 2004). These studies suggest that the small gift, precisely because it is inexpensive and therefore easy to accept, has enormous strategic significance. It simultaneously confirms (for the rep) and masks (for the doctor) the realization that the doctor can be bought.

Direct-to-consumer advertising (DTCA)—which took off in the United States in 1997 when the FDA dropped its requirement that any advertisement for a prescription drug must contain the complete list of adverse reactions—would be likely to increase psychiatric drug use via three main mechanisms: it encourages people to visit doctors for ailments portrayed; it encourages patients to request drugs advertised; and it influences doctors' behavior through patient requests. There is evidence that physicians "are frequently unaware of and denied the degree to which their thinking was biased by patient requests [for antidepressants]" (Tentler et al., 2008), alongside evidence from controlled trials that patient requests for an antidepressant—either brand-specific or in general—"have a profound effect on physician prescribing in major depression and adjustment disorder" (Kravitz et al., 2005, p. 1995). The argument has been made that the most heavily advertised drugs are the newest drugs, by definition, those about which least is known, and also by definition the costliest drugs, thus increasing spending by stimulating their sales (Donohue & Bernd, 2004; Gellad & Lyles, 2007).

The accuracy of DTC ads has regularly been questioned by the FDA, whose mandate includes reviewing ads for accuracy of content. Only people who believe that ads are an easily accessible form of information and education might be surprised that they are frequently misleading. From 1995 to 2004, the FDA sent 1,359 warning letters to drug companies for what it deemed false or misleading advertising. Throughout the early 2000s, four FDA staffers reviewed thousands of ads (Zalesky, 2006). Between 2001 and 2005, the FDA found ads for a hundred and fifty different drugs false or misleading. Misleading messages mostly targeted doctors; 35 percent of the ads misrepresented the degree of risk from the drug, 22 percent promoted unproven uses, and 38 percent made unsupported claims. For example, according to the FDA, a 2007 ad for Geodon (atypical antipsychotic) aimed at doctors neglected to mention the risks of neuroleptic malignant syndrome (a potentially fatal explosive neurological and metabolic attack), tardive dyskinesia (permanent abnormal movement disorders), hyperglycemia, and diabetes. The ad also exaggerated claims of efficacy of Geodon over older, unbranded generic antipsychotics (think back to the CATIE study). To what extent the FDA succeeds in enforcing its requests for drug companies' conformity to the law remains completely unclear, as, despite some massive financial penalties imposed on various manufacturers for not divulging safety data, for misbranding drugs, and for illegal marketing, the same companies are observed to be in violation year after year.[7]

Pharmaceutical companies or their subcontractors enlist academics to form expert panels to construct guidelines and algorithms that assert or argue that newer, more expensive drugs (SSRIs and atypical antipsychotics) are more effective and must become first-line treatments in the absence of definitive data or the presence of contradictory data (Healy, 2006a). In some states, such algorithms are promoted by means of covert, illicit cash payments to state officials responsible to make the drugs eligible for government funding (Moynihan, 2004). In other cases, generous payments—licit and later disclosed—are made to members of state advisory panels that help select the billions worth of drugs that Medicaid programs will reimburse for the poor and disabled (CBS News, 2007). In his later analyses, Healy (2012) has made the more encompassing and worrying argument that industry-paid academic panels as well as independent government-funded councils always appear to agree to recommend the industry's latest drugs for whatever ailment is being considered, for the simple reason that the "evidence" (the studies and clinical trials) these different sources review is, in large measure, industry-generated.

On the one hand, the drug industry's marketing efforts and its massive infusions of money to support psychiatric activities, and on the other hand psychiatry's enthusiastic acceptance of the partnership, have *completely subsumed psychiatry as a satellite branch of the multinational pharmaceutical industry*. Undoubtedly, several branches of medicine are "on the take" (Kassirer, 2005), with many of their practitioners, researchers, and professional associations awash in (mostly undisclosed) conflicts of interests that destroy the credibility of their pronouncements and the trustworthiness of their conduct (Committee on Finance, 2011). Yet, as we have indicated throughout this chapter, psychiatry may be unique in the extent to which intellectual and practical innovations and fashions in that field center around the industry's introduction of new drugs, the "discovery" and marketing of new uses for recently introduced drugs, and the expansion of *DSM* disorder categories both to accommodate and to stimulate the popularity of new drugs. Some partial data from Minnesota appear to illustrate the special impact on psychiatry of the industry's funds. In that state between 1997 and 2005, not only did psychiatrists as a group receive more money from drug companies than any other types of physicians (Harris, 2007; Ross et al., 2007), but within the group of psychiatrists, those who received more than $5,000 wrote on average four times more prescriptions of atypical antipsychotics off-label to children than those receiving less than that amount (Harris, Carey, and Roberts, 2007).

The Paralysis of Science

The virtually complete blurring of marketing and science has paralyzed science—or what has passed as science. Conflicts of interest permeate the FDA and its advisory committees, scientific journals, and the scientific literature. Telling an infomercial from a scientific article requires analysis of primary (usually proprietary) sources (Jureidini, McHenry, & Mansfield, 2008), most of which are only revealed accidentally, during legal proceedings, for example (Steinman, Bero, Chren, & Landfeld, 2006). Commenting only on ghostwriting—the practice of paying academics to lend their names to publications without having seen or collected the data reported (Lacasse & Leo, 2010)—the *PLoS Medicine* editors (2009) lamented that marketing campaigns now center on "evidence" provided by seemingly respectable academic review articles, original research articles, and even reports of clinical trials. What, a cynical reader might ask, can I truly trust as being unbiased? The answer is that, sadly, for some or even many journal articles, we just don't know. (p. 1)

More recently, however, Healy (2012) has provided some extremely sobering estimates, with supporting sources, to answer the *PLoS Medicine* editors' question: "We also now know that close to 30 percent of the clinical trials that have been undertaken remain unreported, and that of the 50 percent that are reported almost all will be ghostwritten and roughly 25 percent of the published trials altered to the extent that a negative result for a drug will have been transformed into evidence the drug works well and is safe. In 100 percent of cases, the data from trials remain inaccessible to scrutiny" (pp. 252–253).

When the editor of the *New England Journal of Medicine* sought a research psychiatrist with no ties to the drug industry to evaluate an SSRI trial, she could find none (Angell, 2000). When the *American Journal of Psychiatry* published a pediatric trial of citalopram (Celexa) that reported positive results, neither the authors nor the editors disclosed (or knew) that a previous unpublished pediatric trial funded by the same sponsor had observed opposite results (Meier, 2004). When an article in *JAMA* warned pregnant women not to stop taking antidepressants because of the risk of re-experiencing depression, most of the thirteen authors did not disclose their financial ties to makers of antidepressants (DeAngelis, 2006). Medical journals appear to struggle to manage disclosure but not necessarily with great success, as virtually no negative consequences are imposed, or even threatened, on violators (Lacasse & Leo, 2010). Occasionally, the editors of prominent journals shoot themselves in the foot in full view of their readership and constituencies, asserting that they fully control the problem while simultaneously failing to screen obvious violations and then awkwardly managing the consequences (Leo, 2009).

It has now become well established that the funding source of a drug's clinical trial is associated with the trial's formal conclusion that the drug should be used. Als-Nielsen and colleagues (2003) showed that in RCTs in eight medical disciplines, regardless of the magnitude of the drug's effect relative to placebo or the presence of adverse effects, trials funded by for-profit organizations were 5.3 times more likely to recommend the drug than trials funded by not-for-profit organizations. In the case of antipsychotics, researcher Stephan Heres and colleagues (2006) examined the outcomes of thirty head-to-head comparisons of different atypical antipsychotics and looked for relationships with sponsorship. In twenty-seven comparisons (90 percent), the outcome favored the sponsor's drug. This pattern "resulted in contradictory conclusions across studies when the findings of studies of the same drugs but with different sponsors were compared" (p. 185). In other words, when Eli Lilly funded a study comparing its Zyprexa with Janssen's

Risperdal, Zyprexa came out ahead. When Janssen funded the exact same comparison, Risperdal came out ahead.

In light of their own observation of "biased interpretation of trial results," Als-Nielsen et al. warned readers to "carefully evaluate whether conclusions in randomized trials are supported by data" (2003, p. 921). Indeed, when Australian child psychiatrist Jon Jureidini and colleagues (2004) published their groundbreaking review of pediatric SSRI trials that concluded that benefits had been exaggerated while risks downplayed, they had (not yet) found a smoking gun (Leo, 2006). They had simply underlined misleading conclusions in the original publications, such as their authors' pronouncing a 10 percent drug-placebo difference as "clinically significant" and downplaying strikingly high rates of serious adverse effects in drug-treated children relative to placebo. But what if the study's data are not published, or a report of the study is published with different data than were actually collected? Psychiatric researcher Erik Turner and colleagues (2008) retrieved seventy-four FDA-registered antidepressant trials of several antidepressants and compared their data to what had appeared in refereed journal publications. They found that thirty-six of thirty-seven trials with positive results had been published, compared to three of twenty-two with negative results. For eleven other trials with negative or questionable results in the FDA database, their journal publications spun the results positively. Overall, 94 percent of published trials showed drugs as superior to placebo, whereas only 51 percent of the full dataset of seventy-four trials showed such positive results. The problem here is simply that the published trial reports are much more easily available and distributed with the approval and review of peer reviewers and prestigious scientific journals and therefore are customarily taken as *the* record of the trial, *the* scientific literature. (Most readers might not know that an FDA record exists and is usually available to them from the FDA website, though it might need to be searched for within a voluminous FDA review of a particular drug.)

The authors of the two major reviews of psychiatric trials we have discussed, Turner and colleagues (2008) and Heres and colleagues (2006), make some seemingly obligatory hedging statements in their articles, wanting to appear to be completely fair by considering all possibilities, or perhaps having acquiesced to an editor or reviewer's request. Turner et al. (2008) state that selective publication of data and trials misleads all those who rely on the scientific literature, but they state that they cannot establish for certain just why negative trials of antidepressants are not published. Similarly, Heres et al. (2006) identify a dozen possible sources of bias in the head-to-head comparisons of antipsychotics but cannot state which might end up favoring the sponsors' drugs and "limit the validity" of such comparisons. It is, of course, entirely appropriate and even desirable for scientists to be cautious in drawing conclusions. Perhaps they are personally unsure about which conclusions should be reached. They may entertain doubts about the purposes of the drug industry and the extent to which the industry might plot to alter outcomes of studies to favor its products. But in this case, researchers' and editors' and conscientious practitioners' willingness to hedge, to consider every possible interpretation, to step back from what is the most probable reality, leaves only one player in this drama that has no doubt, no hesitancy, no incentive to pursue the truth, and no ambivalence about its goals and the behavior of other players—and that is the drug industry.

In our view, what has occurred and what is occurring is the systematic manipulation of the scientific process to reach predetermined conclusions, which means, the paralysis of science as an unbiased enterprise to advance knowledge or even as a pragmatic enterprise to improve the quality of human life. The current trend is toward increased disclosure and transparency in scientific publications and increased verification (for example, via the constitution of clinical trial registries in which the aims and protocols of drug trials are announced in advance) of the drug industry's claims. New rules, however, require broader enforcement, while existing rules have yet to be enforced consistently. In any case, increased scrutiny often leads violators to search new outlets to practice their reproachable but enormously profitable behavior. This being the case, increased transparency is bound to trigger, at least temporarily, even more creative marketing efforts designed to mislead and seduce professionals and the public with the appearance of science.

Conclusion

Does the psychiatric drug treatment of emotional distress and misbehavior constitute a genuine improvement over the practices of the past, or is it merely the recycling of age-old tendencies to palliate distress and control disturbing behavior by psychoactive sedation or stimulation? Are clinical psychopharmacologists members of a scientifically driven discipline or merely the willing executors of mad science, the vast, well-orchestrated advertising campaigns by the pharmaceutical industry to increase market shares of the drug du jour? Our questions purposefully impose a dichotomous template on complex and multilayered issues because the former positions have been too uncritically promoted and accepted as self-evidently true. Still, if simple answers were to be given, we think the evidence overwhelmingly supports the latter positions in both of these questions.

As psychoactive drugs continue to be promoted as harmless and essential products for modern citizens, but as the boundaries between licit and illicit drug use continue to blur, more profound changes may be in the works. For example, the Internet has helped to democratize to some extent the conversation between doctors, patients, and regulators. Online, laypersons now frequently disseminate their views and reviews of psychoactive drugs, unfiltered by professionals, and freely offer each other advice on using this or that drug in this or that way, obtaining it this or that way, or ceasing to take it this or that way. Some consumer-constructed websites (e.g., askapatient. com) offer thousands of individual patient reviews for hundreds of drugs, including real-time graphs and charts of efficacy and adverse effect evaluations from large groups of users (e.g., patientslikeme.com). No comparable data has ever existed before, anywhere.

A first comparison of discourse about two prescribed psychotropic medications (an antidepressant and an antipsychotic) appearing on consumer-constructed and professionally controlled websites on the Internet found that both types of sources "generally reported similar effects" of the two medications "but differed in their descriptions and in frequency of reporting. Professional medication descriptions offer the advantage of a concise yet comprehensive listing of drug effects, while consumer reviews offer the advantage of greater context and situational examples of how effects may manifest in various combinations and to varying degrees" (Hughes and Cohen, 2011). No one can tell where the trend regarding consumer contributions is headed, but these and many other findings we have discussed throughout this book make one thing clear: knowledge about psychiatric drugs is increasingly being constructed completely outside the usual expert disciplines and will involve possibly as-yet-unknowable players.

Public cynicism concerning the integrity of psychiatric knowledge continues to grow, in parallel with the democratization of information and the appeal of self-care and self-directed performance enhancement that have always characterized much of the use of psychotropic drugs throughout history and culture. As a result, psychiatric-professional assertions of unique or specialized knowledge in psychopharmacology will become increasingly contested, just as they have been in this and the previous chapter.

But there is more. Periodic revelations concerning the profession's unjustified, scientifically unsophisticated, and crassly bought enthusiasm over this or that psychoactive drug class, and the sweeping under the carpet of the victims of the enthusiasm may also threaten drug prescription authority—the key legal prerogative presently resting on the assumption of medical and psychiatric expertise and accountability. We find it intriguing that two of the best-known psychiatric critics, the late US psychiatrist Thomas Szasz, and UK psychiatrist David Healy, whose views on the nature of mental illness and the legitimate sphere of state-sponsored psychiatry differ dramatically, have nonetheless both proposed the abolition of medical prescription privileges (and not merely their redistribution to clinical psychologists, for example). Do people really need psychiatrists (or anyone else claiming special knowledge) to give them permission to take the psychoactive drugs they want?

Notes

1. Although we use these two words interchangeably in this chapter, the careful speaker might wish to distinguish them. We borrow here from Thomas Szasz (2007), who notes that according to Thomas Ban (2001), the first person to use the word *psychotropic* was Ralph Waldo Gerard (1900–1974), an American physiologist, in the late 1950s. Under the new moniker, Gerard included only the six then-modern *psychiatric* drugs: "neuroleptics, i.e., chlorpromazine and reserpine . . . antidepressants, i.e., iprionazid . . . and imipramine . . . an anxiolytic, i.e. meprobamate . . . and a mood stabilizer, i.e., lithium carbonate" (Ban, 2001, p. 712). Szasz points out: "All of these drugs were introduced in a 6-year period, 1949–1957. Note that chlorpromazine heads the list and that not one of these drugs is a substance a healthy person uses, or would want to use, as a recreational drug" (p. 173–174). Szasz's point is that *psychotropic* is a modern semantic confusion designed to bracket modern psychiatric drugs from other psychoactive substances, that is, to avoid putting *all* psychoactive drugs—drugs that have a direct effect on mental activity and behavior—on an equal footing for accurate comparison purposes. Google's N-gram database shows that the use of both terms between 1960 to 2000 in American English runs parallel, with *psychoactive* experiencing a relative decline between 1980 and 1990. Our own impression is that authors who use both terms use them interchangeably. However, we think authors usually favor *psychotropic*, especially when discussing *prescribed* psychoactive drugs.

2. This section is drawn from a number of books and articles written by and with British psychiatrist Joanna Moncrieff (Moncrieff, 2008; Moncrieff & Cohen, 2005, 2006, 2009; Moncrieff, Mason, and Cohen, 2009; Moncrieff, Porter, & Cohen, 2012).

3. Although this is far beyond the scope of this chapter and this book, we note that biochemists and molecular biologists increasingly discuss drugs as acting not merely on cells' membrane receptors to change processes inside and around the cell but also—in some as yet not well-understood manner—changing the expression of genes. Gene expression is the process by which a gene's encoded information is used to create proteins that shape or dictate the structures and functions of cells. In principle, by modifying gene expression, the potential effects of drugs on the human body and human functions, short- and long-term, grow exponentially.

4. In the world of illicit psychoactive drug use, drug users have no difficulty attributing unpleasant or pleasant experiences mainly to the drug, with acknowledgments that the setting and the user's preparation may shape the experience. Popular and scholarly writings about marijuana, LSD, or ecstasy illustrate this point. However, in the controlled world of testing of psychoactive drugs to conform to the psychiatric and regulatory vision of these drugs as conventional medical remedies, researchers and regulators have the greatest difficulty to treat them as capable of producing complex and unpredictable experiences from individual to individual. Here, the presumed sameness of the subjects' mental disorders, the moralistic opposition to intoxication, and the channeling of the subjects through evaluation

procedures copied directly from the world of physiological medicine—all combine to dictate the expectation that pleasant or euphoric psychoactive effects originate in drugs and will probably create drug addicts, while unpleasant psychoactive effects probably originate in psychiatrically disturbed subjects and can be tolerated or further treated.

5. In the experience of one of us (DC), however, clonazepam withdrawal is always extremely difficult. Working with over a dozen individuals who had been taking clonazepam for periods ranging from six years to nineteen years, and who had previously tried different methods, sometimes including inpatient hospital-based detoxification, it was found all of them experienced excruciating withdrawal symptoms and none were able to reach their goal of being completely clonazepam-free.

6. Recent repeated associations of chronic benzodiazepine use with the onsent of dementia in careful cohort studies (see, most recently, de Gage and colleagues, 2012) will hasten the demise of these drugs and will lead to increases in the promotion of other tranquilizers and sedatives to physicians and patients. Although benzodiazepines have long been observed to cause memory problems, such problems are reported with virtually all psychotropic drugs on the market today.

7. Since 1991, pharmaceutical manufacturers in the United States have paid the staggering sum of $30 billion to settle allegations of wrongdoing, notably illegal marketing of drugs and deliberate overcharging of government health programs like Medicare and Medicaid (Almashat & Wolfe, 2012). The pace of such criminal and civil suits from the federal government and states has increased: of the 239 settlements and court judgments occurring during that period, 74 (totaling $10.2 billion) occurred between November 2010 through July 2012. As the authors point out, these financial penalties "still continue to pale in comparison to company profits and a parent company is only rarely excluded from participation in Medicare and Medicaid for the illegal activities . . ." (p. 5). While overcharging of public health programs has been the most common alleged violation, illegal (off-label) marketing has resulted in the largest settlements. The three largest settlements involved accusations of the illegal marketing of the antidepressants Paxil and Wellbutrin by Glaxo Smith Kline, the antipsychotic Risperdal by Johnson & Johnson, and the anticonvulsant Depakote by Abbott Laboratories.

References

Abood, R. R. (2011). *Pharmacy practice and the law*. Sudbury, MA: Jones and Bartlett.

Adair, R. F., & Holmgren, L. R. (2005). Do drug samples influence resident prescribing behavior? A randomized study. *American Journal of Medicine, 118,* 881–884.

Almashat, S., & Wolfe, S. (2012, September 27). *Pharmaceutical industry criminal and civil penalties: An update.* Retrieved from www.citizen.org

Als-Nielsen, B., Chen, W., Gluud, C., & Kjaegard, L. L. (2003). Association of funding and conclusions in randomized drug trials: A reflection of treatment effect or adverse events? *JAMA, 290,* 921–928.

American Psychiatric Association. (2005, May 4). Mental illness stigmas are receding, but misconceptions remain. [News release]. Retrieved from http://www.psych.org/MainMenu/Newsroom/NewsReleases/2005NewsReleases/05-24apanewsreleaseonpoll-%20final.aspx

Angell, M. (2000). Is academic medicine for sale? *New England Journal of Medicine, 342*, 1516–1518.

Avorn, J. (2007). Paying for drug approvals—Who's using whom? *New England Journal of Medicine, 356*(17), 1697–1700.

Backer, E. L., Lebsack, J. A., Van Tonder, R. J., & Crabtree, B. F. (2000). The value of pharmaceutical representative visits and medication samples in community-based family practices. *The Journal of Family Practice, 49*(9), 811–816.

Ban, T. A. (2001). Pharmacotherapy of mental illness: A historical analysis. *Progress in Neuro-Psychopharmacology & Biological Psychiatry, 25*, 709–727.

Ban, T. A. (2006). The role of serendipity in drug discovery. *Dialogues in Clinical Neuroscience, 6*, 335–344.

Begley, S. (2010, January 29). The depressing news about antidepressants: Studies suggest that the popular drugs are no more effective than a placebo. In fact, they may be worse. *Newsweek.* Retrieved from www.newsweek.com/id/232781

Begley, S. (1994, February 7). One pill makes you larger, and one pill makes you smaller. *Newsweek.* Retrieved from www.newsweek.com/id/113120/page/1

Benson, K., & Hartz, A. J. (2000). A comparison of observational studies and randomized, controlled trials. *New England Journal of Medicine, 342*, 1878–1886.

Bezchlibnyk-Butler, K. Z., & Jeffries, J. J. (Eds.). (2005). *Clinical handbook of psychotropic drugs* (15th rev. ed.). Seattle: Hogrefe.

Bourgeois, M. (1994, June). De vraies maladies [Genuine diseases]. *Le Monde des Débats, 9.*

Breggin, P. R. (1983). *Psychiatric drugs: Hazards to the brain.* New York: Springer Publishing Company.

Breggin, P. R., & Breggin, G. (1994). *Talking back to Prozac: What doctors aren't telling you about today's most controversial drug.* New York: St. Martin's.

Byck, R. (1976). (Ed.). *Cocaine papers: Sigmund Freud.* New York: New American Library.

Cavanna, A. E., Ali, F., Rickards, H. E., & McCorry, D. (2010). Behavioral and cognitive effects of anti-epileptic drugs. *Discovery Medicine, 9*(45), 138–144.

CBS News. (2007, August 21). Minnesota law sheds light on drug companies.

Chast, F. (1995). *Histoire contemporaine des médicaments* [Contemporary history of medications]. Paris: Éditions La Découverte.

Chew, L. D., O'Young, T. S., Hazlet, T. K., Bradley, K. A., Maynard, C., & Lessler, D. S. (2000). A physician survey of the effect of drug sample availability on physicians' behavior. *Journal of General Internal Medicine, 15*(7), 478–483.

Cohen, D. (1995). Le tabagisme: Norme, déviance, maladie, ou délit? [Tobacco use: Norm, deviance, disease, or crime?] In L. Bouchard & D. Cohen (Eds.), *Médicalisation et contrôle social* [Medicalization and social control] (pp. 121–132). Montreal: Les Cahiers Scientifiques-Acfas.

Cohen, D. (1996). Les "nouveaux" médicaments de l'esprit: Marche avant vers le passé? [*The "new" mind drugs: A forward step into the past?*] *Sociologies et Société, 14*, 17–39.

Cohen, D. (1997a). A critique of the use of neuroleptic drugs in psychiatry. In S. Fisher & R. P. Greenberg (Eds.), *From placebo to panacea: Putting psychiatric drugs to the test* (pp. 173–229). New York: Wiley & Sons.

Cohen, D. (1997b). Psychiatrogenics: The introduction of chlorpromazine in psychiatry. *Journal of Existential Psychology and Psychiatry, 23*, 206–233.

Cohen, D. (2002). Research on the drug treatment of schizophrenia: A critical appraisal and implications for social work education. *Journal of Social Work Education, 38*(2), 1–24.

Cohen, D. (2008, May 4). Christmas comes early—as Lilly reveals first-quarter healthcare grants. Retrieved from http://ahrp.blogspot.com/2008/05/on-may-2007-we-reported-that-eli-lilly.html

Cohen, D. (2011). *Banishing the psychoactive? The Food and Drug Administration's pre-approval review of atomoxetine for Attention-Deficit/Hyperactivity Disorder.* Unpublished manuscript.

Cohen, D., & Jacobs, D. (2007). Randomized controlled trials of antidepressants: Clinically and scientifically irrelevant. *Debates in Neuroscience, 1*, 44–54.

Cohen, D., & Hughes, S. (2011). How do people taking psychiatric drugs explain their "chemical imbalance"? *Ethical Human Psychology & Psychiatry, 13*(3), 176–189.

Cohen, D., & McCubbin, M. (1990). The political economy of tardive dyskinesia: Asymmetries in power and responsibility. *Journal of Mind and Behavior, 11*, 465–488.

Cohen, D., McCubbin, M., Collin, J., & Perodeau, G. (2001). Medications as social phenomena. *Health, 5*(4), 441–469.

Cole, J. O. (1960). Behavioral toxicity. In L. Uhr and J. G. Miller (Eds.), *Drugs and behavior* (pp. 166–183). New York, London: Wiley.

Committee on Finance, United States Senate. (2011, May 25). *Staff report on Sanofi's strategic use of third parties to influence the FDA.* 112th Congress, 1st session, S. Prt. 112–120.

Committee on Finance, United States Senate. (2007, April). Use of educational grants by pharmaceutical manufacturers. 110th Congress, 1st session, S. Prt., 110–121.

Constans, J.-P. (1992). Les neuroleptiques ont-ils condamné à disparition la psychochirurgie? [Did the neuroleptics condemn psychosurgery to disappear?] In: J.-P. Olié, D. Ginestet, G. Jolles & H. Lôo (Eds.), *Histoire d'une découverte en psychiatrie. 40 ans de chimiothérapie neuroleptique* [History of a discovery in psychiatry: 40 years of neuroleptic chemotherapy]. Paris: Doin Éditeurs.

Critser, G. (2005). *Generation Rx: How prescription drugs are altering American lives, minds, and bodies.* Boston: Houghton Mifflin Company.

Cross-National Collaborative Group. (1992). The changing rate of major depression: Cross-national comparisons. *JAMA, 268*, 3098–3105.

Cutler, N. R., Sramek, J. J., Murphy, M. F., Riordan, H., Bieck, P., & Carta, A. (2010). *Critical pathways to success in CNS drug development.* Oxford: Wiley-Blackwell.

Dana, J., & Loewenstein, G. (2003). Doctors and drug companies: A social science perspective on gifts to physicians from industry. *JAMA, 290*(2), 252–255.

De Angelis, C. D. (2006). The influence of money on medical science. *JAMA, 296*(8), 996–998.

De Gage, S. B., Bégaud, B., Bazin, F., Verdoux, H., Dartigues, J-F., Pérès, K., Kurth, T., & Pariente, A. (2012). Benzodiazepine use and risk of dementia: Prospective population based study. *BMJ, 345*, e6231.

DeGrandpre, R. (2007). *The cult of pharmacology: How America became the world's most troubled drug culture.* Durham, NC, and London: Duke University Press.

Deniker, P. (1989). From chlorpromazine to tardive dyskinesia (brief history of the neuroleptics). *Psychiatric Journal of the University of Ottawa, 14*, 253–259.

Donnelly, L. (2010, May 2). Valium prescriptions soar during recession. *The Sunday Telegraph* (London). Retrieved from http://www.telegraph.co.uk/health/healthnews/7662900/Valium-prescriptions-soar-during-recession.html

Donohue, J. M., & Bernd, E. R. (2004). Effects of direct to consumer advertising on medication choice: The case of antidepressants. *Journal of Public Policy & Marketing, 23*(2), 115–127.

Dorsey, E. R., de Roulet, J., Thomson, J. P., Reminick, J. I., Thai, A., . . . Moses, H. (2010). Funding of U.S. biomedical research, 2003–2008. *JAMA, 303*(2), 137–143.

Dunham, H. W., & Weinberg, S. K. (1960). *The culture of the state mental hospital.* Detroit, MI: Wayne State University Press.

Dutton, G. (February 7, 2011). 2011 budget outlook: Trim, cut, then slash. *Genetic Engineering & Biotechnology News.* Retrieved from http://www.genengnews.com/analysis-and-insight/2011-budget-outlook-trim-cut-then-slash/77899360/

Ehrenberg, A. (1995). *L'individu incertain* [The uncertain individual]. Paris: Calmann-Lévy.

Eisenberg, L. (1995). The social construction of the human brain. *American Journal of Psychiatry, 152*, 1563–1575.

Elliott, C. (2003). *Better than well: American medicine meets the American dream.* New York: W. W. Norton.

Elliott, C. (2004). Pharma goes to the laundry: Public relations and the business of medical education. *Hastings Center Report, 34*(5), 18–23.

Elliott, C. (2006, April). The drug pushers. *The Atlantic.* Retrieved from http://www.theatlantic.com/magazine/archive/2006/04/the-drug-pushers/4714/

Elliott, C. (2010). *White coat, black hat: Adventures on the dark side of medicine.* Boston: Beacon.

Even, C., Siobud-Dorocant, E., & Darennes, R. M. (2000). Critical approach to antidepressant trials: Blindness protection is necessary, feasible and measurable. *British Journal of Psychiatry, 177*, 47–51.

Executive Office of the President of the United States. (2011). *Epidemic: Responding to the prescription abuse crisis.* The White House.

Farr, M. (1994, August). Is everybody happy? The pushy politics of Prozac. *This Magazine, 28* (2), 28–33.

FDA. (2012). New molecular entity approvals for 2011. Retrieved from http://www.fda.gov/Drugs/DevelopmentApprovalProcess/DrugInnovation/ucm285554.htm

Fédida, P. (1995, October). Le chimique et le psychique. Un défi pour la psychanalyse [The chemical and the psychical: A challenge for psychoanalysis.] *La Recherche*, no. 280, 95–97.

Fields, R. D. (2009). *The other brain: From dementia to schizophrenia, how new discoveries about the brain are revolutionizing medicine and science.* New York: Simon & Schuster.

Frankenburg, F. (1994). History of the development of antipsychotic medication. *Psychiatric Clinics of North America, 17*, 531–540.

Freyhan, F. (1955). The immediate and long range effects of chlorpromazine on the mental hospital. In *Colloque international sur la chlorpromazine et les médicaments neuroleptiques en thérapeutique psychiatrique Paris, 20, 21, 22 Octobre 1955* (pp. 790–792) [International colloquium on chlorpromazine and neuroleptic medications in psychiatric treatment], Paris: G. Douin et Cie.

From discovery to cure: Accelerating the development of new and personalized interventions for mental illnesses. (2010, August). Report of the National Advisory Mental Health Councils Workgroup. Retrieved from http://www.nimh.nih.gov/about/advisory-boards-and-groups/namhc/reports/fromdiscoverytocure.pdf

Fugh-Berman, A., & Ahari, S. (2007). Following the script: How drug reps make friends and influence doctors. *PLoS Medicine, 4*(4): e150.

Fullerton, C. A., Busch, A. B., Frank, R. G. (2010). The rise and fall of gabapentin for bipolar disorder: A case study on off-label pharmaceutical diffusion. *Medical Care, 48*(4), 372–379.

Gagnon, M.-A., & Lexchin, J. (2008). The cost of pushing pills: A new estimate of pharmaceutical promotion expenditures in the United States. *PLoS Medicine, 5*(1), e1.

Geddes, J., Freemantle, N., Harrison, P., & Bebbington, P. (2000). Atypical antipsychotics in the treatment of schizophrenia: Systematic overview and meta-regression analysis. *BMJ, 32*, 1371–1376.

Gellad, Z. F., & Lyles, K. W. (2007). Direct-to-consumer advertising of pharmaceuticals. *The American Journal of Medicine, 120*(6), 475–480.

Goldsmith, L. & Moncrieff, J. (2011). The psychoactive effects of antidepressants and their association with suicidality. *Current Drug Safety, 6*(2), 115–121.

Goodnough, A. (2011, September 14). In Louisville, a center's doctors cut off Xanax prescriptions. *New York Times.* Retrieved from http://www.nytimes.com/2011/09/14/us/in-louisville-a-centers-doctors-cut-off-xanax-prescriptions.html?ref=abbygoodnough

Goozner, M. (2004). *The $800 million pill: The truth behind the cost of new drugs.* Berkeley: University of California Press.

Greenberg, G. (2010). *Manufacturing depression: The secret creation of a modern disease.* New York: Simon & Schuster.

Greene, J. A. (2004). Attention to "details": Etiquette and the pharmaceutical salesman in postwar America. *Social Studies of Science, 34*(2), 271–292.

Haig, S. (2007, January 2). Attack of the Pharma babes. *Time.* Retrieved from http://www.time.com/time/health/article/0,8599,1573327,00.html

Harris, G. (2007, June 27). Psychiatrists top list in drug maker gifts. *New York Times.*

Harris, G., Carey, B., & Roberts, J. (2007, May 10). Psychiatrists, children, and drug industry's role. *New York Times.*

Healy, D. (2012). *Pharmageddon.* Berkeley, CA: University of California Press.

Healy, D. (2008). *Mania: A short history of bipolar disorder.* Baltimore: The Johns Hopkins University Press.

Healy, D. (2006a). Manufacturing consensus. *Culture, Medicine and Psychiatry, 30*, 135–156.

Hegarty, J., Baldessarini, R., Tohen, M., Waternaux, C., & Oepen, G. (1994). One hundred years of schizophrenia: A meta-analysis of the outcome literature. *American Journal of Psychiatry, 151*, 1409–1416.

Heres, S., Davis, J., Maino, K., Jetzinger, E., Kissling, W., & Leucht, S. (2006). Why olanzapine beats risperidone, risperidone beats quetiapine, and quetiapine beats olanzapine: An exploratory analysis of head-to-head comparison studies of second-generation antipsychotics. *American Journal of Psychiatry, 163*, 185–194.

Horwitz, A. V. (2010). How an age of anxiety became an age of depression. *The Milbank Quarterly, 88*, 112–138.

Hughes, S., & Cohen, D. (2011). Can online consumers contribute to drug knowledge? A mixed methods comparison of consumer and professional reports on psychotropic medications on the Internet. *Journal of Medical Internet Research, 13*(3), e53.

Hurko, O., & Ryan, J. L. (2005). Translational research in central nervous system drug discovery. *Neurotherapeutics, 2*, 671–682.

IMS Health. (2011). *Top therapeutic classes by U.S. sales.* Retrieved from http://www.imshealth.com/deployedfiles/ims/Global/Content/Corporate/Press%20Room/Top-Line%20Market%20Data%20&%20Trends/2011%20Top-line%20Market%20Data/Top_Therapy_Classes_by_Sales.pdf

IMS National Prescription Audit. (2010, April 6). *Top 15 U.S. pharmaceutical products by dispensed prescriptions.*

Insel, T. R. (2010, February 19). A decade after the decade of the brain: Understanding mental disorders as circuit disorders. *Cerebrum.* Retrieved from http://www.dana.org/news/cerebrum/detail.aspx?id=25802

Irani, F., Dankert, M., Brensinger, C., Bilker, W. B., Nair, S. R., Kohler, C. G., Kanes, S. J., Turetsky, B. I., Moberg, P. J., Ragland, J. D., Gur, R. C., & Siegel, S. J. (2004). Patient attitudes toward surgically implantable, long-term delivery of psychiatric medicine. *Neuropsychopharmacology, 29*, 960–968.

Jacobs, D. (1995). Psychiatric drugging: Forty years of pseudo-science, self-interest, and indifference to harm. *Journal of Mind and Behavior, 16*(4), 421–470.

Jacobs, D. H., & Cohen, D. (1999). What is really known about psychological alterations produced by psychiatric drugs? *International Journal of Risk and Safety in Medicine, 12*, 37–47.

Jacobs, D. H., & Cohen, D. (2010). Does "psychological dysfunction" mean anything? A critical essay on pathology vs. agency. *Journal of Humanistic Psychology, 50*, 312–334.

Janofsky, M. (2004, March 18). Drug fighters turn to rising tide of prescription abuse. *New York Times.*

Jureidini, J., Doecke, C. J., Mansfield, P. R., Harby, H. M., Menkes, D. B., & Tonkin, A. L. (2004). Efficacy and safety of antidepressants for children. *BMJ, 328*, 879–883.

Jureidini, J., McHenry, L., & Mansfield, P. (2008). Clinical trials and drug promotion: Selective reporting of Study 329. *International Journal of Risk & Safety in Medicine, 20*, 73–81.

Kassirer, J. (2005). *On the take: How America's complicity with big business can endanger your health.* Oxford & New York: Oxford University Press.

Kessler, R., McConagle, K., Zhao, S., Nelson, C. B., Hughes, M., Eshleman, S., Wittchen, H.-U., & Kendler, K. S. (1994). Lifetime and 12-month prevalence of DSM-III-R psychiatric disorders in the United States. *Archives of General Psychiatry, 51*, 8–19.

Klerman, G. L. (1978). The evolution of a scientific nosology. In J. C. Shershow (ed.), *Schizophrenia: Theory and practice* (pp. 99–121). Cambridge, MA: Harvard University Press.

Koumjian, K. (1981). The use of Valium as a form of social control. *Social Science and Medicine, 15E*, 245–249.

Kramer, P. (1993). *Listening to Prozac: A psychiatrist explores antidepressant drugs and the remaking of the self.* New York: Viking.

Kravitz, R. L., Epstein, R. M., Feldman, M. D., Franz, C. E., Azari, R., Wilkes, M. S., Hinton, L., & Franks, P. (2005). Influence of patients' requests for direct-to-consumer advertised antidepressants. *JAMA, 293*, 1995–2002.

Krohe, J. (1994, September). An epidemic of depression? *Across the Board, 31*, 23–27.

Krupka, L., & Vener, M. (1985). Prescription drug advertising: Trends and implications. *Social Science and Medicine, 20*, 191–197.

Kutchins, H., & Kirk, S. (1988). The business of diagnosis: DSM-III and clinical social work. *Social Work, 33*, 215–220.

Lacasse, J., & Leo, J. (2010). Ghostwriting at elite academic medical centers in the United States. *PLoS Medicine, 7*(2), e1000230.

Lader, M. (1978). Benzodiazepines: Opium of the masses? *Neuroscience, 3*, 159–167.

Landis, S. (2010, February 22). A decade after the decade of the brain: Basic science and gene findings drive research. *Cerebrum.* Retrieved from http://www.dana.org/news/cerebrum/detail.aspx?id=25802

Lane, C. (2007). *Shyness: How normal behavior became a sickness.* New Haven, CT: Yale University Press.

Leake, C. D. (1958). *The amphetamines: Their actions and uses.* Springfield, IL: Charles C. Thomas.

Lehmann, H. E. (1989). The introduction of chlorpromazine to North America. *Psychiatric Journal of the University of Ottawa, 14*, 263–265.

Lehmann, H. E. (1993). Before they called it psychopharmacology. *Neuropsychopharmacology, 8*, 291–303.

Leo, J. (2009). *JAMA*, free speech, and conflicts of interest. *Society, 46*, 472–476.

Leo, J. (2006), The SSRI trials in children: Disturbing implications for academic medicine. *Ethical Human Psychology & Psychiatry, 8*, 29–41.

Leo, J., & Lacasse, J. R. (2008). The media and the chemical imbalance theory of depression. *Society, 45*, 35–45.

Lieberman, J. A. (2006). Comparative effectiveness of antipsychotic drugs. *Archives of General Psychiatry, 63*(10), 1069–1072.

Light, D. W., & Warburton, R. (2011). Demythologizing the high costs of pharmaceutical research. *BioSocieties, 6*, 34-50. doi: 10.1057/biosoc.2010.40

Lopez-Muñoz, F., Ucha-Udabe, R., & Alamo, C. (2005). The history of barbiturates a century after their introduction. *Neuropsychiatric Disease and Treatment, 1*, 329–343.

Mahecha, L. A. (2006). Rx-to-OTC switches: Trends and factors underlying success. *Nature Reviews. Drug Discovery, 5*, 380–385.

Meier, B. (2004, June 21). A medical journal quandary: How to report on drug trials. *New York Times*, A1.

Metzger, K. L., Shoemaker, J. M., Kahn, J. B., Maxwell, C. R., Liang, Y., Tokarczyk, J., Kanes, S. J., Hans, M., Lowman, A., Dan, N., Winey, K. I., Swerdlow, N. R.,

& Siegel, S. J. (2007). Pharmacokinetic and behavioral characterization of a long-term antipsychotic delivery system in rodents and rabbits. *Psychopharmacology, 190,* 201–211.

Meyers, C. (1985). *Histoire des drogues et médicaments de l'esprit* [History of drugs and medications for the mind.] Paris: Erès.

Moncrieff, J. (2008). *The myth of the chemical cure: A critique of psychiatric drug treatment.* London: Palgrave MacMillan.

Moncrieff, J., & Cohen, D. (2009). How do psychiatric drugs work? *BMJ, 338,* b1963.

Moncrieff, J., & Cohen, D. (2006). Do antidepressants cure or create abnormal brain states? *PLoS Medicine, 3*(7), e240.

Moncrieff, J., & Cohen, D. (2005). Rethinking models of psychotropic drug action. *Psychotherapy & Psychosomatics, 74,* 145–153.

Moncrieff, J., Cohen, D., & Mason, J. (2009). The subjective effects of taking antipsychotic medication: A content analysis of Internet data. *Acta Psychiatrica Scandinavica, 120,* 102–111.

Moncrieff, J., Porter, S., & Cohen, D. (2012). *The psychoactive effects of psychiatric medications.* Unpublished manuscript.

Moore, T. J., Cohen, M. R., & Furberg, C. D. (2007). Serious adverse drug events reported to the Food and Drug Administration, 1998–2005. *Archives of Internal Medicine, 167* (16), 1752–1759.

Moynihan, R. (2004). Drug company targets US state health officials. *BMJ, 328,* 306.

Moynihan, R., & Cassels, A. (2005). *Selling sickness: How the world's biggest pharmaceutical companies are turning us all into patients.* New York: Nation Books.

NAMI's pharma funders: Serial off-label promoter Astra-Zeneca tops the list. (2010, April 29). Retrieved from http://pharmamkting.blogspot.com/2010/04/namis-pharma-funders-serial-off-label.html

Naranjo, P. (1979). Hallucinogenic plant use and related indigenous belief systems in the Ecuadorian Amazon. *Journal of Ethnopharmacology, 1*(2), 121–145.

National Institute on Drug Abuse. (2011, May). Prescription drug abuse. Retrieved from http://www.nida.nih.gov/tib/prescription.html

Nesi, T. (2008). *Poison pills: The untold story of the Vioxx drug scandal.* New York: St. Martin's Press.

Oldani, M. J. (2004). Thick prescriptions: Toward an interpretation of pharmaceutical sales practices. *Medical Anthropology Quarterly, 18*(3), 325–356.

Patel, N. C., Crismon, M. L., Hoagwood, K., & Jensen, P. S. (2005). Unanswered questions regarding antipsychotic use in aggressive children and adolescents. *Journal of Adolescent and Child Psychopharmacology, 15*(2), 270–284.

Petersen, M. (2008). *Our daily meds: How pharmaceutical companies transformed themselves into slick marketing machines and hooked the nation on prescription drugs.* New York: Farrar, Strauss, and Giroux.

Pickering, H., & Stimson, G. (1994). Prevalence and demographic factors of stimulant use. *Addiction, 89,* 1385–1389.

Pieters, T., & Snelders, S. (2009). Psychotropic drug use: Between healing and enhancing the mind. *Neuroethics, 2,* 63–73. doi: 10.1007/s12152-009-9033-0

PLoS Medicine Editors. (2009). Ghostwriting: The dirty little secret of medical publishing that just got bigger. *PLoS Medicine, 6*(9), e1000156.

Porter, R., & Teich, M. (1997). *Drugs and narcotics in history*. Cambridge: Cambridge University Press.

Pringle, E. (2009, April 21). Drugging kids with no verifiable disease. Retrieved from www.lawyersandsettlements.com/blog/drugging-kids-with-no-verifiable-disease.html

Ramonet, I. (1995, August). Citoyens sous surveillance [Citizens under surveillance]. *Manière de voir, 27,* 10–13.

Rasmussen, N. (2006). Making the first anti-depressant: Amphetamine in American medicine, 1929–1950. *Journal of the History of Medicine and Allied Sciences, 61*(3), 288–323.

Reist, D., & VandeCreek, L. (2004). The pharmaceutical industry's use of gifts and educational events to influence prescription practices: Ethical dilemmas and implications for psychologists. *Professional Psychology: Research & Practice, 35*(4), 329–335.

Restak, R. (1994). *Receptors.* New York: Bantam.

Rimer, S. (1993, December 13). With millions taking Prozac, a legal drug culture arises. *New York Times.* Retrieved from www.nytimes.com/1993/12/13/us/with-millions-taking-prozac-a-legal-drug-culture-arises.html?scp=1&sq=&st=nyt

Robins, L. N., & Regier, D. N. (Eds.). (1991). *Psychiatric disorders in America: The epidemiologic catchment area study.* New York: The Free Press.

Rosen, D. M. (2008). *Dope: A history of performance enhancement in sports from the nineteenth century to today.* Westport, CT: Praeger.

Rosenberg, T. (2007, June 17). When is a pain doctor a drug pusher? *New York Times Magazine.* Retrieved from www.nytimes.com/2007/06/17/magazine/17pain-t.html

Ross, J. S., Lackner, J. E., Lurie, P., Gross, C. P., Wolfe, S., & Krumholz, H. M. (2007). Pharmaceutical company payments to physicians: Early experience with disclosure laws in Vermont and Minnesota. *JAMA, 297*(11), 1216–1223.

Rothman, D. (1994, February 14). Shiny happy people: The problem with "cosmetic psychopharmacology." *New Republic,* 34–38.

Scott, P. (2008, October). Was the Prozac revolution all in our heads? *Men's Health,* 144–149.

Screening the Public for Depression. (1995). *American Journal of Psychiatry, 152*(11), A42.

Smith, M. (1981). *Small comfort: A history of the minor tranquilizers.* New York: Praeger.

Steinman, M. A., Bero, L. A., Chren, M., & Landfeld, C. S. (2006). The promotion of gabapentin: An analysis of internal industry documents. *Annals of Internal Medicine, 145,* 284–293.

Stengers, I. (1995). Le médecin et le charlatan [The physician and the quack]. In T. Nathan & I. Stengers (Eds.), *Médecins et sorciers* [Physicians and sorcerers] (pp. 115–161). Paris: Les Empêcheurs de Penser en Rond.

Strassman, R. (1995). Hallucinogenic drugs in psychiatric research and treatment. *Journal of Nervous and Mental Disease, 183,* 127–138.

Szasz, T. (1974). *Ceremonial chemistry: The ritual persecution of drugs, addicts, and pushers.* Garden City, NY: Anchor Press.

Szasz, T. (2001). *Pharmacracy: Medicine and politics in America.* Westport, CT: Praeger.

Szasz, T. (2007). *Coercion as cure: A critical history of psychiatry.* New Brunswick, NJ: Transaction Publishers.

Tandon, R., Keshavan, M. S., & Nasrallah, H. A. (2008). Schizophrenia, "just the facts": What we know in 2008—Part 1: Overview. *Schizophrenia Research, 100,* 4–19.

Tentler, A., Silberman, J., Paterniti, D. A., Kravitz, R. L., & Epstein, R. M. (2008). Factors affecting physicians' responses to patients' requests for antidepressants: Focus group study. *Journal of General Internal Medicine, 23,* 51–57.

Tracy, S. W., & Acker, C. J. (Eds). (2004). *Altering American consciousness: The history of alcohol and drug use in the United States, 1800–2000.* Amherst, MA: University of Massachusetts Press.

Turner, E. H., Matthews, A. M., Linardatos, E., Tell, R. A., & Rosenthal, R. (2008). Selective publication of antidepressant trials and its influence on apparent efficacy. *New England Journal of Medicine, 358*(3), 252–260.

Tyrer, P., Oliver-Africano, P. C., Ahmed, Z., Bouras, N., Cooray, S., Deb, S., Murphy, D., Hare, M., Meade, M., Reece, B., Kramo, K., Bhaumik, S., Harley, D., Regan, A., Thomas, D., Rao, B., North, B., Eliahoo, J., Karatela, S., Sonil, A., & Crawford, M. (2007). Risperidone, haloperidol and placebo in the treatment of aggressive challenging behaviour in intellectual disability: Randomized controlled trial. *Lancet, 371*(9606), 57–63.

US Department of Justice. National Drug Intelligence Center. (2010, May 25). *National drug threat assessment 2010.* Publication available at www.usdoj.gov/ndic

Voyer, P., Préville, M., Cohen, D., Berbiche, D., & Béland, S. (2010). The prevalence of benzodiazepine dependence among community-dwelling seniors according to typical and atypical criteria. *Canadian Journal on Aging, 29,* 205–213.

Wazana, A. (2000). Physicians and the pharmaceutical industry: Is a gift ever just a gift? *JAMA, 283*(3), 373–380.

Weil, A. (1970). *The natural mind: A new way of looking at drugs and the higher consciousness.* Boston: Houghton Mifflin Company.

Wood, A. J. J., & Darbyshire, J. (2006). Injury to research volunteers: The clinical-research nightmare. *New England Journal of Medicine, 354* (18), 1869–1871.

Wright, R. (1994, March 14). The coverage of happiness. *The New Republic,* 24–29.

Zalesky, C. D. (2006). Pharmaceutical marketing practices: Balancing public health and law enforcement interests; moving beyond regulation-through-litigation. *Journal of Health Law, 39*(2), 235–264.

Zarifian, E. (1994). *Des paradis plein la tête* [Brimming with paradises]. Paris: Odile Jacob.

Zarifian, E. (1995, October). Les limites d'une conquête [The limits of a conquest]. *La Recherche, 280,* 74–78.

8

The Structure of Mad Science

A critical attitude needs for its raw material, as it were, theories or beliefs which are held more or less dogmatically. Thus science must begin with myths, and with the criticism of myths, neither with the collection of observations, nor with the invention of experiments, but with critical discussion of myths and of magical techniques and practices.

Karl Popper, *Conjectures and Refutations, p. 50.*

Introduction

In this book we have, indeed, taken a critical attitude toward the conventional understandings and treatments of madness over the last fifty years in America. We sought to examine the three major psychiatric "revolutions" that scholars often use to define and characterize the mental health system. These revolutions are often proclaimed to be the results of enlightenment, humanitarianism, and scientific progress. For each revolution we found that the particular rhetoric used by the psychiatric establishment to claim progress in the management of madness was and is pseudoscientific. It does not describe a science based on independent inquiry, transparency, objectivity, or the skeptical scrutiny of assumptions and evidence, but a distorted science, a make-believe science, one used to advance a welter of particular institutional agendas and cultural schemes. Instead of a science of madness, we documented a mad science.

Examining Our Own Assumptions

As scholars and researchers, we recognize that our personal unexamined assumptions affected how we shaped this book. As we indict the self-interest of countless actors in the mad science enterprise, our own self-interest must be scrutinized. Indeed, each of us has not only written critically about these issues for decades but has built an academic career on critical writings, especially ones challenging the disease model of distress and misbehavior and practices based on this model. We think that we have accurately communicated the recognized absence of biological verification of the Western scientific model of disease—disease as cellular or molecular pathology—applied to distress and misbehavior. Nonetheless, perhaps we bring a presumptive bias against disease as a first-line explanation for any complex, negatively perceived human behavior.

Still, our book does not privilege our own data but rather our serious effort to assess what psychiatry itself has presented as its best evidence for the disease model of distress and misbehavior. We have looked at the disease model and found the scientific evidence wanting. In drawing our conclusions, we did not seek out obscure studies conducted by outsiders. Rather, we analyzed what psychiatry has promoted as its *best* evidence, the most notable studies published in the leading journals of medicine and psychiatry, what psychiatric leaders and promoters in government and elsewhere have stated and written publicly. Although many critical books about psychiatry and the disease model have been published, especially recently,[1] we think our book is the first to examine systematically the links among three major arenas that typify psychiatric practice and thinking today: coercion in institutional and community settings, *DSM* diagnoses, and drugs. We are not aware of any important, substantive, independent studies that we have overlooked.

Perhaps we hold psychiatry to unreasonable expectations of scientific rigor, when some merely claim psychiatry to be a clinical art that tries to use science. For example, when Louis Menand in *The New Yorker* (March 1, 2010) raised the question, "Can psychiatry be a science?" the APA's president at the time, Alan Schatzberg, responded (March 22, 2010) by stating that no medical specialty, including psychiatry, is a science. "Psychiatry," Schatzberg wrote, "rests on a foundation of scientific findings . . . but must employ both clinical judgment and their empathic skills in diagnosing and treating patients." Revealingly, Schatzberg omitted to mention involuntary hospitalization and treatment—which no other medical specialty but psychiatry uses. Although his depiction of some psychiatric practices as art makes sense to us and could benefit patients and society were it taken *literally*, it is definitely not the depiction that psychiatry itself promotes and presents. We think that, here again, we have not misrepresented psychiatric sources. Self-servingly, when trying to explain failure to deliver on promises of factual understandings, novel treatments and improved outcomes, individual psychiatrists might claim occasionally to be only practicing an art—or an art mixed with guesswork, placebos, and something else. But, beyond any doubt the profession's consistent message has been that its accomplishments rest on the best scientific thinking. Furthermore, it is by claiming psychiatry as a medical science that authorities justify funding its activities and enforcing the coercive recommendations of its practitioners.

Although our story of the last fifty years of the mental health movement is not a tale of progress—if such is possible in the realm of human affairs—we have not argued in this book that the mental health system is monolithic.

We are too steeped in systems thinking to ignore that social systems (open systems by definition) change over time, sometimes radically and unpredictably. Moreover, although we observe that groupthink and herd behavior characterize much of what passes as mental health practice, the fact is that the mental health institutional infrastructure manages to accommodate critics like ourselves, who have been funded by governmental institutions such as public state universities and federal research institutes as well as private foundations. Realistically, we believe this accommodation is extremely small, but it does suggest a potential for change. Of course, as this book demonstrates, change in and of itself may not represent progress in the eyes of different stakeholders. But we do confess to worrying about the increased efficacy of institutions that rely on control by coercion and use mystification to expand their jurisdiction and power. Is it unwarranted to be anxious about *that* sort of progress—the possibility of a nightmarish therapeutic state in which all misbehavior or ineptitude is defined by presumed defective physiology and managed by empowered quasi-medical bureaucrats? This is no fantasy. America and its legal, political, and mental health authorities have previously come together to handle human "defectives" by legitimating involuntary sterilization of innocent citizens. As late as 1927, during a time ironically called the Progressive Era, one of America's most famous Supreme Court justices, Oliver Wendell Holmes Jr., wrote the opinion for a court majority (that included Justice Louis Brandeis and the chief justice, former president William Howard Taft) to uphold the right of a state to sterilize mental defectives. By 1941, about 36,000 men and women had been sterilized or castrated (Black, 2003, p. 121–123).

One final potential bias to consider is that we are social workers, not psychiatrists or other medical doctors. We think that this bias, really our professional training as social workers, shows in our consistent attention to interactions and transactions between individuals and their environments over time. Having said this, we think, first, that being social workers gives us pertinent inside knowledge of the field of mental health services, treatment, and research, if only because more social workers are involved in delivering mental health services in the United States than any other profession. Second, while we have no expertise in treating patients for their physical illnesses, each of us has been professionally trained to work and has worked as a clinical social worker with people who are very distressed, who misbehave badly, or both, which we've argued throughout this book is the real stuff of madness—if madness can be said to be made up of any thing. Also, together we've amassed over seventy-five years of teaching mental health courses in graduate schools of social work to thousands of students and practitioners (and learning from them), and as academics we've published scores of articles in journals of all of the mental health disciplines. In sum, we are not exactly outsiders to the madness enterprise.

Recapitulations

Any assessment of the psychiatric enterprise over the last fifty years depends primarily on assessing the success of deinstitutionalization and community treatment, descriptive diagnosis, and the prescription of psychoactive drugs.

The Language of Madness

Our analysis of the psychiatric state of affairs past and present is a linguistic attempt at persuasion, an argument by three individuals, each with his own fallible nature, earnestness, background, experiences, knowledge, and biases regarding the book's subject matter. "Authoritative" historians of madness are not that different from us; they are as earnest, conscientious, and flawed. They may fail to recognize where they imply (absent any demonstrations) that madness is self-evidently a medical problem by using medically tainted language. As we described, despite their differences (see Scull, 1985), virtually all infuse their texts with medicalized terms such as *mental illness, disorder,* or *disease,* as analogs for madness, even when they recognize the inability of these concepts to capture the range of heterogeneous behavioral content that is subsumed under the disjunctive category of madness. Their message to their readers is therefore likely to be: you are reading an account of the laborious journey to the scientific discovery of the true nature of madness as medical illness amenable to medical supervision.

However, an alternative vision of madness recurs throughout history. It accepts of course the mental and behavioral consequences of well-defined diseases such as pellagra, neurosyphilis, Alzheimer's dementia, or alcohol poisoning resulting in *delirium tremens.* It portrays madness not as a medical issue (disease/illness) or a phenomenon of nature as much as a human locus for a wide variety of existential struggles and deviant human actions. That conception requires a willingness to see the vast majority of mad persons, those whose behavior has not been scientifically linked to pathological processes, as poorly, sometimes very poorly, prepared actors (or sometimes evil actors) in a complex world, who try their best to deal with problems in living, sometimes very grave ones. We suggest throughout this book that this conception remains a wholly valid contender, despite its old-fashioned appearance, because, after more than ten decades of determined research and the expenditure of untold sums, no one can verify that madness is a medical disease. But even were we to accept psychiatry's basic premises about madness, we would be forced to conclude that its approaches to the mad are steeped in coercion (by which we mean deliberately and forcefully interfering in their lives), mystification (by which we mean propagating false or unverifiable statements about their problems and their solutions), and intoxication (which means according to standard dictionary definitions, "stupefaction or excitement by the action of a chemical substance," and "poisoning by a toxic substance"). These have extremely little connection with scientific inquiry or medical treatment.

Language is a human construction. Words do not necessarily represent a tangible reality and often rest on "perceptual metaphors," all the while giving listeners directions for response. The use of *disease* in reference to madness suggests that we should respond to many disparate behaviors as if they *were* diseases (e.g., schizophrenia) or the personal and social harm *caused* by diseases (e.g., suicide caused by post-psychotic depression). These words instruct their speakers to view some actors in the drama of life as nonvolitional and to excuse them from responsibility for behaviors that otherwise would be considered vexing or inept but motivated. Simultaneously, these words instruct their speakers to view other actors as healers motivated *only* by the desire to help, surely an absurd proposition. The language of disease permeates all aspects of the psychiatric enterprise and distorts how we think about deviance, distress, and suffering, and about responding to these.

That is why psychiatric language has been essential to that profession's economic and political success. For psychiatrists and all the allied mental health professionals, the mere application of the language of disease has managed to give madness a scientific verity, because the language's abstractions were easily treated as if they had a concrete existence. This was accomplished through the simple substitution of one metaphor for another, with people attributing more material reality to each new expression. Perhaps it went something like this: From about the late Middle Ages (circa 1350 CE) we have had useful if murky terms in the English language such as *madness, lunacy,* and *craziness* (*Merriam-Webster.com, 2011*) for troubling or troubled behavior. When the social order expected more formal codification to enforce the organized control of persons who could not resist their labeling by these terms, the terms were changed to the legal and perhaps more definitive-sounding *insanity*. Later, under the control of medical managers of the insane, that term was changed to our contemporary terms, *mental disease, illness,* and *disorder*. No change ever involved demonstrating the material referent of the words, but each change deeply shaped—while also reflecting—society's understandings and responses to human travails. So it was with the change to illness and to medical conceptions of madness, which has beguiled even historians perhaps because we are all still steeped in it. It is difficult for anyone to disentangle the embedded assumptions in the language from the story that is told. And to complicate matters further, the stories serve professional, institutional purposes.

The metaphor of disease is extremely seductive, not only because it distances a person from volition and responsibility while absolving "helpers" of political fallout when they take sides in interpersonal conflicts, but because it refers to something immediately recognizable. Without comment we ask our readers to reflect on the following few words and how they are viscerally experienced simply when reading them: *illness, brain disease, research, doctor, patient, diagnosis, prescription, treatment, therapy, evidence-based, medication, safe, effective, hospitalization.* We think this vocabulary transforms the awesome threat of madness—confusion and bewilderment—into the still challenging but more understandable and controllable threat of disease. It is as if these words (just like the words marketing firms employ to claim laundry detergents can, impossibly, clean "whiter than white") do much of their work just by being intoned regularly.

The Enduring Role of Coercion

Coercing the mad into madhouses to separate and detain them occurred long before physicians were authorized to manage that enterprise, and coercion continues to distinguish "scientific" psychiatry to our day. Though many people might know that madmen and madwomen used to be confined, beaten, tied, shocked, or whirled into submission, fewer might realize that the physical control of "dangerous" mental patients remains today a central if not the only function of the public mental health system, with more people being coerced now than ever.

About half a million people were involuntary residents of state and county asylums and mental hospitals by the mid-1950s. Today, about three times that many experience shorter periods of involuntary detention in psychiatric wards and other mental health facilities for examination and evaluation of their dangerousness to self or others. They are part of the approximately four million people who experience coercive measures from mental health workers, including those treated involuntarily in the community, the place once proffered as the obviously more humane alternative to long-term hospitalization of the mad. Coercion runs deep and wide throughout psychiatry and the mental health system, creating an unavoidable yet strangely silent climate of intimidation and acquiescence among clients and professionals and the media, whose job used to be to alert us to human rights abuses and scrutinize the functioning of the state.

Beginning slowly in the 1950s and extending throughout several decades, with encouragement from federal and state governments, the inmates of state mental hospitals were forcefully discharged to communities, even when they wished to remain institutionalized. The ostensible rationale was to remove them from coercive and inhumane total institutions and usher them into more therapeutically effective community-based programs. Assertive community treatment, one of the best-known such programs, was developed by a few mental health professionals steeped in the use of force on psychiatric inmates in one particular Wisconsin institution for the mad between the 1950s and 1970s. However, the only consistent outcome for patients uncovered by ACT proponents then and now is that of reduced hospital stays. This was not achieved by improving patients' functioning or reducing their distress and misbehavior but by forcing ACT patients to stay in the community while allowing comparison patients to be hospitalized. Understandably, "reduction in hospital stays" made policy makers, agency administrators, and government funders happy because it appeared to save money. It also allowed ACT promoters to enjoy continued authority because uncritical observers implicitly assumed that ACT accomplished other objectives, such as providing humane, noncoercive, effective interventions. Yet no consistent improvement in autonomous motivated behavior regarding education, vocation, or "symptoms" can be attributed to ACT, nor can it be distinguished from other less expensive and less coercive community programs used nationwide (reduced hospital stays disappeared when ACT programs did not force patients to stay in the community for treatment). Needless to say, ACT has been anointed as an evidence-based treatment.

Extremely few authors today discuss openly the extent of psychiatric coercion in America (Oaks, 2011). The first recorded involuntary confinement in an American mad hospital occurred in 1752. Two hundred and fifty-five years later, psychiatrist Robert Drake explained that the majority of the severely mentally ill opt out of mental health care because "They're afraid of the coerciveness of the system" (cited in Wiencke, 2007, p. 4). Today, coercion has been reinvented and institutionalized as a scientifically valid therapeutic approach for managing madness and as a proper subject for scientific investigation by psychiatric clinicians. Coercion might be presented as an unpleasant but necessary extra push to make patients use the range of available effective treatments for their mental illnesses. Our analysis, however, leads us to conclude that *outside coercion, public psychiatry has no effective approaches* to handle the existential difficulties of those who don't ask for help with their travails but whom nevertheless psychiatry claims under its jurisdiction. Coercion is the only intervention to have endured since the birth of psychiatry. We suggest that coercion (sometimes verbally airbrushed into the term *leverage*) and the threat of coercion persist because coercion is *all there is* for those who are behaviorally disobedient or wish to be left alone.

Once an acknowledged ethical and legal problem in psychiatry given its use against the helpless, the hopeless, or the legally innocent (Szasz, 2007), coercion is now a therapeutic tool, and discussions of coercion increasingly focus on the technical strength and effectiveness of its leverage effects (Monahan, 2008) and whether those who are coerced might not necessarily perceive it as such. Further, as we discussed in chapter three, some psychiatric authorities are beginning to argue that no medical justification is really needed for what psychiatric coercers do since this is identical to what other state sanctioned coercers, such as the police, do to maintain civil order. The police maintain that they catch and punish lawbreakers. However, psychiatry has originally and consistently maintained that *it* coerces not to punish but to treat, because *it* deals with problems constituting a special subset of *medical disease* that impairs its victims' ability to judge and discern rationally, thus requiring coercion when all else fails.

Coercion directly affects the freedom of mental health professionals. To receive payments from government programs and insurance companies, practitioners must generate *DSM* diagnoses, constraining the reluctant or skeptical to conform even though the diagnostic system—now openly recognized as deeply flawed, even caricatural—does arguably little to help their work. Designating some interventions as "evidence based" through a nonscientific, consensus-authority based arrangement also restricts professionals to use only these, if they want to keep their professional credibility. This would be especially the case in slow-to-change agencies dependent on public funds. Other interventions that are not yet anointed as acceptable by experts but which may prove to be or are useful to particular clients are discouraged. Few professionals will risk employing such interventions or risk sanctions by some supervisory agency. If the attitude prevails that "we already know what works best," innovation becomes even less probable, unless it promises to accommodate to or take a subsidiary position toward dominant interventions (inevitably, drugs).

More importantly, the recognition in public psychiatric practice that coercion is always at hand if persuasion fails creates an atmosphere of surveillance and expected compliance, making it difficult for a professional and a client to develop a meaningful working alliance. Deeply troubled persons will be careful to censor their thoughts and feelings, even if expressing them might be essential to their well-being, because they fear involuntary measures that could lead to psychiatric detention, involuntary drugging, and occasionally involuntary electroshock (Snyders, 2009). As stated earlier, involuntary measures keep many of the mad from seeking help in the first place (Hahm and Segal, 2010).

Instructed by tradition and by law, mental health professionals, too, will be hypervigilant for any sign from the patient of thoughts of suicide or harm in order to safeguard the patient's existence. Despite the fact that most state statutes concerning civil commitment are discretionary rather than mandatory (that is, professionals are not automatically *required* to take measures in response to perceived dangerousness), in our experience, extremely few mental health professionals actually know the letter of these laws.[2]

We see no legitimate role for coercion in the helping enterprise. It is obvious that societies must use coercion and force in particular circumstances. Our police and military have the authority to maintain civil order and defend against threats to our survival, while our legal and political systems are charged with supervising its appropriate use. We question why psychiatry, under the guise that it is a medical discipline, persists in using coercion in the mental health system and why other medical disciplines, who reject coercion in their own practice, turn a blind eye to it in psychiatry. Before homosexuality's sudden redefinition from feared condition and mental disorder to merely a variant of normal sexual preference, was it proper to coerce homosexuals to change their sexual behavior?

The Emptiness of Descriptive Diagnosis

Compared to the historical uncertainties about the nature of madness, the disease model of madness offered the rubric of medicine to classify, understand, and control various misbehaviors as one would do with symptoms of brain diseases. To mimic research and practice of physical medicine, psychiatry needed a method of identifying and categorizing types of mental illnesses. The initial invention and subsequent attempted refinements of the *DSM* embodies this effort to name and classify.

The first edition of the *DSM* was ignored, the second scorned, and by the 1970s the *DSM* had become a battleground of contending interest groups and ideologies. A subgroup of biologically oriented research psychiatrists wrestled control of the *DSM* from the dominant psychoanalytic faction, claiming that diagnosis must become more scientific (as they understood the term) if psychiatry as a profession was to endure and thrive. This new leadership cadre emphasized making the classification system more reliable (i.e., consistent), conveniently ignoring the far more important criterion of validity (i.e., establishing the reality of the disorders). They created "descriptive diagnosis," exemplified by the 1980 *DSM-III* and its subsequent editions. It simply assumed that mental disorders existed and focused on getting clinicians to agree on who fit into which *DSM* diagnosis. For thirty years, the leaders of the APA claimed that descriptive diagnosis succeeded in making the *DSM* more scientific. They convinced policy makers and the public to trust their claims. The medical model of madness became further institutionalized, supported, and promoted by NIMH, mental health professionals, Big Pharma, insurance companies, and virtually everyone else.

Yet, as the unfolding controversies over the *DSM-5* illustrate, descriptive diagnosis has been an utter scientific failure. It led neither to more reliable or valid diagnoses, nor to any sort of scientific breakthrough in identifying hoped-for biomarkers of the elusive disorders that would begin to validate the medical model of madness. Moreover, in an effort to ape medical reasoning, by removing contextual clues about person's situations and circumstances to produce neutral- and objective-sounding "diagnostic criteria sets," understanding living persons became a quaint and irrelevant enterprise in the new psychiatry, where studying contrived *DSM* diagnoses substituted for studying persons and the possible functions of their disturbing behaviors. Much of this failure has remained hidden behind hopeful promises that the causes and cures for madness are just around the next biomedical corner. More deleteriously, descriptive diagnosis has allowed for widespread financial conflicts of interest among the APA, government, mental health practitioners, and leading researchers. By making it exceedingly easy to name new disorders and expand the scope of existing ones, the latter editions of the *DSM*s have manufactured an epidemic of mental illness and a huge expansion in the uses of lucrative but questionably useful psychochemicals. Improving the psychiatric diagnostic system was supposed to bring accuracy to psychiatric judgments, and for a while it was a public relations triumph. But instead of serving as a scientific cornerstone for research and practice, the *DSM* has become a mainstay of mad science, in which professional interests and power regarding diagnosis trump logic and scientific evidence.

The Madness of Medications

The modern prescribed psychoactive drugs are associated with nearly identical outcomes as all biological psychiatric treatments have always been. At best, about 30 percent of people diagnosed with the major clinical madnesses of our time (persistent depressed mood, called Major Depressive Disorder, persistent mood punctuated by euphoric mood, called Bipolar Disorder, and extremes of despair and deviance, called Schizophrenic Disorder) appear to show sustained improvement while taking these treatments. This proportion is very similar to that obtained today and in the past in observational or controlled studies by placebos, by seclusion and restraints, by excision of various bodily organs, by prolonged barbiturate-induced comas, by lengthy baths and showers, by surgical mutilations of the brain, by epileptic seizures induced by chemical or electrical shocks, by conversation, by seemingly irrelevant activities, or by the mere passage of time. The latest drug treatments—the SSRI antidepressants, the mood stabilizers, and the second- and third-generation antipsychotics administered under whatever conditions and in whatever combinations their adherents have proposed—have had no additional positive impact whatsoever on any measurable indices of pain and burden associated with madness and may have had negative impacts.[3]

This total failure has been the dirty little secret of psychiatric drug treatment for decades, but starting in 2005 with publications from the largest drug trials using real-world patients, doctors, and outcomes, funded by the NIMH and conducted by the drug industry-soaked clinical and research elite of American psychopharmacology, it could no longer remain shrouded. Some leaders of the mental health movement professed surprise at the findings, and some admitted that prescribers had accepted exaggerated claims of drugs' effectiveness in the absence of evidence. But the findings came as no surprise whatsoever to careful observers of the drug treatment scene. The disconnect between findings from reasonably well-conducted studies and lay and professional claims about the powers of the latest psychotropic medications suggests that much prescribed psychoactive drug use is today as it has always been: fundamentally ceremonial, fulfilling deep social needs, and needing no scientific justification whatsoever (Szasz, 1974).

The history of psychoactive substance use throughout time and throughout the world highlights the elemental fact that some users appreciate the effects of a drug, some users don't, and still more users have no particular responses. Instead of building upon this observation, drug experts and authorities invented artificial divides between "approved medications" and "dangerous drugs." Not only were the same drugs separated linguistically, they were made unequal politically. Authorities then justified desires for approved drugs by postulating that these drugs corrected chemical imbalances in their users, thereby ameliorating mental illnesses and enhancing population health—and should be prescribed by duly licensed physicians. As for the unapproved drugs, experts warned that these caused chemical imbalances, thereby creating mental illnesses and disrupting the fabric of society—and should be proscribed by any reasonable person. No genuine science, medicine, or public health could ensue from such a ridiculous dichotomy.

To maintain the dichotomy, a scientific and administrative apparatus was established, within which psychiatry was offered a retainer. The apparatus included the procedures and experiments testing psychoactive drugs' effectiveness in treating *DSM*-defined madnesses, all of them modeled to duplicate procedures used to evaluate conventional medical treatments for medical diseases. The Food and Drug Administration promised to verify the integrity of these procedures to ensure "safe and effective" prescribed psychoactive drugs, while the Drug Enforcement Agency promised to wage war on those who persisted on using unapproved psychoactive drugs. The puzzling fact that unapproved drugs could cross over into approved territory, or vice versa, or occupy both spaces simultaneously, seemed to puzzle no one.

Already blinded by unquestioned assumptions of madness as disease, experts confused the effects of stupefying drugs producing quiet on oppressive asylum wards with a revolutionary new medical understanding of psychosis. They confused dazzling images of our living brains with discoveries of the physiological substrates of the specific mental illnesses served up by new editions of the *DSM*. They took doctored reports of drugs' effectiveness as scientific validations of the guesses or marketing slogans proposed to explain the (presumed) drug effectiveness. They chose not to see how drug industry largesse made them indentured servants. Finally, because most of them had given up engaging in disciplined conversation with distressed persons (but could not fathom abandoning coercion), they lost the ability to conceive of psychiatric practice and research as anything other than prescribing drugs and waiting for new drugs. In these ways, American biological psychiatry became a state- and corporate-funded cult of psychoactive drug use.

That people might find psychoactive drugs helpful to them is obvious and cannot be contested. Nonetheless, and incredibly so, much of this power of psychoactive drug use went completely unnoticed and unmentioned—let us say, repressed—in the prodigious psychopharmacological research effort.

By definition, psychoactive drugs change people's thoughts, feelings, and behavior. Yet, psychopharmacology continually assumed that if the bearer of a psychiatric diagnosis reacted positively to a drug, this confirmed the presence of disease. That psychoactive drugs sedate, calm, tranquilize, desensitize, stupefy, awaken, arouse, or excite people who take them, and thereby may help some people temporarily or permanently to traverse daunting circumstances, disappeared from the official psychiatric understanding of psychiatric medications. As a result, this official understanding also neglected the rigorous detection of drug-induced harm in psychiatric practice.

The Structure of Mad Science

In the academic literature on any complex subject, careful readers can find examples of the misinterpretation of data, conclusions only partially supported by the evidence, and inadequate methodologies. Occasionally, someone uncovers deliberate falsification of data or unscrupulous behavior by a researcher, although recently there has been an alarming increase in reports of such behavior (Zimmer, 2012). These discoveries usually make newspaper headlines. Names are noted, careers are ruined, institutions are tainted, and the truth-seeking of science is reaffirmed.

This is *not* the story we have told in this book. When it comes to the understanding and treatment of madness, the distortions of research are not rare, misinterpretation of data are not isolated, and bogus claims of success are not voiced by isolated researchers seeking aggrandizement. In our detailed analyses of community treatment, diagnosis, and drugs, these characteristics of bad science are endemic, institutional, and protected. They are what we have labeled "mad science." Here are some of its major ingredients and the institutional arrangements that promote it.

Amnesia and the Recycling of Problems

The mental health field displays an uncanny tendency to sweep under the carpet vexing issues that threaten the status quo, only to treat them as novel problems once they resurface. We have discussed, for example, how by the early 1980s the architects of *DSM-III* had managed to deflect the scientific gaze off the central problem in psychiatric diagnosis—the lack of validity—onto the more manageable, less threatening problem of lack of reliability. By 2010, however, no less than the chair of the *DSM-IV* task force could lament that the *DSM*'s imperialism had created "false epidemics" of childhood disorders and could assert that the very definition of the key concept in the *DSM*, and arguably in all of psychiatry—*mental disorder*—was "bullshit" (Greenberg, 2011). We have cited the informed director of the NIMH professing surprise that the best conducted trials of optimally administered drug treatments had shown that these had reduced neither symptoms nor impairment. Yet such results characterized the longer-term fate of every major biological psychiatric treatment in the last hundred years. We have seen that coercion as the key mechanism ensuring compliance with treatments for the seriously disturbed has continually been downplayed publicly or rendered benign through verbal anesthesia and promoted as another helpful mental health technique called *leverage*, while its widespread employment never wavered.

The Medical Imprimatur

Psychiatry via the APA and NIMH has continuously proclaimed that, despite conflicting evidence, great scientific strides were made in community treatment, diagnosis, and drug treatments. These claims would have no shelf life without their acceptance and repetition by the mental health professional organizations and practicing clinicians. This acceptance rests on a few factors.

The first is the sheer power and prestige of the medical enterprise in the United States. Psychiatry used its links to medicine to capitalize on the technical breakthroughs and successes of this powerful social institution. Everyone has at least some vague appreciation of brain imaging, microsurgery, and other impressive technical advances in physiological medicine. The medical imprimatur stamped on psychiatric coercion, misdiagnosis, and ineffective drugs as the latest technological advances for helping the mad goes a long way in producing uncritical acceptance.

Second, psychiatric claims are not easily verified by other scholars, clinicians, or the public. Both the methods of scientific studies and the complex and arcane statistical analyses of data that fill the medical and psychiatric journals are a challenge to comprehend, even for the best-trained professionals, as articles in *The Economist* (2012) and elsewhere recently noted (Zimmer, 2012). Only a handful of psychiatrists, psychologists, social workers, or other mental health clinicians have the time, skills, or motivation to scrutinize the deluge of claims published weekly. Most rely only on popular media sources for soundbites of progress.[4] And when the media broadcast "advances," why should the clinicians be skeptical? In fact, they have seemed quick to become boosters, exploiting their membership in an enterprise that appears to be advancing.

Finally, professionals and the public are not simply gullible to shaky claims but have found many ways to benefit from them. The mental illness metaphor, whatever its possible uses for thinking, speaking, and coercing, is accepted as a statement of fact. But even if it is not, clients and professionals widely use it to justify insurance reimbursement from third parties, to get services to those who they think need help, and to earn a living. They collude with psychiatry to do something that the rest of medicine cannot do: to diagnose as an illness "behavior that society doesn't like," allowing assumed pathology to

311

replace morality. The public, confounded and discomfited by these behaviors, goes along with the ruse, relinquishing or outsourcing responsibility for one's behavior to experts. Irwin Savodnik, a UCLA psychiatrist and philosopher, has written that "the erosion of personal responsibility is, arguably, the most pernicious effect of the expansive role psychiatry has come to play in American life" (Savodnik, 2006, p M3).

Distorted Science and Exaggerated Claims

As we have described, many psychiatric studies take on the trappings and the appearance of scientific investigations, even when they are seriously flawed or interpreted much more positively than justified. Concerning diagnosis, it is the very rare study that actually tests average clinicians' agreement on *DSM* diagnoses for the same patients. Instead, the reliability literature is awash with tests of structured scales and checklists of presumed mental illnesses. Moreover, the vast majority of these studies are conducted among groups of clients or in narrowly focused research settings where it is expected that the problem being studied will be the chief presenting complaint (i.e., where there are likely to be high base rates of behaviors that are the diagnostic criteria of a particular disorder category). These studies are the equivalent of shooting fish in a barrel. Finally, without valid methods to verify the existence of "mental disorders," what exact purpose besides conformity or indoctrination is served by teaching clinicians to agree with published diagnostic criteria sets?

The durations of clinical drug trials are truncated to avoid showing that the drugs are ineffective over more than a couple of months of use. Double-blind procedures are rarely tested. Inconvenient subjects who respond to placebo early on are dropped. Only inert placebos, never active placebos known to evoke more powerful responses, are used as comparisons to drugs with sometimes stupefying behavioral effects. Adverse effects are investigated and reported with approximately one-tenth the energy devoted to assess hoped-for beneficial effects. It is a rare study that compares a drug treatment with a well-administered psychosocial alternative. The methodologically sound use of *no treatment* comparison groups is considered to be unethical in psychiatric research, and such groups are never used in experiments. But if one is attempting to determine whether a treatment is effective, than it would be crucial to know if that treatment (which typically produces some toxic adverse effects) is better than doing nothing at all (recalling medicine's commitment to "First, do no harm"). Finally, when results are unacceptable or deemed too financially threatening to sponsors, results have been doctored or suppressed.

We have illustrated throughout the book how even studies that are repeatedly cited to confirm claims of scientific progress are seriously flawed. Of course, all studies, no matter how meticulously conducted, have limits. Still, studies with profoundly serious flaws are presented as highly credible breakthroughs, sponsored by NIMH, authored by esteemed scientists at prestigious universities, and supported by the research community. That community praises the findings and exaggerates their significance: reliability is greatly improved; community treatment is effective and noncoercive; medications are safe and effective. The psychiatric lobbyists insert these conclusions into repositories of "evidence-based practices," "practice guidelines," or "best practices," thereby institutionalizing some of the weakest science (Medical Guesswork, 2006).

The exaggerated claims today are often about neuroscience. The public and professionals appear to suspend judgment in the face of "the seductive allure of neuroscience explanations" (Weisberg, Keil, Goodstein, Rawson, & Gray, 2008). About five hundred brain-imaging studies are published each year, and researchers for thirty years have been promising that "snapshots of the living brain" will unlock the mysteries of madness and will be used for diagnosing mental disorders (Carey, 2005). Although many of these studies may help scientists to understand more about brain functioning, to date, no standardized brain imaging tools exist for diagnosis or treatment in psychiatry. (No biomarker appears as a diagnostic criterion for any primary mental disorder in the *DSM*.) Harvard psychiatrist and former director of NIMH, Steven Hyman, admits that "the community of scientists was excessively optimistic about how quickly imaging would have an impact on psychiatry... people forget that the human brain is the most complex object in the history of human inquiry" (cited in Carey, 2005). The writer Diane Ackerman, in *An Alchemy of Mind*, captured this strange optimism well while offering an apt analogy for what brain imaging offers the understanding of persons:

> ... we may lift the lid off the brain with PET, MRI, fMRI, or MEG and peer inside, but that still leaves us voyeurs, distant viewers.... We measure its blood flow, hunger for glucose and oxygen, its radioactivity or magnetism. Regions light up and offer us some illumination. But the porch light can be on without telling you who is at home. When it comes to brain mapping "our knowledge is akin to looking out of the window of an airplane," neuroscientist William Newsome, of Stanford University, explains. "We can see patches of light from cities and towns scattered across the landscape, we know that roads, railways, and telephone wires connect those cities, but we gain little sense of the social, political, and economic interactions within and between cities that define a functioning society." (Ackerman, 2004, p. 251)

Big Science

Jonathan Cole, a prominent Columbia University sociologist and former provost, resigned in protest from the National Research Council's committee charged with evaluating PhD programs in the United States, just before the committee's final report (sponsored by the National Academy of Sciences) was due to be published in 2010, after seven years of committee effort. Cole (2011) concluded that it "was not worthy of publication" and had succumbed to "faulty assumptions, poor analysis, political pressure from the academy, and unexamined preconceptions." Cole's protest highlights an all-too-common disappointment with large scientific undertakings. The members of the committee, Cole believes, were unwilling to acknowledge that their study had failed (recall Donald Campbell and Karl Popper's methodological urgings):

> There are many examples .... of large studies thought too big to fail, despite insufficient data. One can find such failures, which lead to policy changes based on poor data, in medical experiments about drugs, public-health studies, and a variety of assessments of health risks . . . A crowd psychology emerges within committees where individuals don't want to be perceived as spoilers. Discussion of why a study has failed is truncated—to the detriment of learning from our mistakes. An attitude has developed in American society, and it plagues research efforts as well.
>
> The mantra is, "It's better than nothing. But is it?" (p. B12)

Has psychiatry simply become better than nothing? Is it too big to fail? Consider the size and character of psychiatric research. Nearly all studies published in the major psychiatric journals are big studies, involving sizeable teams of researchers at multiple clinics and hospitals across the nation, funded by big sponsors such as the pharmaceutical industry, the NIH, and foundations, and recruiting very large samples of patients. Like the NRC study described by Cole, the studies take years of planning and years of data collection. Decision making is done by teams and committees, which are carefully selected and supervised by the study directors and by the funding bodies. This is Big Science in psychiatry, and many institutions and individuals have a significant and personal stake in making it a success.

Big Science, however, is an insider's game. The leading players move easily among positions in the major arenas or psychiatric power. Top university scientists have their research funded by NIMH, are later appointed to review panels at NIH, are selected to serve on important APA committees such as the *DSM* task force, all the while earning increasing amounts of money serving as consultants or speakers for multiple pharmaceutical companies. Universities thrive on the large grants from NIH, foundations, and Big Pharma, as does the APA and other organizations such as NAMI. These individuals and institutions, woven tightly together by personnel, money, and self-interest have an additional shared goal, namely to consistently portray the vast enterprise as a scientific success and to ensure that it doesn't fail, no matter what.

The insiders' preferred world view is, of course, the biomedical model of madness: mental disorders are prevalent and spreading, caused by soon-to-be-discovered brain defects (themselves caused by soon-to-be-discovered genetic variations); palliation, prevention, and cures are just around the corner or already available but used by too few; and all that is needed to eradicate madness is more money, more time, and fewer critics. All evidence to the contrary, this worldview has been a runaway success.

The success results partly from the ways Big Science can annihilate potential opposition. By controlling almost all sources of funding, no rival scientific efforts gain traction. Funded and published studies are too big to replicate except by the insiders themselves. Outsiders, especially if they have no clinical appointments within medical institutions, may have a very difficult time conducting outcome studies on patients. This is especially so for studies on controversial topics, such as evaluating the outcomes of electroconvulsive treatment or involuntary commitment (McCubbin, Dallaire, Cohen, & Morin, 1999). The power-elite insiders control appointments to decision-making committees, to grants review panels, and to what gets published in the main journals. Academic enthusiasts of assertive community treatment, for example, receive federal and state funding to create ACT programs, and they also implement them and design the training manuals and tools to ensure that replications cohere to the ACT model. Then these same individuals evaluate the programs for effectiveness. Because of all of these ACT-related activities, these insiders become the experts. Thus they sit on the consensus committees that "objectively" validate their own treatments as evidence-based practices. All this allows them to buttress the status quo, reinforcing the view that they are promoting the "correct" view of madness and its management, reassuring the public that the experts have it under control and brushing off outcroppings of dissent.

As we write these lines one example occurs in the latest data brief from the US Centers for Disease Control and Prevention (CDC) bearing on usage of antidepressants in the United States (Pratt, Brody, & Gu, 2011). The report documents an increase from 1988–1994 to 2005–2008 of approximately 400 percent in the use of antidepressants in the general population, finding use in one in six women and one in sixteen men over the age of twelve years. The increase is observed in both genders, all age groups, and in the major races and ethnicities (though white users largely predominate). We have made many sorts of comments on these trends in this book. The authors of the CDC brief, however, chose to make a single comment, and it bears on their subfinding that "only" one-third of individuals with severe depressive symptoms were using antidepressants:

> According to American Psychiatric Association guidelines, medications are the preferred treatment for moderate to severe depressive symptomatology. The public health importance of increasing treatment rates for depression is reflected in *Healthy People 2020*, which

includes national objectives to increase treatment for depression in adults and treatment for mental health problems in children. (p. 5, references omitted).

The authors of this brief ignore the mountain of data on the near-equivalence of antidepressants (i.e., the numerous different substances gathered under that inappropriate moniker) to placebos in addressing feelings of depression. They ignore concerns that led the FDA to place black box warnings on antidepressants' labels starting in 2004 warning of agitation, agressivity, and suicidal ideation, especially in children. They cite guidelines produced by the most interest-conflicted professional organization in the United States on the subject of whether people ought to take antidepressants for what ails them. And for the final seal of approval to get even more people on antidepressants, they cite an official government policy. For sheer errancy or inanity, it would be hard to top this Big Science comment under the imprimatur of the CDC.

Has mainstream psychiatric thinking permeated all agencies devoted to protecting us from disease? Are there no countervailing sources of dissent within the established madness institutions? Psychiatry, unfortunately, may not be an only child in the medicine family to be harmed by the central planning of the biomedical industrial complex in this regard. The journalist Gary Taube (2007) conducted an exhaustive review of the research literature on nutrition and health and questions whether the research is deemed worthy of being called science.

> The institutionalized vigilance . . . is nowhere to be found in the study of nutrition, chronic disease and obesity, and it hasn't been for decades. For this reason, it is difficult to use the term "scientist" to describe those individuals who work in these disciplines, and indeed, I have actively avoided doing so in this book. It's simply debatable, at best, whether what these individuals have practiced for the past fifty years, and whether the culture they have created, as a result, can reasonably be described as science, as most working scientists or philosophers of science would typically characterize it. . . . Practical considerations . . . have consistently been allowed to take precedence over the dispassionate, critical evaluation of evidence and the rigorous and meticulous experimentation that are required to establish reliable knowledge. . . . The urge to simplify a complex scientific situation . . . has taken precedence over the scientific obligation of presenting the evidence with relentless honesty. (p. 451)

The leaders of the bureaucracies in which many scientists work are not accustomed to honesty when it might reveal weaknesses and cause trouble, nor are they good at promoting innovation. Their organizations are much more adept at protecting their flanks by the control of information. The few signs of countervailing influences come not from contending organizations but from the relatively uncontrollable Internet. Communities of dissent now have direct access to the public. These include networks of former psychiatric patients, blogs offering pointed criticisms of establishment thought, broadly distributed critical e-mails from whistleblowers and insiders, and websites brimming with detailed personal reviews of medications. Of course, the Internet is also itself an arena for battles between established sources and upstarts, especially as concerns "health information" (Hughes & Cohen, 2011).

But Big Science in psychiatry is trying hard to be absorbed into neuroscience, largely abandoning sociology and psychology, drawing the wagons around a biomedical fortress at NIMH. Thomas Insel, the director of NIMH, (as reported by Kaplan, 2011), explained that the new direction seeks to identify biomarkers of individual responses to drugs in order to develop "preemptive treatments . . . to prevent disability." He is following guidance provided by a report of a high-level National Mental Health Advisory Council, *From Discovery to Cure: Accelerating the Development of New and Personalized Interventions for Mental Illness.* The co-chair of that council, John March from Duke Clinical Research Institute, describes the report as advancing the "transformative neurodevelopment research in mental illness." In the report all mental illnesses are considered brain disorders and virtually all are called "developmental disorders." March wants the NIMH to invest in "translational neuroscience" based on drugs being developed by NIH, as Big Pharma has signaled its withdrawal from psychiatric drugs since most lucrative patents from the 1990s are expiring or have expired. March describes this new direction as "incredibly exciting." He states that the report "points the field toward the molecular origins of mental illness in early development" and he adds, "it becomes possible for the first time to envision preemptive treatments, a world without mental illness. How wonderful is that?" (cited by Kaplan, 2011).

Conflicts of Interest

There is now a broad recognition that psychiatry and psychiatric research—the heart of mad science—is awash in money that distorts honest inquiry. In medicine, in general, it is estimated that 25 percent of practitioners take cash payments from drug and medical device companies, and nearly 66 percent receive routine "gifts" from them (Pear, 2012). Among psychiatric leaders and researchers, the proportion is probably greater. The federal government has enacted regulations mandating as of 2012 drug companies receiving funds under Medicare and Medicaid programs to collect data on all payments and gifts to doctors and hospitals and to make this information publicly available. The research enterprise should be an arena that prizes free and open inquiry, independence of thought, and unbiased research. Instead, as we and many others have described, psychiatry has become engulfed in a thicket of distortions. On Big Pharma's payroll are most prominent psychiatrists as speakers, consultants, researchers, and marketeers in every state. It funds the APA and its major conferences; shapes the research agendas of scientists; censors what data may be published and when; manipulates studies to ensure positive results; pays for ghostwritten articles; hides its sponsorship of spokespersons and events; forges corrupting ties with universities; attacks critics; floods the professional and public media with ads for drugs; constrains and manipulates the FDA; and ensures that expensive but ineffective drugs remain the dominant treatment in psychiatry as they are sought by millions of people. At the cost of dozens of billions of dollars, Big Pharma and its allies in the biomedical industrial complex finance mad science and own a profession.

The entanglement of researchers and clinicians in financial conflicts of interest means that the interests and welfare of consumers and the public are ignored. Senator Charles Grassley's recent congressional investigations of the madness establishment were a welcomed exposé of the corruption of science.

The Therapeutic State

Big Pharma and Big Science are supported by a much larger entity: Big Government. The federal government's size, power, and influence make it the number-one funder of mad science and buyer of Big Pharma's products. For instance, the federal Medicare and Medicaid programs for older adults, the disabled, and poor purchase more than $100 billion a year of drugs and devices (Pear, 2012). With regard to the biomedicalization of human distress and suffering, the pharmaceutical industry and the federal government function as corporate partners in supporting the therapeutic state.

The federal government collaborates with the APA on many fronts, serves as patron of institutional psychiatry via the NIMH, and utilizes the myth-enhancing *DSM* in its proclamations. Moreover, through regulation and funding of medical and social services in conjunction with the states and through its "public health" policies identifying "mental health" goals, it has institutionalized, sanctioned, and legitimized the disease model of madness. Through policies governing health care, Medicaid, Supplemental Security Income (SSI), and Social Security Disability Insurance (SSDI), and making both public and private health insurance programs offer "parity" coverage for the mentally ill, the federal government has provided enormous financial incentives to states, hospitals, clinics, and providers of mental health services to interpret human distress as symptoms of brain disease. The boom in rates of mental disability for adults and children are striking. Angell (2011) notes an increase of 250 percent for adults between 1987 and 2007, and a thirty-five-fold increase for children. The offer of insurance coverage for psychiatric help and cash supplements for those in poverty if they are "disabled" is seductive and exploited by all players in the system. Robert Samuelson in the *Washington Post* calls Social Security's disability program a budget-busting, expensive "political quagmire" (Samuelson, 2012). The mechanisms for creating these huge increases in mental disability are the focus of many of our chapters: confusing the illness metaphor with reality, accepting brain disease as the ultimate cause of misery sans evidence, reifying arbitrary *DSM* categories, and creating the illusion that safe and effective medications are available. The government has become a full partner with psychiatry in medicalizing human problems.

The problem is this: people who need assistance are labeled as mentally ill in order to receive income supports, health care, and social services. Why do so many people need assistance? The economy is stalled or spiraling down, fewer unskilled jobs are available and unemployment has increased, inflation-adjusted wages for the average middle-class family have not increased in two generations, record numbers of families have lost their homes, and services from nonprofits and local and state governments have been sharply cut in the Great Recession. Millions of adults and children, normally living in relatively precarious circumstances, are now under enormous social stress. This stress does not result from the increasing incidence of brain defects, but from economic and policy defects. These people need opportunities and assistance, and social workers and mental health clinicians would like to help them with some of their problems so that they might seize opportunities or bear discomfort more constructively until circumstances improve. But to help an increasing number of these individuals today can only be done after fulfilling one enormously silly requirement: diagnose them with some form of mental disability or mental disorder. As one psychiatric blogger noted (thelastpsychiatrist.com, 2011):

> If, however, you abolish SSI then you will reduce psychiatry to the size of neonatal endocrinology [very small]. If you uncouple social services from "medical disability"—not abolish them, just find some other, better, more logical way to distribute them—you'll change America forever. . . . Psychiatry serves at the pleasure of the government.

Change of all kinds prompts resistance. The familiar, even if uncomfortable, often trumps the unknown; uncertainty causes understandable feelings of anxiety. Institutions as well as people are suspicious and defensive of calls for reform, even when they can expect the change to be beneficial. They might lie and confabulate to keep things the same. None of this is surprising. Even scientists trained in critical thinking, as Thomas Kuhn (1962) argued in his famous book, *The Structure of Scientific Revolutions*, resist findings suggesting that their theories are inadequate.

This is certainly the case in trying to suggest an alternative to the medical and public health model of madness. Biomedicine is a great success story.

Epidemics of infectious disease were averted or prevented, fatal afflictions became treatable or were eradicated, infant mortality was reduced and life-span accordingly increased. Science has triumphed over nature by producing knowledge that has greatly improved the quality of life for billions of individuals. There is no question about this. Thus, we understand why it is so alluring to view madness as a brain disease that awaits a miraculous cure.

But the available empirical research literature, corroborated by even the most enthusiastic supporters of the notion that disturbances of behavior are diseases, provides no convincing evidence that this is so. Yet the public is as quick as NIMH and the APA to nourish this illusion. The seduction is easy to appreciate. The medical explanation of human travails provides comfort, solace, and hope. It suggests that personal distress, inadequacy, and failure are really due to internal neurological defects that once fixed will eradicate these failings, much as antibiotics cure bacterial infections. It promises that people will not be held responsible for their failings. It promises John March's happy myth of "a world without mental illness." This illusion also helps all the institutions and bureaucracies that must count and categorize people and their troubles in the process of trying to help and support them. Even invalid classifications grounded in myth can ease the work of organizations, particularly once they become dependent on them to rationalize their operation. There is also a dark side to using mental illness as the focus of scientific efforts, and that is to scapegoat those who are called mentally ill. In the second debate of the candidates in the 2012 US presidential campaign, President Barack Obama actually mentioned the "mentally ill" on three occasions, surely an unusual occurrence in such a forum. Twice, he proposed keeping guns out of the hands of "the mentally ill."[5] Although, as we have cited earlier, the APA claims that 25 percent of the US population in any given year, and 50 percent over their lifetime, will be mentally ill, we suspect that the president was not slyly introducing a new gun control strategy.

Imagining Alternatives

Despite the described difficulties of mad science and how its results have become institutionalized in mental health policy and practice, there are alternative ways of thinking about and reimagining the provision of services for people in need. Some of these alternatives already exist, although at the margins of mental health practice. We offer here a few suggestions for a different roadmap for charting a more reasonable and humane future for those in the current mental health system.

Individuals and families in distress have always turned to others for advice, explanations, and solutions. Historically, help was sought from members of the extended family, neighbors, village elders, spiritual healers, witchdoctors, and priests. The assistance provided by these traditional sources of help was sometimes effective and gratefully received. At other times, the effects were illusive, questionable, or harmful. Faith in the healer, good fortune, and placebo effects undoubtedly aided helping efforts. By the late twentieth century, however, such traditional sources of help were devalued, as the biomedical industries encouraged people to turn first to medical professionals. Assistance with personal and family problems was moved under the jurisdiction of the new mental health professions and the medical establishment. Interpersonal supports were transformed into medical interventions, talismans into pharmaceuticals.

During this cultural transformation, the definition of *normal* was narrowed, and the perimeter of pathology was expanded. In the old normal, one recognized that existence is a struggle, an effort to be engaged with the world. Everyone's life had its ups and downs; people had strengths and weaknesses; and all experienced times of loss, disorientation and restoration, failure and resilience. Some dealt better than others with these challenges. This was viewed as part of the textured variation and diversity of human life. But, as we have described in this book, much of this diversity of life, some of it quite troublesome, has been redefined as an ominous sign of incipient brain disease. To a great extent, the public accepts this medicalized view that traumas, fears, dilemmas, conflicts, and misbehaviors are not inevitable parts of the human comedy but expungable illnesses. The new implicit definition of a normal or "healthy" person is someone who will harbor no serious worries or animosities, no undue sadness over losses or failed ambitions, no failures or disabilities, no serious disappointments with children or spouses, no doubts about themselves or conflicts with others, and certainly no strange ideas or behaviors. Those who fall short of these lofty expectations become candidates for psychiatric labeling. By reframing personal troubles or differences, especially serious ones, as psychiatric illness, as expressions of brain disease, people can be released from individual responsibility for imperfections of mood and behavior. They are given a temporary pass. Unusual behavior is a result of disease; foul moods the outcome of chemical imbalances.

It is incontrovertible that many, if not all, people face distress of many types and from diverse sources. People try to cope with distress in many different ways, some by seeking professional help. This is natural and prudent, because many may benefit from such professional help and support. Nothing we have argued in this book is an attempt to ignore or deny these elemental facts. Seeking professional help, especially voluntarily and in an informed manner, can be a positive method of coping. Psychotherapy (structured conversations or activities focused on the client) with caring, capable, and committed helpers of all stripes, even nonprofessionals, can be extremely helpful. Psychoactive drugs may be perfectly effective, if informed and willing clients choose them based on clearly announced profiles of effects.

The fact is, however, that assistance for those who need and want it can be offered without using the *DSM*'s list of contrived mental disorders. A fidgety boy or an adult who thinks the devil is out to kill him does not need to be labeled as suffering from a brain disease called Hyperactivity Disorder or Delusional Disorder. They are more usefully and honestly called . . . a fidgety boy and a person with incredible, scary beliefs. People who are distressed or misbehaving can be helped without inferring some, as yet undiscovered, neurological defects. Exhibiting an arbitrary number of ambiguous "symptoms" from a *DSM* checklist and, thereby, qualifying for a mental disorder label and insurance reimbursement, is neither necessary nor perhaps the best way to allocate assistance. Our current system has many drawbacks. First, labels of mental disorder imply that the needed help is "medical," which currently results overwhelmingly in a prescription for one or more medications written quickly by physicians who are not paid to investigate realistically what is the matter with the patient (Carlat, 2010; Greenberg, 2010; Harris, 2011). Second, the labels incorrectly imply that a specific medication can be effectively used with all people having the same label (Moncrieff & Cohen, 2005). Third, it disregards the vastly different skills and personal resources that each person may have that bear directly on their capacities to contend with their own weaknesses and fears (Saleeby, 1992). Forcing those who are most socially vulnerable—the poor, the uninsured, the marginal, or inept—to submit to becoming officially mentally ill in order to receive financial assistance, health care, social services, educational services, and other forms of assistance is medically and socially improper and unnecessary. This sorting may be bureaucratically useful and politically safe, but both scientifically and as a matter of social policy it is deeply flawed. We realize that changing that entrenched system, with so many stakeholders gripping firmly to the illusion that human suffering is merely a matter of disease, is a tall order. But the only possible way that Dr. March's wish for a world without "mental illness" will be achieved is by abandoning that very term.

The alternative view is that the array of misbehaviors, mistaken and disturbing feelings experienced by those now labeled with brain disorders are better viewed as normal human experiences in all their varieties, as described by scholars in sociology, psychology, anthropology, history, philosophy, and other disciplines that study the human condition, than by neuroscience. We realize that this view is not as seductive, comforting, or immediately useful, even if it is more accurate. Such an expanded view does not dismiss human agency or personal responsibility. It recognizes that individuals are inextricably rooted in and influenced by the social environments in which they struggle and flourish. It acknowledges the power of cultural and social learning and accepts the imperfections of the human condition. It also embraces the power of individuals and communities to provide compassionate assistance to others when needed. There are no silver bullets for the human condition, only collective and personal striving to cope.

As a result we think that psychiatry must abandon one of the two foundational roles allocated to it. First, the two professional roles that have been sanctioned by society for psychiatry must be decoupled: the pseudomedical coercive police or social management of behavioral deviance (involuntary treatment and involuntary hospitalization)[6] from the therapeutic or helping role for people seeking to ameliorate their minor and serious problems in living (voluntary treatment). This would put psychiatry on par with all other medical and helping professions, who are judged as providing help, or not, by the recipients of their services.

Because the scientific evidence for the reality of mental diseases is non-existent, no rationale for such entities causing harm to others should be advanced, and so psychiatry's police and social management role must be integrated back into the already-existing legal system, where bad behavior toward others beyond a certain level of intensity is deemed either a civil or criminal offense subject to penalties ranging from probation to community service to fines to imprisonment and, ultimately in American society at present, to death. This approach makes clear to all that bad behavior deemed directly harmful to others has consequences and that outside of the legal (not psychiatric) finding that the individual lacks *mens rea* (a guilty mind) and therefore is not responsible, the proper penalty is imposed. This in no way should prevent someone who wishes voluntarily to be helped to change behaviors that might have caused the harm from seeking and receiving help either during or after their punishment.

With regard to individuals who are at risk of harming themselves or threatening suicide, which is understandably deeply frightening to others, helping professionals should continue to reach out vigorously and offer help but not engage in forced treatment. With adults[7] there are ethical concerns about whether professionals should act solely on their own assessment of an identified self harmer, without full knowledge of why that person chooses to self harm. This is particularly the case since the extensive research literature on suicide suggests that involuntary treatment in any form can neither predict when or if someone will kill themselves, nor prevent a committed person from the act of suicide (Sher, 2004). Involuntary treatment may, of course, delay that act. We think that mental health professionals should offer only voluntary help, free of coercion (since coercive "help" does not work). Only in this way can helper and client honestly confront what is known and unknown about volitional human behavior, and only in this way can troubled human beings seek self-understanding and realistic options to deal with the complexities of existence.

The regulation of psychoactive drugs could also use some bold rethinking. It's obvious that medical practitioners do not engage in any sort of sophisticated biomedical reasoning when they prescribe these drugs to distressed people and may actually engage in illogical reasoning. Further, the collective judgment of psychiatric practitioners has been hijacked by the drug industry, and little exists to ensure that individual prescribers' decisions aim to protect individual patients' best interests. Prescribers, it seems, are the very last players to catch on to knowledge about the ill effects of the drugs they prescribe. With polypharmacy becoming the norm and any class of drugs being prescribed for any presenting problem, the question is raised why a psychiatric diagnostician stands between a patient and a drug. Whatever diagnosis-treatment pairings do exist (e.g., antipsychotics initially for psychosis, antidepressants initially for depression, etc.) can be easily memorized by the average junior high school student. Moreover, with direct-to-consumer ads now ubiquitous, prescription drugs have fully become consumer products. Finally, the Internet has already revolutionized access to and dissemination of information about medications and can revolutionize how prescribers and users can minimize unintended harm to users (Healy, 2012). This means that knowledge about drugs—about taking, continuing to take, or ceasing to take them—is now distributed and being constructed far beyond the offices or authority of traditional medical experts.

For these and other reasons, one of the principal arrangements for providing access to psychoactive medications to people has not served them well. In fact, granting physicians a monopoly on prescribing drugs is probably causing excess harm and needs to be seriously challenged. Our own preference is to abolish prescription privileges. We don't think they should be merely redistributed, say, to clinical psychologists, who have lobbied their state legislatures since the 1990s to obtain them. We cannot justify that any profession should possess a state-enforced monopoly to grant or deny people permission to use psychoactive drugs. Overall, prescription privileges have hindered the discovery of psychoactive drugs' potential benefits by hindering personally creative ways to employ drugs (self-medication). Prescription privileges also help to perpetuate patients' exposure to toxic effects and excessive drug combinations that patients otherwise would probably never attempt on their own. Although we guess that medical prescription privileges are widely seen as a "natural" arrangement for which no alternatives could possibly exist, the facts are that an explicit argument *for* the existence of this arrangement cannot be found, and the notion that they comprehensively "protect the public" has never, ever been critically tested (Cohen, 2008). Thomas Szasz and David Healy are two psychiatrists who differ fundamentally on their understanding of madness and the proper spheres of psychiatry as a profession. However, it happens that both have analyzed—the first from a libertarian perspective and the second from a public health perspective—the prescription psychoactive drug system. Both have proposed abolishing prescription privileges (Healy, 1997, 2012; Szasz, 1992).

Regardless of who is licensed to prescribe drugs, safety should be the primary formal concern of the FDA, and perhaps its only concern. The 1962

Kefauver amendments mandated the FDA to establish both efficacy and safety of drugs before their approval for marketing. We think the FDA has failed miserably in its mandate to establish the efficacy of psychiatric drugs currently on the market. From the perspective of a potential or actual user of these drugs, establishing their efficacy via randomized clinical trials has been a colossal waste of money and resources. Worse, clinical trials have radically restricted the understanding of psychoactive drugs as substances with psychoactive (and other) effects and created the absurd impression that every psychoactive drug that someone might find useful must fit to a "disease." And all this occurred despite the "efficacy" established by the drug's premarketing investigation having practically no bearing on how the drug will be prescribed once it's on the market. "Efficacy" is to clinical trials as "protecting the public" is to prescription privileges—a ruse.

If people were allowed to determine for themselves how to use chemical aids for the vicissitudes of life—with all the guidance, advice, and recommendations that experts and authorities wish to provide them and should be able to provide them—any *genuine psychological benefits* deriving from drug use are more likely to be discovered and then nurtured by users. Without the arbitrary obstacles and barriers erected to benefit pharmaceutical companies that have been documented in this book, information about drugs, their uses, their effects, their advantages, and their disadvantages should flow more freely. Individual consumer preferences, rather than clinical or regulatory commercial prerogatives or strategies, should determine the value of a psychoactive drug. Adverse effects—so defined by *whoever* would wish to so define them, rather than by industry-sponsored researchers and bureaucracies aided and abetted by the FDA—should be immediately publicized. This would reduce use of bad drugs, just as investors recoil from a bad stock *if the system isn't manipulated to withhold or suppress information about the genuine value of stocks.* In sum, no one would need to take a useless or harmful drug merely because only an overwhelmed and disinformation-vulnerable doctor controlled access to pharmaceuticals.

So-called clinical trials could be broadened to include many other ways to evaluate the impact of drugs ingested for long periods of time on complex biopsychosocial beings. This would help to establish safety as the genuine central concern of a drug regulatory system. As to ascertaining benefits of drugs, clinical trials would have to define these benefits from *users'* perspectives rather than employ contrived outcome measures of short-term "symptomatic improvements" decided upon by psychiatric investigators. The range of tested drugs would, of course, have to encompass more than just the chemicals that drug companies can patent, to include the countless psychoactive drugs that may have important benefits for people experiencing psychological distress. Of course, this proposal is not nearly as practical as it is logical, as it comes up against the century-old wall of drug prohibition. As Szasz (2004) aptly reminds,

> In the absence of a free market competition between legal and illegal psychoactive drugs—say, lithium and opium—the benefits of psychiatric drugs, as the patient defines benefit, will remain unknown and unknowable. (p. 178)

If one were interested in conducting genuine real-world trials of psychotropic drugs, one should compare realistic options, including drugs with other forms of help, tailored to broad groups of individuals with varying preferences. To accomplish this, different stakeholders (the federal and state government, insurance companies, *Consumer Reports*, family lobbies, independent or charitable foundations) must get involved in funding clinical trials—especially since establishing so-called efficacy for a "disorder" would not drive the entire process of bringing a drug to market. Moreover, as former *British Medical Journal* editor Richard Smith (2005) has already suggested, medical journals should agree not to publish company-funded clinical trials, only critical reviews of such trials, and only if their data are publicly available for reanalysis. Such reforms would help to free disciplined psychoactive drug use (i.e., drug use as therapy) from its current pseudoscientific pretensions, its disease justifications, and its medico-legal guardians. Enhanced by a rapidly developing technological matrix, it's possible that a truly consumer-oriented "cosmetic psychopharmacology" would bloom. Though *we* think cosmetic psychopharmacology remains a mythical, hopeless pursuit, society might have an easier time to regard it as such. The availability of psychoactive drugs by prescription is a monopolistic arrangement that remains extraordinarily sheltered from critical examination. Perhaps this is so because the arrangement sweeps—under the veneer of medical experts directing diseased people toward efficacious treatments too dangerous to understand by anyone but the self-styled experts—a mountain of painful, exceedingly complex personal and social ethical and practical choices. Our society is hesitant to tackle these choices forthrightly because they rest on ill-clarified values concerning the availability of chemical performance enhancement in education, working, and sports.[8]

How Change May Come

Despite all of our concerns just expressed about the difficulties ahead for alternate ways to handle madness, we still remain optimistic. As far as we can tell mad science has failed: it informs us that madness has grown, not shrunk, with about one in five American adults diagnosable as mentally ill today. We don't know much more—and perhaps less—about madness after the famed decade of the brain than we did before. Medications must obviously be beneficial for some people who take them, but that is not saying much, given the extent of iatrogenic harm and the baseline level of appreciation of any and all psychoactive substances by their users.

We think, keeping in mind our conviction that all forms of psychiatric coercion must be disavowed and disallowed, the first step is to get this information out to the population at large. Some of this has already begun and is accelerating, and unsurprisingly it is being led by some mainstream psychiatric insiders who provide a steady flow of articles and books about much that is wrong with psychiatry and the way it handles its charges. This expands public awareness, fueling further debates, which in turn encourage further critical examinations. We believe that this cycle cannot but be self-reinforcing (as previous cycles of reform that we have criticized have been). We can imagine a future time when a forward-thinking foundation or a Silicon Valley billionaire funds a series of well-crafted commercials adeptly communicating to ordinary people the scientific and moral emptiness of the mental health enterprise in our society.

When the information and the wasteful expenditure of public funds are more broadly disseminated, we believe that both mad and "normal" citizens will be energized. The so-called grassroots mental health recovery movement is the first sign that mad people can take care of themselves if they so desire. The surgeon general's report on mental health (US Department of Health and Human Services, 1999) recognized that the recovery movement is helping the mad to have "a more optimistic view of the possibility of recovering." Official recognition of this movement by psychiatric authorities has likely resulted from "the contemporary wave of writings [with] their critical mass, organizational backing, and freedom of expression from outside the institution" (pp. 97–98). This, together with the massive failure of institutional psychiatry to successfully deal with the problem of madness, triggered a lobby powerful enough to gain the attention of experts and authorities. We believe, however, that the official recognition of the recovery movement occurred also because its main spokespersons did not directly question the reality of mental illness and only mildly challenged the medical management of mental patients. So, as long as the foundational belief in madness as mental disease is apparently assented to by this movement, institutional psychiatry can appear gracious to recognize some of its tenets, that mad individuals can be helped to "build full meaningful, and productive lives . . . [by] a focus on life goals, consumer involvement, a diversity of treatment options, an emphasis upon consumer choice, and individually tailored services" (Kidd et al., 2010, p. 343). Again, *we* think that this agenda ultimately must be met with the absence of coercion and without superfluous diagnoses (unless helpers and their contracting clients wish to use "diagnoses" they agree upon).

We are also impressed by the fact that knowledge that was once the prerogative of medical professionals is now discussed with a high level of intelligence and wisdom by ordinary consumers who are seeking to acquire information and to share information with others. We've briefly reviewed in an earlier chapter how the aggregate, first-person reviews of prescribed psychoactive medications by consumers may resemble much of what official and "authoritative" medical accounts disseminate, with the useful added dimension of providing contextual clues and insights to people trying to make treatment decisions. As technological progress increases the ability to use these freely available databases and to allow even more focused and individualized contributions from laypersons, many pseudoscientific pretensions of clinical psychopharmacology might be laid bare.

We believe that these cracks in the fortress of the medical model can be used to engage both the mad and their families to move further away from the current system. This is absolutely essential, because the system will not be changed entirely from within. Power is not voluntarily relinquished, but those in power respond when the formerly powerless coalesce around critical issues that cannot be ignored. If the extent of the failure of psychiatric practice is made clear to the mad, their families, and friends, the critical dialogue may become more earnest. There is, of course, the unpredictable but remote possibility that the psychiatric system produces its "Gorbachev," a widely acknowledged leader and spokesperson who says plainly and loudly that the emperor has no clothes, that while many people could use help for their distress or have their disturbance contained to preserve our peace of mind, there is no mental illness.

The current worldwide economic crisis and the related serious debates about health-care costs will directly affect the issues of change in the mental health system. Since most mental health costs are paid for by public monies, the system appears unlikely to sustain the current infrastructure based on the medical model, although societies have in the past and in our time pursued wrongheaded policies that nearly ruined them. If our analysis is correct, moving toward an increasingly demedicalized, voluntary approach could reorient the services needed (even a moderate reduction in involuntary hospitalizations will reduce expenditures by billions of dollars, though it could increase expenditures by other social control systems).

Our suggestions may seem radical, but we think that both ethics and science are on our side. There can be no cutting-edge science in this field as long it rests on the unverified but reified concept of mental disease or mental disorder. Society's response to personal distress and misbehavior should be guided by the ideals of compassion, justice, tolerance, education—and yes, protection of society. Human existence, the struggle for survival and for fulfillment, entails an effort to improve the troubled and fallible world of human beings. That effort must be tempered by the oft-confirmed realization that solutions lead rarely to their intended consequences. And even then, they entail other, unimagined consequences that must be resolved, creating other new problems . . . *ad infinitum*. In place of gleaming but illusory promises of medical cures for madness, we would all be better served by recognizing the inevitable precariousness of the human condition. To move society forward in the service of others who request help, the best that human beings are capable of is taking courageous steps based on honest critical analysis and debate, and constant scrutiny to minimize harm and monitor unintended consequences.

Notes

1.   Some of these books include the following: *Psychiatry: The Science of Lies* (Szasz, 2010), *Unhinged: The Trouble with Psychiatry—A Doctor's Revelations about a Profession in Crisis* (Carlat, 2010), *Anatomy of an Epidemic: Magic Bullets, Psychiatric Drugs, and the Astonishing Rise of Mental Illness in America* (Whitaker, 2010), *The Emperor's New Drugs: Exploding the Antidepressant Myth* (Kirsch, 2010), *Pharmageddon* (Healy, 2012), *Manufacturing Depression: The Secret of a Modern Disease* (Greenberg, 2010), and *The Myth of the Chemical Cure: A Critique of Psychiatric Drug Treatment* (Moncrieff, 2009).

2.   State laws vary, but jurisprudence has established that professionals' actions do not depend directly or entirely on the patient's behavior. Rather, they depend on a variety of factors, including: the duration of the relationship established with the patient; the implicit and explicit promises professionals have made; the type of consent provided by patients; the usual responsibilities of the setting in which the relationship occurs; and other factors. A competent technical description of one large state's commitment laws is found in Behnke et al., 2000. A first-person account by a practicing psychiatrist of coercion and commitment in the psychiatric emergency room is found in Linde, 2010.

3.   In a remarkably thorough and well-documented book, Robert Whitaker (2010) argues that the modern psychiatric drug treatments have created an enormous swell of iatrogenic injury in the form of neurobiological dysfunctions. Thus, the antipsychotics have damaged the dopaminergic systems, and SSRI antidepressants have damaged the serotonergic and monoaminergic systems, of people who take them for long periods of time. Whitaker also argues that these neurological dysfunctions explain the increase in counts of what he calls mental illness, principally as inferred from the number of people receiving social security funds for mental or behavioral disability in the United States since the widespread use of these drugs. We think that Whitaker's arguments concerning iatrogenic damage are persuasive, but we question calling drug-induced injury "mental illness."

4.   French researchers from University of Bordeaux and one of the authors of this book (DC) teamed up to analyze how the media echoed scientific findings. They identified the ten scientific studies on ADHD most-often echoed by English-language newspapers during the decade of the 1990s, as well as sixty-seven subsequent scientific studies that investigated the same questions until 2011. While 223 newspaper articles covered the first 10 studies, only 57 articles covered the subsequent related studies. More important, the authors found that the findings in eight of the top ten studies were either refuted or strongly attenuated in the subsequent studies. This

fact, however, was acknowledged in only a single of the fifty-seven news-paper articles covering these subsequent studies. The authors conclude: "Because newspapers preferentially echo initial ADHD findings appearing in prominent journals, they report on uncertain findings that are often refuted or attenuated by subsequent studies. If this media reporting bias generalizes to health sciences, it represents a major cause of distortion in health science communication" (Gonon et al., 2012).

5. According to the transcript of the October 16, 2012 debate, published by the Commission on Presidential Debates, President Obama's three mentions were the following: 1) "So my belief is that, (A), we have to enforce the laws we've already got, make sure that we're keeping guns out of the hands of criminals, those who are mentally ill;" 2) "And so what I want is a—is a comprehensive strategy. Part of it is seeing if we can get automatic weapons that kill folks in amazing numbers out of the hands of criminals and the mentally ill;" 3) "We're not going to eliminate everybody who is mentally disturbed, and we've got to make sure they don't get weapons." (Retrieved from http://www.debates.org/index.php?page=october-1-2012-the-second-obama-romney-presidential-debate)

6. This would necessitate abandoning all statutory authority for involuntary hospitalization and treatment.

7. Children, the largest coerced minority in the world, have exceedingly few rights to make autonomous decisions. Regarding their self-harming behaviors or actions, like any of their other actions, children should continue to be subjected to parental authority and "treated" according to that authority's best judgment, except where that authority is deemed judicially not to operate in the child's best interest, in which case the standard legal procedures as exist today would be applied.

8. Perhaps this critical examination might be triggered by what we think are three important and extremely unusual newspaper publications, all appearing in late 2012 in the *New York Times* and the *Washington Post*. The first is a series of six brief position papers arguing the pros and cons of having various prescription medications available to patients over the counter, without a doctor's prescription. The position statements appeared in the *Times'* Room for Debate forum on September 16, 2012, under the title "Getting Your Prescriptions, Without A Prescription," and thoughtful reader comments were appended (Available from http://www.nytimes.com/roomfordebate/2012/09/16/getting-your-prescriptions-without-a-prescription). The second *Times* article, written by reporter Alan Schwartz, appeared on October 9, 2012, with the title "Attention Disorder or Not, Pills to Help in School" (Available from http://www.nytimes.com/2012/10/09/health/attention-disorder-or-not-children-prescribed-pills-to-help-in-school.html?pagewanted=all). This article laid bare, for the first time as far as we know in a major media outlet, the reality that both psychiatric diagnoses and medical prescription for drugs are merely convenient pretexts for making various psychoactive drugs available to users for their own ends. Over seven hundred reader comments were quickly appended to that article. The third, an opinion piece by Brad Allenby, a professor of ethics and engineering at Arizona State University, appeared in the *Post* on October 26, 2012, under the title "Lance Armstrong's Fall: A Case

for Allowing Performance Enhancement" (available, along with nearly eight hundred reader comments, from http://www.washingtonpost.com/opinions/lance-armstrongs-fall-a-case-for-allowing-performance-enhancement/2012/10/26/6f7cccf0-1d41-11e2-b647-bb1668e64058_story_1.html).

References

Ackerman, D. (2004). *An alchemy of mind: The marvel and mystery of the brain.* New York: Scribner.

Angell, M. (2011). The epidemic of mental illness: Why? *New York Review of Books,* June 23.

Behnke, S. H., Winick, B. J., & Perez, A. M. (2000). *The essentials of Florida mental health law: A straightforward guide for clinicians of all disciplines.* New York: Norton Professional.

Black, E. (2003). *War against the weak.* New York: Four Walls Eight Windows.

Carey, B. (2005, October 18). Can brain scans see depression? *New York Times.*

Carlat, D. (2010). *Unhinged: The trouble with psychiatry--A doctor's revelations about a profession in crisis.* New York: Free Press.

Cohen, D. (2008). Automédication. Abolition de l'ordonnance en psychiatrie? [Self medication. Abolishing prescription in psychiatry?] In Folie/Culture & Revue Santé Mentale au Québec (Eds.), *La pensée critique en santé mentale* [Critical thought in mental health], pp. 71-84. Québec: Édiscript.

Cole, J. (2011, April 29). Too big to fail. *The Chronicle Review,* pp. B12–14.

Gonon, F., Konsman, J.-P., Cohen, D., & Boraud, T. (2012). Why most biomedical findings echoed by newspapers turn out to be false: The case of attention deficit hyperactivity disorder. *PLoS One, 7*(9), e44275.

Greenberg, G. (2010). *Manufacturing depression: The secret history of a modern disease.* New York: Simon & Schuster.

Greenberg, G. (2011, January). Inside the battle to define mental illness. *Wired.* http://www.wired.com/magazine/2010/12/ff_dsmv/

Hahm, H. C., & Segal, S. P. (2010). Failure to seek health care among the mentally ill. *American Journal of Orthopsychiatry, 75,* 54–62.

Harris, G. (2011, March 5). Talk doesn't pay, so psychiatry turns to drugs. *New York Times.*

Healy, D. (2012). *Pharmageddon.* Berkeley: University of California Press.

Healy, D. (1997). *The antidepressant era.* Cambridge, MA: Harvard University Press.

Hughes, S., & Cohen, D. (2011). *A qualitative analysis of psychotropic medications discourses in consumer-generated and professionally controlled text on the Internet.* Unpublished manuscript.

Kaplan, A. (2011, February 9). NIMH shifts focus to molecular origins of mental illness. *Psychiatric Times.*

Kidd, S. A., George, L., O'Connell, M., Sylvestre, J., Kirpatrick, H., Browne, G., et al. (2010). Fidelity and recovery-orientation in assertive community treatment. *Community Mental Health Journal, 46,* 342–350.

Kirsch, I. (2010). *The emperor's new drugs: Exploding the antidepressant myth.* New York: Basic Books.

Kuhn, T. S. (1962). *The structure of scientific revolutions.* Chicago: University of Chicago Press.

Linde, P. R. (2010). *Danger to self: On the front line with an ER psychiatrist.* Berkeley: University of California Press.

McCubbin, M., Dallaire, B., Cohen, D., & Morin, P. (1999). Should institutions that commit patients also be gatekeepers to information about civil commitment? Implications for research and policy. *Journal of Radical Psychology, 2*(1).

Medical guesswork. (2006, May). *Business Week.*

Merriam-Webster.com (Ed.) (2011). Merriam-Webster.com.

Monahan, J. (2008). Mandated community treatment: Applying leverage to achieve adherence. *Journal of the American Academy of Psychiatry and the Law, 36,* 282–285.

Moncrieff, J. (2009). *The myth of the chemical cure: A critique of psychiatric drug treatment.* London: Palgrave Macmillan.

Moncrieff, J., & Cohen, D. (2005). How do psychiatric drugs work? *British Medical Journal, 338*(b.1963).

Oaks, D. W. (2011). The moral imperative for dialogue with organizations of survivors of coerced psychiatric human rights violations. In T. W. Kallert, J. E. Mezzich, & J. Monahan (Eds.), *Coercive treatment in psychiatry: Clinical, legal and ethical aspects.* New York: John Wiley and Sons.

Pear, R. (2012, January 16). U.S. to force drug firms to report money paid to doctors. *New York Times.*

Pratt, L. A., Brody, D. J., & Gu, G. (2011). *Antidepressant use in persons age 12 and over: United States (2005–2008).* Retrieved from http://www.cdc.gov/nchs/data/databriefs/db76.htm

Saleeby, D. (1992). *The strengths perspective in social work practice.* New York: Longman.

Samuelson, R. J. (2012, February 12). Budget quagmire revealed by Social Security disability program. *Washington Post.*

Savodnik, I. (2006, January 1). Psychiatry's sick compulsion: Turning weaknesses into diseases. *Los Angeles Times,* pp. M1, M3.

Scull, A. (1985). Humanitarianism or control? Some observations on the historiography of Anglo-American psychiatry. In S. Cohen & A. Scull (Eds.), *Social control and the state* (pp. 118–140). Oxford, UK: Basil Blackwell Ltd.

Sher, L. (2004). Preventing suicide. *QJM, 97,* 677–680.

Smith, R. (2005). Medical journals are an extension of the marketing arm of pharmaceutical companies. *PLoS Medicine, 2*(5), e138.

Snyders, M. (2009) Minnesota mental health patient Ray Sandford forced into electro-shock therapy. *Minneapolis City Pages* (20 May), p. 1.

Szasz, T. (1974). *Ceremonial chemistry: The ritual persecution of drugs, addicts, and pushers.* New York: Bantam Books.

Szasz, T. (2007). *Coercion as cure.* New Brunswick, NJ: Transaction Publishers.

Szasz, T. (2010). *Psychiatry: The science of lies.* Syracuse: Syracuse University Press.

Szasz, T. (2004). *Words to the wise: A medical–philosophical dictionary.* New Brunswick, NJ: Transaction Publishers.

Szasz, T. (1992). *Our right to drugs: The case for a free market.* Syracuse, NY: Syracuse University Press.

Taube, G. (2007). *Good calories, bad calories: Fats, carbs, and the controversial science of diet and health.* New York: Anchor Books.

thelastpsychiatrist.com. (2011). Retrieved from http://thelastpsychiatrist.com/2011/06/the_epidemic_of_mental_illness.html

The Economist (2012, September 10). An array of errors. pp. 91–92. http://www. economist.com/node/21528593

US Department of Health and Human Services. (1999). *Mental health: A report of the surgeon general.* Retrieved from www.surgeongeneral.gov/library/ mentalhealth/home.html

Weisberg, D. S., Keil, F. C., Goodstein, J., Rawson, E., & Gray, J. R. (2008). The seductive allure of neuroscience explanations. *Journal of Cognitive Neuroscience, 20,* 470–477.

Whitaker, R. (2010). *Anatomy of an epidemic: Magic bullets, psychiatric drugs, and the astonishing rise of mental illness in America.* New York: Crown.

Wiencke, M. C. (2007). Choice over coercion. *Dartmouth Medicine, 32*(2) 4.

Zimmer, C. (2012, April 16). A sharp rise in retractions calls for reform. *New York Times.*

Zimmer, C. (2012, October 2). Misconduct widespread in retracted science papers, study finds. *New York Times*, D2.

Index

Centers for Disease Control and
  Prevention (CDC), 315–316
chemical imbalances, belief in, 251–252
children
    antipsychotic drugs and, 19
    bipolar disorder and, 19–21. *See also*
      Wagman, Benjamin
    disease mongering and, 19–20
    pharmaceuticals and, 17, 18
    serious emotional disturbances and,
      4–5
chlordiazepoxide (Librium), 270
chlorpromazine, 220, 263–264, 287n1
chronicity, 99–100, 113n3
citalopram (Celexa), 222
Civilization and Its Discontents
  (Freud), 130
classification, 127–128, 141
Clinical Antipsychotic Trials of
  Intervention Effectiveness (CATIE),
  220–222, 226–227, 233–234, 266
clinical treatment effect, 113n6
clonazepam (Klonopin), 270–271
clonidine, 218
clozapine, 254, 265
coca, 241
cocaine, 242, 248
Cochrane Collaboration, 94, 113–114n6
"Code of Chronicity, The" (Ludwig and
  Farrelly), 99–100
coercion
    ACT and, 106–109
    concern regarding, 301
    development of ACT and, 100
    emergence of, 75
    endurance of, 304–307, 311
    forms of, 87–88
    impact of, 84–85
    justification for, 78–79, 305–306
    overview of, 26–28
    purpose of, 76–77
    reliance on, 80, 109–111
    statistics on, 86–87
    See also confinement, forced; hospi-
      talization: involuntary; treatments:
      involuntary
*Coercion and Aggressive Community
  Treatment* (Dennis and Monahan),
  108
Coercive Treatment in Psychiatry
  (Monahan), 108

coffee, 235, 241
Cohen, D., 247, 258
Cole, Jonathan, 313–314
combat conditions, 51. *See also* military
  service
Committee on Finance, 279
community care
    coercion and, 87–88
    military service and, 51, 52
    overview of, 26–28
    shift toward, 52–53, 54, 81, 304
    See also assertive community
      treatment (ACT)
comorbidity, 113n3, 171–172
*Concepts of Insanity in the United
  States* (Dain), 56, 64
confinement, forced, 41–42, 83–84. *See
  also* asylums; coercion; hospitalization:
  involuntary
conflicts of interest, 282, 307–308,
  317–318
continuing medical education,
  278–279
controlled trials, 259–261. *See also*
  randomized controlled trial (RCT)
convulsive treatments, 264–265
Coppel, Anne, 213
cosmetic psychopharmacology,
  248–249, 326
Costello, Jane, 18
cure, meaninglessness of, 274–275

Dain, Norman, 56, 64
Dartmouth Assertive Community
  Treatment Scale (DACTS), 108
Davis, J. M., 108
DEA (Drug Enforcement Agency), 243,
  309
DeGrandpre, Richard, 213–214, 243
deinstitutionalization, 26–28, 53, 69, 81,
  82–83, 133, 304
Delay, Jean, 263
dementia praecox, 128, 265. *See also*
  schizophrenia
Deniker, Pierre, 263
Dennis, D. L., 108
depakote, 218, 288n7
DePaulo, J. Raymond, Jr., 232–233
depression
    drug treatments and, 212, 220,
      222–224, 271